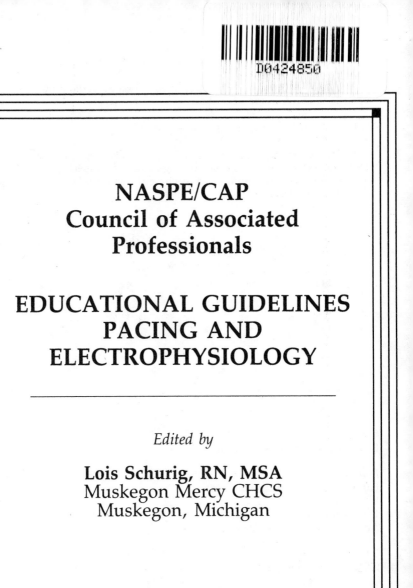

D0424856

NASPE/CAP
Council of Associated Professionals

EDUCATIONAL GUIDELINES PACING AND ELECTROPHYSIOLOGY

Edited by

Lois Schurig, RN, MSA
Muskegon Mercy CHCS
Muskegon, Michigan

Library of Congress Cataloging-in-Publication Data to Come

Educational guidelines: pacing and electrophysiology / edited by Lois
   Schurig. — Edition one.
       p.   cm.
   Includes bibliographical references and index.
   ISBN 0-87993-592-8
   1. Cardiac pacing—Outlines, syllabi, etc. 2. Electrophysiology—
Outlines, syllabi, etc. 3. Cardiac pacing—Study and teaching.
4. Electrophysiology—Study and teaching. I. Schurig, Lois.
RC684.P3E38 1994
617.4'12059—dc20   94-12051
                                                               CIP

Copyright © 1994
Futura Publishing Company, Inc.

Published by
Futura Publishing Compnay, Inc.
P.O. Box 418
135 Bedford Road
Armonk, New York 10504

L.C. No. 94-12051
ISBN No. 0-87993-592-8

Every effort has been made to ensure that the information in this book is
as up to date and accurate as possible at the time of publication. However,
due to the constant development in medicine, neither the author, nor the
editor, nor the publisher can accept any legal or any other responsibility
for any errors or omissions that may occur.

All rights reserved. No part of this book may be translated or reproduced
in any form without written permission of the publisher.

Printed in the United States of America on acid-free paper.

Contributors

Robert Audette RN BA CCRN Good Samaritan Hospital, Suffern, New York

Joni Baxter BSN Sacred Heart and Deaconess Medical Centers, Spokane, Washington

Karen Belco RN BSN Baylor College of Medicine, Houston, Texas

Alan D. Bernstein EngScD, FACC Newark Beth Israel Medical Center, Newark, New Jersey

Rosemary Bubien RN MSN UAB School of Medicine, Birmingham, Alabama

Elizabeth Darling RN MSN Krannert Institute of Cardiology, Indianapolis, Indiana

Katharine Irene Faitel RN, BSN Sinai Hospital, Detroit, Michigan

Margaret Millis Faust RN BSN Nashville, Tennessee

Richard C. Forney Ph.D. Robert L. Batey Cardiology Center, Bradenton, Florida

Jennifer A. Fraser RN Peterborough Regional Pacemaker Center, Peterborough, Ontario Canada

Nancy H. Fullmer RN The Emory Clinic, Atlanta, Georgia

John Gentzel RN CCP Memorial Hospital, Colorado Springs, Colorado

Carol Gilbert RN BSN Sinai Samaritan Medical Center, Milwaukee, Wisconsin

Melanie T. Gura RN BSN Robinson Memorial Hospital, Hudson, Ohio

Chea Haran RN BSN ARNP Advanced Cardiac Pacemakers Inc., Miami, Florida

Carol Higgins RN MSN CCRN McLaren Regional Medical Center, Flint, Michigan

Marleen E. Irwin RCRT The General Hospital (Grey Nuns) of Edmonton, Edmonton, Alberta Canada

Patricia A. Manion RN BSN CCRN McLaren Regional Medical Center, Flint, Michigan

Mary Neubauer RN BS CPH2 Morristown Memorial, Morristown, New York

Tomas Ozahowski RN Dartmouth-Hitchcock Medical Center, Lebanon, New Hampshire

Brenda Rosenbery RN BSN Providence Hospital, Detroit, Michigan

Kathleen Ann Ruggiero RN Buffalo Cardiology and Pulmonary Association, Buffalo, New York

Jeanne M. Scewchik RN Cleveland Clinic, Cleveland, Ohio

Lois Schurig, RN, MSA Muskegon Mercy CHCS, Healthcare Unlimited, Muskegon, Michigan

Susan L. Song RN BSN Pacemaker Center, USC School of Medicine, Los Angeles, California

Kathleen Strong RN MS Horton Hospital, Middletown, New York

Mark Sweesy BS RCPT R. L. Bakey Cardiology Center, Bradenton, Florida

Beverly Taibi RN Buffalo Cardiology and Pulmonary Associates, Buffalo, New York

Jo Ellen Thomson RN Evanston Hospital, Evanston, Illinois

Michelle G. Tobin RN Cleveland Clinic, Cleveland, Ohio

Rosemary Fabiszewski-Volosin RN MSN Cooper Hospital University Medical Center, Camden, New Jersey

Charles Witherell RN CS MSN San Francisco, California

Vicki Zeigler MSN, RN Division of Cardiovascular Nursing, Children's Hospital of the Medical University of South Carolina, Charleston, South Carolina

Introduction

Historical Perspective

Back in 1986, a sign was posted on the message board at the annual scientific sessions of the North American Society of Pacing and Electrophysiology (NASPE) held in Boston, Massachusetts. The message read "Anyone who would like to participate in writing the educational guidelines for pacing and electrophysiology. . . ." The speciality at this time was in its infancy and the NASPE/CAP (Council of Associated Professionals) had not been completely defined. About 15 people were present at the initial session for the educational guidelines. During the meeting the group brainstormed general areas of knowledge. Each member present was assigned an area to research based on their knowledge, area of interest, and experience. Few of the group members had publishing experience, but this did not deter further progress. The work continued for about 2 years until a draft of the content was completed.

In September of 1988, about 35 members of the writing conference convened in Toronto for a *marathon* session in an effort to finalize the guidelines. As one can tell, the group had grown in number as well as expertise. The conference lasted 3 days and nights. It was quite an experience. Talk about a *marathon* weekend. The days went from 7 am until about 10 pm give or take a few hours. Brief nourishment breaks were permitted. The 35 separated into two working groups. One was assigned the educational guidelines and the other the bylaws or Functions and Organization (F&Os) for NASPE/CAP. There was one computer available and a few members rotated the position of secretary. (This was not an easy job at the rate minds were changed.) When the weekend came to a close, the collective efforts of the group had generated two draft documents: 1) Educational Guidelines for Pacing and Electrophysiology and 2) F&Os.

The next step was the approval process. This included review by the advisors of NASPE-CAP, circulation of the drafts to all members of the committee, circulation to the NASPE CME committee, and a content editing prior to submission to the NASPE board for approval. Once this process was completed, the guidelines were submitted to the journal *PACE* for publication. The first edition was published in the November 1990 issue of *PACE*. Step one was completed, define the educational guidelines for pacing and electrophysiology. The guidelines had been published and the F&Os had also been approved by the executive committee of NASPE/CAP and the NASPE board. During the process, NASPE/CAP grew in membership and its role in the NASPE organization also became more defined.

NASPE/CAP Educational Guidelines Position Statement

The field of cardiac arrhythmias over the past two decades has witnessed rapid technological changes in patient care and treatment. Although physicians primarily direct patient care and treatment, a clear need has been developed for well–trained, knowledgeable support personnel. These personnel include, but are not limited to, registered nurses, physician assistants, and cardiovascular technicians whose practices involve different aspects of pacing and electrophysiology. These individuals, who come from widely diverse backgrounds and who have developed a professional identity different from that of the physician, with different educational needs, have come to be known as the associated professionals (AP).

Education of the AP in the field of pacing and electrophysiology traditionally had been accomplished in an erratic manner. The majority of learning occurred through self teaching, instruction by physicians, and the educational efforts of industry. This has resulted in the development of many accomplished and capable APs. We do, however, recognize that this form of teaching is less than ideal, not standardized and produces variable results.

The Council of APs Ad Hoc Committee on Educational Guidelines defined the curriculum by reviewing current literature, medical/technical texts, and interviewing experienced APs in the field of pacing and electrophysiology. The resulting recommendations suggest the minimal level of knowledge required by the AP for safe practice and thus were designated to facilitate the development of teaching programs.

Educational Guidelines Manual

Due to the diversity of the individual practices of AP, it was recognized that different categories of guidelines were necessary. The categories were divided into the following:

1. Core Curriculum—defines a base of knowledge common to both pacing and electrophysiology.
2. Pacemaker Curriculum—defines a base knowledge specific to the specialty of pacing.
3. Electrophysiology Curriculum—defines base knowledge specific to the specialty of electrophysiology.

Not all categories are applicable to every AP, but rather are presented as guidelines for training and education of individuals in the field of pacing and electrophysiology. It is expected that familiarity with the three curriculum will provide a common base of knowledge essential to everyone in the field and will thus enhance patient care. It should also establish the foundation for a credentialing process specific to the knowledge and responsibilities of the AP in their scope of practice.

It should be understood that a skill component is critical for this field. Achievement of a skill level is beyond the scope of this text and can be accomplished in a formal educational setting or in established pacing and electrophysiology laboratories.

How to Use the Manual

Each chapter in the manual has been designed to facilitate presentation of the information in a concise format. The major topics are listed in the label of the chapter followed by a brief introduction. Objectives have been written for each chapter to focus the reader. They will be used later for the credentialing process. A glossary and abbreviations section highlights the key words from the text that are helpful to know prior to reading the entire chapter.

The design of the education content is in outline form to highlight the most significant facts related to the subject of the chapter. It consolidates the presentation of an extensive amount of information. The purpose is to identify key characteristics of the subject to focus the reader and provide ample references to expand the subject. The guideline committee believed for the first edition, that this was the optimal method to contain such a volume of knowledge into one text. The references support the text content and provide the reader with the means to conduct a self paced learning tutorial. The references (over 475) cover the last 8 years. Older references were retained due to their historical value and in many cases they identified the start of new technological advances, enhanced the scope of pacing and electrophysiology, and established the principles for both specialties.

Note: No one ever said this was going to be an easy process. Good luck with your endeavors and please utilize the NASPE/CAP members for assistance. Any of the members can be reached by calling the NASPE office in Upper Newton Falls, Massachusetts.

Acknowledgments

The NASPE/CAP writing committee would like to acknowledge the support, encouragement, and assistance given to us by the NASPE organization—Carol McGlinchey, Barbara Krause, and Doris DeNisco and their staff. In grateful appreciation, we would like to thank the advisors for NASPE/CAP who stood by us through the tides of change and the long hours of work behind this manual—Drs. James Maloney, Paul Gillette, Bernard Goldman, and Victor Parsonnet. We would like to acknowledge and thank the NASPE reviewers who donated many hours of their time to complete a critical appraisal of this text—Drs. Paul Gillette, Nora Goldchlager, Peter Guzy, Gerald Naccarelli, David Steinhaus, and Melvin Scheinman. We would like to thank each of the contributing authors for their willingness to share their knowledge and expertise. It has taken hundreds of work hours to complete this manual which is based on the cummulative knowledge of the authors during more than 343 years working in cardiac arrhythmology (The recognition, evaluation and management of cardiac arrhythmias). We would like to thank Janet Shaub for her expert assistance in carefully and accurately typing the majority of this manual. This work would not have been completed without her efforts.

In conclusion, I would like to personally thank the members of my family—husband Mike and son Steven—for their support and fortitude during the many years it has taken to get this manual to press. It has truly been a test of endurance for us all, but it has been a task worth doing.

Thank you again to all who have participated in completion of this work.

Contents

Contents

Contents

Part 1

CORE CURRICULUM

PART I

CORE CURRICULUM.

CHAPTER 1

Fundamentals of Electronics

Alan D. Bernstein

Subsections:
A. Basic Quantities
B. Derived Quantities
C. Units of Measurement
D. Relationships
E. Circuit Components
F. Signal Components
G. Electronic Subsystems
H. Ohm's Law
I. Current, Voltage, and Resistance
J. Energy and Power
K. Electrical Circuits

By its nature, cardiac pacing is an interdisciplinary field, involving physics, electrical engineering, computer science, and materials technology as well as cardiology, surgery, and cardiac electrophysiology. The essential function of the pacing system itself is to stimulate the heart by passing an electric current through susceptible tissue.

Understanding the *normal* electrical interaction between a pacing system and the heart requires an acquaintance with some of the basic concepts of electricity. Understanding what appears to be *abnormal* pacing-system behavior may require familiarity with additional electrical-engineering concepts. In particular, distinguishing between a true pacing system malfunction and a pseudomalfunction often requires an understanding of special design features of the pulse generator in use, such as adaptive timing intervals or response to sensing during refractory periods. Careful attention to unusual design char-

From: Schurig L. *Educational Guidelines: Pacing and Electrophysiology.* Armonk, NY: Futura Publishing Co, Inc, © 1994.

acteristics may well forestall unnecessary surgery to replace a normally functioning but inappropriately programmed pulse generator.

It is the purpose of this chapter to outline some of the basic concepts of electricity and electronic circuits that are pertinent to optimizing pacing-system operation and interpreting apparent problems.

Objectives

1. Identify important basic electrical quantities, such as charge, current, and voltage.
2. Explain the relationship between current, voltage, and resistance as described by Ohm's law.
3. List the units of measurement for important quantities such as charge, current, voltage, resistance, energy, power, and battery capacity.
4. Make proper use of the Latin and Greek prefixes that make units of measurement smaller or larger.
5. Describe the function of electronic-circuit elements such as resistors, capacitors, and inductors.
6. Describe the function of electronic-circuit subsystems, or modules used in pulse generators and other devices, such as amplifiers and filters.

Glossary and Abbreviations

Afterpotential: The polarization voltage that persists for a time after electrical stimulation of the heart because of charge stored temporarily in the electrode/tissue interface. This voltage can be detected by the sensing circuit in the other channel of a dual-chamber pacemaker, which could interpret it erroneously as a spontaneous depolarization.

Ampere (Amp): The basic unit of electric current. 1 Amp = 1 Coulomb/sec.

Ampere-hour: A unit of battery capacity. It has the dimensions of electric charge.

Amplifier: An electronic subsystem, or module, that increases the amplitude of a signal without changing it in any other way.

Amplitude: The strength of an electrical signal. Usually measured in volts.

Battery capacity: Measured in watt-hours, which are units of charge. As battery capacity is depleted, the internal resistance of the battery (an intrinsic property of the device) increases, limiting the charge that can be drawn from the battery as current.

Bidirectional pulse: A pair of contiguous pulses of opposite polarity.

Biphasic pulse: A pulse that has two distinct phases, or sections. (See bidirectional pulse.)

Capacitance: The relationship between the charge stored in a capacitor and the voltage applied across the capacitor. Measured in farads.

Capacitor: An electronic-circuit component that stores potential energy in an electric field. It can be thought of as storing charge; the amount of charge that can be stored is the product of the capacitance (measured in farads) and the applied voltage. A rapidly-varying signal will pass through a capacitor more readily than a slowly-varying signal.

Charge: The basic electrical quantity, made up of an excess or scarcity of free electrons; measured in coulombs. Charge cannot be created or destroyed (the concept of conservation of charge); thus charge that flows from a battery as current must be balanced by charge returning to the battery at the same rate.

Chronaxie: In the Lapicque approximation of the threshold of stimulation, the stimulus duration at the point where the stimulus amplitude is equal to twice the rheobase.

Circuit: (1) A closed pathway, or loop, through which charge can flow as current. (2) A combination of elements such as resistors, capacitors, and transistors.

Conductor: A substance (such as a metal) that presents low resistance to the flow of current: an ideal conductor has no resistance.

Constant-current pacemaker: A pacemaker with an output circuit that produces a current that does not vary during the course of the stimulus. Most implantable pacemakers have voltage-source output circuits (see constant-voltage pacemaker), with which both the voltage and the current of the stimulus decay continuously during the stimulus.

Constant-voltage pacemaker: A misnomer for a voltage-source pacemaker with an output circuit consisting of essentially a capacitor that discharges through the pacing lead. Both the voltage and the current of the stimulus decay continuously during the stimulus.

Coulomb: The fundamental unit of electrical charge.

Crosstalk: The detection by one channel of a dual-chamber pacemaker of the afterpotential associated with stimulation by the other.

Current: The rate of passage of electric charge through any point in a circuit; measured in amperes.

Current density: The amount of charge flowing through a unit area of a conductive medium per unit of time. It is most commonly expressed in milliamperes per square centimeter. Current density is the operative criterion for capture in cardiac stimulation, which is why electrodes with smaller surface area require lower voltages at the stimulation threshold.

Diode: A circuit component used to limit current flow to a single direction. It presents a high resistance to current flow in one direction and a low resistance to current flow in the other.

Electrode/tissue interface: The physical junction between a stimulating electrode and stimulation-susceptible tissue. It behaves like a circuit possessing both resistive and capacitive components. (See impedance and polarization voltage.)

Energy, potential: When charge is moved against electrical forces it gains potential energy, or the ability to do work. Energy is measured in joules. The same unit is used to describe physical work: 1 Joule = 1 Newton × 1 meter (force multiplied by distance). Related to power (rate of energy supply or absorption) by the relationship 1 Joule = 1 Watt-second. Electrical energy can be converted to other forms of energy. During radio-frequency ablation, for example, electrical energy is absorbed by a resistive medium (tissue) in which it is converted to thermal energy. Although it may be changed from one form to another, energy can be neither created nor destroyed (law of conservation of energy). The energy of a *rectangular* stimulation pulse can be calculated as the product of voltage, current, and stimulus duration. (Volts × milliamperes × milliseconds = microjoules.)

Exponential decay: The pattern of decreasing voltage across, and current through, a resistive load (such as the electrode/tissue interface) when connected to a charged capacitor, as during stimulation of the heart. The decrease is rapid at first, becoming increasingly slower as time progresses.

Farad: The basic unit of capacitance.

Filter: An electronic subsystem that inhibits unwanted frequency components of a signal. In pacemaker pulse generators, a filter may be used to isolate the rapid-deflection component of an intracardiac-electrogram signal.

Frequency: Rate of occurrence of a periodic phenomenon. Measured in hertz (equivalent to cycles per second). Low-frequency audible tones are heard as having low musical pitch; high-frequency tones have high pitch.

Henry: The basic unit of inductance.

Hertz: The basic unit of frequency. Equivalent to cycles per second.

Hybrid circuit: A combination of integrated circuits and discrete components (individual capacitors, etc.).

Impedance: Analogous to resistance, but takes into account the response of capacitors and inductors to signals that vary with time at various frequencies. The magnitude of impedance is measured in Ohms, but there is also a "phase" component (which can be measured in degrees) that reflects the time delays between current and voltage that are produced when a time-varying signal encounters a capacitor or inductor. For example, changes in the current flowing through a capacitor precede the corresponding changes in voltage. When the voltage and current are constant, the impedance that relates the two is reduced to resistance, because in those circumstances a capacitor behaves like an open circuit (infinite resistance) and an inductor behaves like a short circuit (zero resistance). Because of the capacitive component of the electrode/tissue interface, impedance (rather than resistance) is necessary to describe the relationship between current and voltage during cardiac stimulation. Frequently, however, the ratio of instantaneous voltage to instantaneous current at the beginning of the stimulus is (erroneously) given as the lead "impedance," ignoring everything that occurs during the remainder of the stimulus.

Inductance: The property of an inductor by which it stores electrical potential energy in a magnetic field. Measured in henrys.

Inductor: An electronic-circuit component (such as a coil of wire) that stores electrical potential energy in a magnetic field. The inductance is measured in henrys. A slowly-varying signal will pass through an inductor more readily than will a rapidly varying signal.

Insulator: A substance that presents infinite resistance to the flow of current.

Integrated circuit: A combination of circuit elements such as transistors and resistors, constructed as a single miniature unit.

Joule: The basic unit of energy. Sometimes expressed equivalently as watt-seconds.

Lapicque approximation: For rectangular stimulation pulses, an equation that describes the relationship of the stimulus amplitude (voltage or current) to the stimulus duration at the threshold of stimulation. It has the form of an hyperbola, and can be completely characterized by the rheobase (the stimulus amplitude at infinite stimulus duration) and the chronaxie (the stimulus duration at the point where the stimulus amplitude is equal to twice the rheobase). A mathematical expression approximating the strength-duration curve.

Light-emitting diode (LED): A type of diode that emits light when sufficient current flows through it in the forward (low resistance) direction.

7

Newton: A metric unit of force. One Newton (Nt) is equal to 0.225 lb.

Ohm: The basic unit of measurement of resistance. One Kilohm is equivalent to 1,000 Ohms.

Ohm's Law: The proportionality relationship between voltage and current. It can be expressed as voltage = current × resistance.

Open circuit: Two points in a circuit between which there is infinite resistance. Ohm's law predicts that no current can flow between the two points.

Parallel resistance: When two resistors are connected in parallel (side by side), the voltage across each is the same and the currents are additive. The resistance of the combination is lower than that of either resistor alone, and may be calculated by means of the equation

$$R(net) = (R1 \times R2)/(R1 + R2).$$

Polarity: Positive or negative. Often used (misleadingly) in pacing as a synonym for electrode configuration.

Polarization voltage: During stimulation, charge is stored temporarily in the electrode/tissue interface, which acts like a combination of resistance and capacitance. As this charge leaks off through the tissue resistance, a voltage is produced across that resistance as predicted by Ohm's law. Until sufficient charge leaks off, the electrode cannot be used effectively for sensing spontaneous electrical events. (See afterpotential and crosstalk.)

Power: The rate at which energy (whether electrical or otherwise) is delivered or absorbed. Measured in watts (1 watt = 1 joule/sec). For constant current and voltage, power can be calculated as the product of current and voltage.

Prefixes: Multipliers that change the size of a unit of measurement. Latin prefixes make units smaller: deci = 1/10, centi = 1/100, milli = 1/1,000, micro = 1/1,000 1,000

Greek prefixes make units larger: Kil, Kilo = 1,000, Meg, Mega = 1,000,000

Examples: 1 Kilohm (K) = one thousand ohms, 1 microjoule (μJ) = one millionth of a Joule, 1 millivolt (mV) = 0.001 V

Radio-frequency ablation: Ablation of the arrhythmogenic substrate or the normal conduction system, an anomalous conduction pathway, or an ectopic focus of excitation by means of the conversion of electrical energy delivered at frequencies on the order of .3 to 1.0 KHz. The electrical energy is converted into thermal energy as it is absorbed by the tissue, resulting in evaporation and desiccation of cells.

Resistance: The property of an electronic-circuit component (a resistor) through which current flows is proportional to the applied voltage. Measured in Ohms. If 5 Volts (V) are applied to a 1K resistance, the resulting current flow as predicted by Ohm's law is 5 milliamperes (mA).

Resistivity: A property of a material defined as the resistance of a piece of that material of unit length and unit cross-sectional area. Thus, the resistance of a piece of that material is equal to the resistivity multiplied by the length and divided by the cross-sectional area.

Resistor: An electronic-circuit component through which current flow is proportional to the applied voltage as described by Ohm's law.

Rheobase: In the Lapicque approximation of the threshold of stimulation, the stimulus amplitude at infinite stimulus duration.

Semiconductor: A material whose resistivity is not the same in all directions. It can be made into a diode or transistor.

Series resistance: When two resistors are connected in series (end to end), the current through each is the same and the voltages are additive. The resistance of the combination is higher than that of either resistor alone, and may be calculated by means of the equation R(net) = R1 + R2.

Short circuit: Two points in a circuit between which there is zero resistance. Ohm's law predicts that no voltage difference can exist between the two points.

Signal: A time-varying voltage. An example is the intracardiac-electrogram voltage processed by a pulse-generator's sensing circuit.

"Slew rate": A term referring to a property of a particular type of integrated circuit known as an operational amplifier. Often used (misleadingly) in pacing to refer to the maximal *slope* (i.e., the rate of change with time) of the rapid-deflection component of the intracardiac-electrogram signal.

Strength-duration curve: A plot of the stimulus amplitude (voltage or current) as a function of the stimulus duration at the threshold of stimulation. Capture may be achieved during electrical diastole at all combinations of amplitude and duration that lie above the curve, but at no combinations that lie below it.

Transistor: A semiconductor device that can function as a switch or amplifier.

Voltage: Electrical potential energy per unit of charge. Measured in volts (1 volt = 1 Joule per Coulomb). Related to current and resistance by Ohm's law.

Watt-second: A unit of energy equivalent to the joule.

Zener diode: A type of diode that allows current to flow in the normally inhibited direction when the applied voltage exceeds a critical value (called the Zener voltage). It is used to shunt current past a pulse-generator's circuits during external defibrillation to prevent damage to the circuits, but the current is shunted to the pacing lead, where it may produce a dangerously high current density at the cardiac electrode/tissue interface.

Education Content

Note: Due to the technical nature of the information in this chapter, we recommend that the reader study the glossary first. Sections A through G categorize the glossary terminology. Additional reading material is listed at the end of the chapter.

Also refer to Part One, Chapter 7 and Part Two, Chapters 14, 17, and 18.

A. Basic Quantities
1. Charge
2. Current
3. Voltage
4. Energy
5. Power

B. Derived Quantities
1. Current density
2. Resistance
3. Capacitance
4. Inductance
5. Current density
6. Battery capacity
7. Impedance

C. Units of Measurement
1. Ampere
2. Ampere-Hour
3. Charge
4. Coulomb
5. Farad
6. Henry
7. Hertz
8. Joule
9. Newton
10. Ohm
11. Voltage
12. Watt-second
13. Refer to prefixes in glossary

D. Relationships
   1. Ohm's law – see H, below
   2. Power and energy – see J, p 15

E. Circuit Components
   1. Resistors
   2. Capacitors
   3. Inductors
   4. Diodes
   5. Zener diodes

F. Signal Concepts
   1. Signals
   2. Amplitude
   3. Frequency

G. Electronics Subsystems
   1. Amplifiers
   2. Filters

H. Fundamental Electrical Relationships
   1. Ohm's law
       a. Ohm's law describes the relationship between a resistance R, the voltage V across it, and the current I that flows through it. The relationship can be expressed in any of three completely equivalent ways
           1. $V = IR$
           2. $I = V/R$
           3. $R = V/I$
   2. Energy
       a. All forms of energy, whether mechanical or electrical, potential or kinetic, have the physical dimensions of work: the applied force multiplied by the displacement, or the distance moved in the direction of the force. The fundamental metric-system unit of energy is the Joule (J).
       b. In pacing, the energy E of a *rectangular* stimulus (whose voltage and current remain constant throughout the stimulus) can be calculated by multiplying the stimulus voltage V, stimulus current I, and stimulus duration T. ($E = VIT$)
       c. If the voltage is given in V, the current in mA, and the stimulus duration in ms, the resulting calculated energy is in microjoules (μJ). For typical stimuli, with voltage and current decaying exponentially during the course of the stimulus, if this equation is ap-

11

plied to leading-edge values of voltage and current, the resulting value will be an overstimulation of the stimulus energy.

    d. For three important reasons, stimulation energy is of little more than academic interest. First, the stimulation energy is not subject to direct adjustment by a pacemaker-programming device. Second, battery capacity is usually measured, not in units of energy, but in units of electric charge (Ampere-hours). Third, although the threshold of stimulation can be described by any of several amplitude variables (charge, voltage, current or energy) together with the stimulus duration, voltage and current are the most practical and convenient quantities for this purpose.

3. Lead "impedance"

    a. In pacing, the term lead "impedance" usually refers to the instantaneous ratio of applied voltage to measured current at a single instant shortly after the onset of the stimulus. This value, as obtained by pacemaker data telemetry, includes the dc (direct current) resistance of the lead conductors.

        1. Telemetered values of lead "impedance" may be imprecise: random error on the order of 30% has been reported.

        2. Lead "impedance" tends to be somewhat higher with bipolar electrode systems than with unipolar systems.

4. The threshold of stimulation

    a. The stimulation threshold is the *combination* of minimal amplitude (charge, voltage, current, or energy) and stimulus duration that consistently results in cardiac depolarization outside the physiologic refractory period.

        1. Among the factors that determine the threshold as measured are:

            a) The dc resistance of the leads from generator to electrode

            b) The shape and surface area of the electrode

            c) The material of which the electrode is made

            d) The electrical polarization (capacitive effect) that occurs at the electrode/tissue interface when a stimulus is produced

            e) The thickness of non-excitable (scar) tissue separating the electrode from excitable myocardium

            f) The electrode site

            g) Time after implantation

            h) Electrolyte levels and disease processes

            i) Characteristics of the equipment used to measure the stimulus amplitude (i.e., the shape of the stimulus and the point at which the amplitude is measured)

    b. In the absence of steroid elution, the normal development of the electrode/tissue interface following implantation is characterized by:

1. A low initial threshold

2. A rise in threshold over the first 2–6 weeks, followed by

3. A gradual decrease in threshold to a chronic value perhaps 2–4 times the initial threshold, reached 2–3 months after implantation

   c. Stimulation-threshold measurements should be measured in a consistent fashion throughout follow-up, beginning with measurements using a pacemaker-systems analyzer compatible with the implanted pulse generator, using the same stimulus duration (if voltage adjustments are to be made) or voltage (if stimulus-duration adjustments are to be made). Lead "impedance" can sometimes be obtained directly; otherwise it can be calculated using Ohm's law as the ratio of threshold voltage V to threshold current I where both voltage and current thresholds are obtained *at the same stimulus duration,* because the lead "impedance" normally varies with stimulus duration.

5. "Strength-duration" curve

   a. A graphical plot of stimulus amplitude (voltage or current) as a function of stimulus duration. Any programmed combination of amplitude and duration that lies *above* the curve results in cardiac capture outside the physiologic refractory period; any combination that lies *below* the curve results in failure to capture.

      1. With loss of capture, proportionate increases in stimulus amplitude affect the likelihood of regaining capture at *any* value of the stimulus duration, but increasing the stimulus duration alone may be ineffective if it is already fairly large (greater than 1 ms) to begin with.

      2. In programming a pulse generator, a safety margin for capture is often achieved by choosing a combination of voltage and stimulus duration such that the programmed voltage is twice the voltage at threshold for that value of the stimulus duration.

      3. Because the amount of charge required for capture at the threshold of stimulation is lowest for the lowest available stimulus duration, and because battery capacity is measured in units of charge, better battery longevity can be achieved by using a shorter stimulus and a high voltage than with a longer stimulus at a lower voltage, even if both combinations of output parameters offer the same safety margin for capture.

I. Current, Voltage, and Resistance

   1. The fundamental relationship among these three quantities is Ohm's law, described above.

      a. Resistance in series: When two resistances are connected in series (end to end), the current through each is the same but the voltage across the combination is the sum of the voltages across the individual resistances. Thus when a conductor fracture occurs in a pacemaker lead, most of the applied (i.e., battery) voltage drops across the high-resistance gap, leaving only a very low voltage across the heart, inadequate to achieve capture. When fluid fills this gap, its resistance may still be too high for pacing, but sensing may be intact: the pacemaker's sensing amplifier draws very little current, so the voltage drop across the gap is low (as predicted by Ohm's law), and the sensing amplifier "sees" most of the signal voltage generated by a spontaneous cardiac depolarization.

b. Resistances in parallel: When two resistances are connected in parallel (side by side), the voltage across each is the same but the current through the combination is the sum of the currents through the individual resistances. Thus, when an insulation defect occurs in a unipolar pacemaker lead or in the septal insulation of the bipolar lead, most of the current from the pulse generator flows through the insulation break, leaving only a very low current through the heart, inadequate to achieve capture.

J. Energy and Power

1. Energy has been discussed above. Power is defined as the rate of generation or absorption of energy, and in the metric system of units is measured in watts; 1 watt = 1 joule per second. Power P can be calculated from voltage V, current I, and resistance R by the equivalent formulas

$$P = VI \qquad P = I^2R \qquad P = V^2/R$$

2. The amount of power dissipated in the heart during pacing far exceeds the power required for operation of the pacemaker circuits. In terms of pacemaker-battery capacity, the amount of the charge transferred as current during pacing far exceeds the amount transferred during sensing and for other tasks performed by the electronic circuitry.

K. Electric Circuits

1. An electric circuit is a closed loop: current flows from the battery, through the pacemaker circuits and, during stimulation, the heart, and back to the battery again. Electric charge can neither be created nor destroyed, but as the battery's capacity is used up, its internal resistance (a basic property of the device, not a removable component) increases and the voltage available at the battery terminals falls, ultimately to the point where the battery is useless.

a. In a unipolar electrode configuration, the pacing current begins at the pulse generator housing, flows through tissue to the cardiac electrode, and returns through the lead to the pulse generator. (Current is defined as the flow of *positive* electric charge, opposite to the direction of flow of free electrons; pacing is usually achieved using *negative*, or cathodal stimuli, hence the direction of current flow is as described).

b. In a bipolar electrode configuration, the pacing current begins at the pulse generator, flows through the lead to the proximal (ring) electrode, through the heart, and back from the distal (tip) electrode to the pulse generator.

References

Ausubel K and Furman S. Recent developments in pacemaker technology. New York: Clinical Medicine Research Institute, 1987.

Bayless W. The elements of permanent cardiac pacing. Critical Care Nurse. 8(7):31–41. 1988.

Barold S and Winner J. Techniques and significance of threshold measurement for cardiac pacing. Chest. 70(6):760–766. 1976.

Bernstein AD, Parsonnet V. Engineering aspects of pulse generators for cardiac pacing. In Electrical Therapy for Cardiac Arrhythmias. N Goldschlager, S Saksena, (Eds.). Philadelphia: WB Saunders Co., 21–34. 1990.

Dohrmann M and Goldschlager N. Myocardial stimulation threshold in patients with cardiac pacemakers: effect of physiologic variables, pharmacologic agents and lead electrodes. Cardiology Clinics. 3(4):527–537. 1985.

Ellenbogen K, ed. Practical Cardiac Diagnosis: Cardiac Pacing. Boston: Blackwell Scientific, 1992.

Furman S, Hurzeler P, Mehra R. Cardiac pacing and pacemakers IV. Threshold of cardiac stimulation. Am Heart J. 94(1):115–124. 1977.

Furman S, Hayes D, Holmes D. A Practice of Cardiac Pacing. New York: Futura Publishing Co, Inc., 1989.

Preston T and Barold S. Problems in measuring threshold for cardiac pacing, recommendations for routine clinical measurement. Am J Cardiol. 40: 658–660. 1977.

Moses H, Taylor G, Schneider J, Dove J. A Practical Guide to Cardiac Pacing. Boston: Little, Brown, 1987.

Tarjan PP. Engineering aspects of modern cardiac pacing. In Cardiac Pacing and Electrophysiology. N El-Serif and P Samit, (Eds.). Philadelphia: WB Saunders, 484–493. 1991.

CHAPTER 2.AB

Cardiac Anatomy and Physiology

Carol Higgins
Pat Manion

Subsection:
A. Cardiac Anatomy and Physiology
B. Hemodynamics of the Cardiovascular System

This chapter includes descriptions of general location and function of the heart. Gross anatomy of the heart, including chambers, valves, wall structure, and vasculature will be discussed, along with the structure of a myocardial cell.

Hemodynamics describes the ongoing process of physiologic balance that is influenced by cardiac, hormonal, vascular, and respiratory forces. This process is explained based on the anatomy and physiology of the cardiovascular system. The regulatory functions of the cardiac, hormonal, vascular, and respiratory system are described.

Information is supplied constantly to and from the cardiovascular system to maintain optimum function on a stroke-by-stroke basis. These changes occur to meet the changing demands of the cells as the need for oxygen increases and decreases. The role of the pituitary and renal hormones are described with their relationship to the cardiovascular system.

From: Schurig L. *Educational Guidelines: Pacing and Electrophysiology*. Armonk, NY: Futura Publishing Co, Inc, © 1994.

Objectives

1. Identify the chambers, valves, and major blood vessels of the heart.
2. Describe the function of the papillary muscles and chordae tendineae as related to valvular function.
3. Identify the pericardium, epicardium, myocardium, and endocardium.
4. Differentiate between the right and left heart in relation to function, chamber size, and pressures.
5. Describe location of coronary arteries.
6. Describe syncytium.
7. Describe each portion of the cardiac cycle.
8. Identify the correct sequence of events of cardiac systole.
9. Differentiate between preload and afterload.
10. Describe systemic vascular resistance.
11. Identify the mechanism seen in the activation of:
    A. Baroreceptors
    B. Chemoreceptors
12. Describe the relationship between intravascular volume and ADH secretion.
13. Identify three factors that influence myocardial oxygen consumption.

Glossary and Abbreviations

AV: Atrioventricular

Ao: Aorta

Afterload: Resistance which the heart pumps against.

BSA: Body surface area (height × weight = BSA in square meters)

CO: Cardiac output – measured in liters/minute (amount of blood moved by the heart in 1 minute).

CI: Cardiac index—the relation of cardiac output to the body surface area (CO ÷ BSA).

CX: Circumflex branch of left coronary artery

Diag: Diagonal branch

Diastolic blood pressure: Pressure in the ventricle during diastole (resting phase of the cardiac cycle).

Homeostasis: A state of balance or equilibrium maintained by autoregulation of physiologic processes.

IVC: Inferior vena cava

LA: Left atrium

LAD: Left anterior descending branch of left coronary artery

LM: Left main coronary artery

LV: Left ventricle

OMB: Obtuse marginal branch of left Cx

PA: Pulmonary artery

Preload: Stretch of the myocardial muscle filber determined by the volume received by the atrium from venous return to the heart. Generates ventricular filling pressures.

Pulse pressure: Difference between the systolic and diastolic blood pressure.

PVR: Pulmonary vascular resistance

RA: Right atrium

RCA: Right coronary artery

RV: Right ventricle

S_1: First heart sound

S_2: Second heart sound

SV: Stroke volume—measured in cc/beat (amount of blood moved by the heart in one contraction).

SVC: Superior vena cava

SVR: Systemic vascular resistance or peripheral vascular resistance

Syncytium: Interconnections of cardiac muscle fibers.

Systolic blood pressure: Peak pressure reached during ventricular contraction.

Education Content

A. Cardiac Anatomy and Physiology

  1. Cardiac anatomy

    a. General function of the heart

      1. Double pump, working in unison

      2. Right heart

        a) Receives unoxygenated blood from venous system

        b) Sends unoxygenated blood to lungs

      3. Left heart

        a) Receives oxygenated blood from lungs

        b) Sends oxygenated blood to systemic circulation

    b. Gross structure of heart and greater vessels

      1. Location of heart

        a) Within mediastinum, between lungs

        b) Base

          1) Two atria

          2) Behind body of sternum

        c) Apex

          1) Two ventricles

          2) Positioned downward and to left of sternum

      2. Chambers

        a) Atria: thin walled, low pressure chambers

          1) Right atrium (RA) receives unoxygenated blood from the body through the superior vena cava (SVC) and inferior vena cava, and from the heart muscle through the coronary sinus.

          2) Left atrium (LA) receives oxygenated blood from the lungs through the pulmonary veins.

          3) Atria are divided by atrial septum

        b) Ventricles: The "pumping" chambers

          1) Right ventricle (RV) receives unoxygenated blood from right atrium (RA) and pumps it through the pulmonary artery (PA) to a low pressure system, the lungs.

          2) The left ventricle (LV) receives oxygenated blood from the LA and pumps it through the aorta (Ao) to a high pressure systemic circulation.

          3) The LV walls are thicker muscle than the RV walls.

          4) The ventricles are divided by the intraventricular septum.

3. Valves
    a) Atrioventricular (AV) Valves: Allow unidirectional blood flow from atria to ventricles
        1) Tricuspid valve has anterior, posterior, and septal leaflets and connects RA and RV.
        2) Mitral valve has a posterior (mural) and anterior (aortic) leaflet and connects LA and LV.
        3) When the pressure in the ventricles falls below the pressure in the atria (ventricular diastole) the AV valves open and blood flows from atria to ventricles.
    b) Semilunar valves: Allow unidirectional blood flow from ventricles to PA and Ao
        1) Pulmonary valve has an annulus (ring), three commissures, and three cusps.
        2) Pulmonary valve connects RV to PA.
        3) Aortic valve has an annulus and normally three cusps.
        4) Aortic valve connects LV to Ao.
    c) Heart Sounds:
        1) Sound 1 (Lub, S_1) is closure of tricuspid and mitral valves
        2) Sound 2 (Dub, S_2) is closure of aortic and pulmonic valves.
        3) Murmur: blood being forced through a nonelastic (stenotic) valve or turbulent flow through a normal or an incompetent valve.
4. Papillary muscle and chordae tendineae
    a) Papillary muscles
        1) Arise from inner walls of ventricles
        2) Attach to chordae tendineae
    b) Chordae tendineae
        1) Tendinous strings connecting papillary muscle to AV valves
    c) Purpose
        1) Ventricular contraction increases the pressure in the ventricles which forces AV valves to close.
        2) Simultaneous contraction of the papillary muscles causes tension on Chordae tendoneae.
        3) Prevents AV valves from ballooning backward into atria.
        4) Preventing retrograde flow of blood from ventricles to atria.
2. Coronary arteries
    a. Originate in sinuses of Valsalva, at root of aorta just above aortic valve
    b. Fill during ventricular relaxation
    c. Right coronary artery (RCA)

1. Winds around in right AV groove
2. Forms posterior descending artery in posterior interventricular groove in about 80% of hearts
3. Supplies sinoatrial (SA) Node in 55% of hearts
4. Supplies AV node in approximately 90% of hearts
5. Supplies right atrial and ventricular heart muscle
6. Supplies inferior and posterior wall of left ventricle
7. Supplies posterior portion of interventricular septum

   d. Left main coronary artery bifurcates into two major coronary arteries: left anterior descending (LAD) and circumflex (CX)

   e. LAD
1. Travels down anterior interventricular groove
2. Supplies anterior part of interventricular septum
3. Supplies anterior wall of LV
4. Supplies the bundle of His

   f. CX
1. Winds around the left AV groove
2. Supplies SA node in 45% of hearts
3. Supplies AV node in 10% of hearts
4. Supplies posterior surface of LV via obtuse marginal branch (OMB)

3. Venous return from cardiac muscle
   a. Great and small cardiac veins
   b. Coronary sinus, drains into the right atrium and represents 85% of the venous blood from the left ventricle
   c. Thebesian veins, drains into the right and left atria and limited into the right ventricle and represents 40% of the venous blood from the atria

4. Histology
   a. Walls of the heart
1. Epicardium
   a) Outermost layer
   b) Thin, serous membrane
   c) Part of serous pericardium
2. Myocardium
   a) Middle layer
   b) Working muscle of heart
3. Endocardium
   a) Innermost layer
   b) Lines myocardium with endothelial tissue

      c) Endothelial tissue also covers valves and is continuous with the blood vessels emptying into and exiting the heart.

    4. Fibrous tissue

      a) Separates atria from ventricles

      b) Provides framework for cardiac valves

  b. Pericardial sac

    1. Fibrous tissue

    2. Layers

      a) Visceral pericardium is epicardial layer of heart muscle

      b) Parietal pericardium lines pericardial sac

    3. Pericardial fluid

      a) Small amount of fluid between layers of pericardium

      b) Eliminates friction as the heart contracts and relaxes

  c. Cardiac muscle

    1. Sarcomere

      a) Functional contractile unit of muscle fiber in heart

      b) Overlapping actin and myosin filaments with sarcomere

    2. Intercalated discs

      a) Separate individual myocardial muscle cells

      b) Conduct electrical impulses from one cell to the next very rapidly

    3. Cardiac muscle fibers

      a) Composed of many sarcomeres

      b) Join and divide many times forming interconnections

    4. Stimulation of cardiac muscle causes:

      a) Actin and myosin slide past each other as binding sites change

      b) Rapid uncoupling and recoupling occurs

      c) Sarcomeres shorten

      d) Cardiac muscle contraction occurs

    5. Syncytium

      a) Interconnections of cardiac muscle fiber

      b) Wave of contraction spreads rapidly

      c) Results in almost simultaneous contraction

B. Hemodynamics of the Cardiovascular System

  1. Systemic blood pressure determined by:

    a. Circulating blood volume

    b. State of relaxation or contraction of peripheral arteries and veins (arterial morphology)

   c. Vascular patency
   d. Cardiac output
2. Cardiac output
   a. Electrical stimulation generates muscle activity (mechanical events)
   b. Atrial systole (contraction)
      1. Completes ventricular filling
      2. "Atrial kick" provides 20% of LV filling volume. Will be variable depending on compliance and timing factors.
   c. Atrial diastole (Relaxation)
      1. RA fills from SVC and IVC, coronary sinus, and thebesian veins
      2. LA fills from the pulmonary veins
   d. Ventricular systole
      1. Isovolumic contraction
         a) Ventricular muscle begins to contract
         b) Ventricular pressures increase
         c) AV valves close
         d) Increased pressure, no change in volume
      2. Rapid ventricular ejection
         a) Ventricular muscle continues to contract
         b) Aortic and pulmonic valves open
         c) Blood is ejected into Ao and PA
   e. Ventricular diastole
      1. Isovolumic relaxation
         a) Decrease in ventricular pressures
         b) No change in ventricular volume
         c) Aortic and pulmonic valves close
      2. Rapid ventricular filling
         a) Atrial pressures higher than ventricular pressures
         b) AV valves open
         c) Blood passively enters ventricles
         d) Atrial systole then completes ventricular filling phase
         e) Maximum coronary artery perfusion occurs during ventricular diastole
   f. Calculation: CO = SV × HR
      1. Normal resting Cardiac output: 4–8 Liters/minutes
      2. Cardiac Index: $\dfrac{CO}{BSA}$
         a) Normal resting CI: 2.4–4 Liters/minutes/M^2
         b) Better value to use for clinical decision making
   g. Determination of cardiac output

1. Preload
2. Afterload
3. Myocardial contractility
4. Heart rate

3. Myocardial oxygen consumption (MVO_2)
   a. Balance should exist between oxygen supply and oxygen demand.
   b. Myocardial oxygen supply
      1. Patency of coronary arteries
      2. Coronary filling time (length of ventricular diastole)
      3. Pressure of oxygen dissolved in arterial blood (PO_2)
      4. Amount of hemoglobin
      5. Ability of hemoglobin to transport O_2
      6. Coronary artery perfusion pressure
   c. Myocardial oxygen demand
      1. Heart rate
      2. Myocardial contractility
      3. Afterload
      4. Wall tension

4. Myocardial contractility
   a. Preload
      1. Volume of blood in ventricles at the end of ventricular diastole
      2. Stretches the ventricular muscle
      3. The greater the stretch the greater the force of contraction
      4. Compliance also plays a role in the ability of the chamber to stretch
   b. Afterload (systemic vascular resistance)
      1. The resistance that the ventricles must overcome in order to eject their blood
      2. Resistance is overcome during phase of isovolumic contraction
      3. Overcoming afterload, as well as wall tension, heart rate and contractility consumes most of the O_2 delivered to myocardium
      4. Decreased afterload allows ventricles to eject blood with less effort
      5. Increased afterload forces ventricles to increase the workload, can result in pulmonary edema or a poor ejection fraction (EF)
   c. Alterations in contractility
      1. Diastolic abnormalities
         a) Decreased preload
            1) Due to decreased venous return (Hypovolemia, vasodilatation)

       2) Decreases cardiac output

       3) Hypotension

   b) Increased preload

       1) Due to decreased contractility

       2) Due to valvular dysfunction

          • Mitral and/or tricuspid insufficiency

          • AV valve stenosis

          • compliance

       3) Decreases cardiac output

       4) Right and/or left ventricular failure

  2. Systolic abnormalities

    a) Decreased myocardial contractility

    b) Valvular dysfunction – pulmonic and/or aortic stenosis (increase afterload)

5. Heart rate

  a. If stroke volume is normal (approximately 70 cc):

    1. Increased heart rate can increase cardiac output:

    Example: SV of 70 cc × HR of 140 = CO 9800 cc

    2. Decreased heart rate can decrease cardiac output:

    Example: SV of 70 cc × HR of 40 = CO of 2800 cc

  b. If stroke volume is decreased:

    Example: decreased myocardial contractility, hypovolemia

    1. Increased heart rate can maintain normal cardiac output:

    Example: SV of 40 × HR of 120 = CO of 4800 cc

    2. Normal heart rate can result in decreased cardiac output:

    Example: SV of 40 × HR of 80 = CO of 3200 cc

  c. A very rapid heart rate can decrease cardiac output because of shortened diastolic filling time, thereby reducing stroke volume:

    Example: SV of 20 × HR of 180 = CO of 3600 cc

  d. If stroke volume is increased:

Example: Athletic heart, even a very slow heart rate can provide a normal cardiac output:

Example: SV of 120 cc × HR 40 = CO of 4800 cc

6. Role of autonomic nervous system on the cardiovascular system
  a. Sympathetic stimulation
   1. SA node and AV node
     a) Increases rate
     b) Increase AV nodal conduction
   2. Atria
     a) Increases contractility
   3. Ventricles
     a) Increases contractility
   4. Blood vessels
     a) Generally cause vasoconstriction
     b) May dilate coronary arteries
  b. Parasympathetic stimulation (vagus nerve)
   1. SA node and AV node
     a) Decreases rate
     b) Decreases AV nodal conduction
   2. Atria
     a) Decreases contractility
   3. Ventricles
     a) Decreases contractility
     b) Distribution less than in atria
   4. Blood vessels
     a) Vasodilitation
7. Internal homeostasis
  a. Heart rate
   1. Will increase to:
     a) Meet increased metabolic demands for oxygen (fever, exercise, infection)
     b) Maintain normal cardiac output in presence of decreased stroke volume (MI, CHF, hypovolemia)
     c) Compensate for decreased oxygen in blood (anemia, hypoxemia)
   2. Will decrease to:
     a) Meet decreased metabolic demands (sleep)
     b) Maintain normal cardiac output in people with large stroke volumes (athletic heart)
  b. Myocardial contractility

1. Frank-Starling law of the heart
   a) When ventricular end-diastolic pressure (preload) increases, diastolic fiber length is increased, which increases the force of recoil (contractility) which in turn increases stroke volume.
c. Myocardial hypertrophy
   1. Results from chronically increased preload or afterload
      a) Hypertension (systemic or pulmonary)
      b) Semilunar valve stenosis
      c) Left to right shunts
   2. Compensatory mechanism to maintain cardiac output
d. Vascular tone
   1. Arterioles
      a) Major factor in regulating blood flow
      b) Offer most resistance
      c) Vascular smooth muscle comprises the majority of arterial walls and controls vascular tone.
   2. Sympathetic stimulation
      a) Vasoconstriction in small arteries and arterioles – increasing systemic blood pressure
      b) Increases venous return to the heart which increases cardiac output
e. Baroreceptors (pressure receptors)
   1. Located in aortic arch, carotid sinus, atria, pulmonary arteries, SVC, and IVC. (The LV has mechanoreceptors and C fibers)
   2. Sensitive to changes in blood pressure
   3. Increased blood pressure causes:
      a) Inhibition of sympathetic nervous system
      b) Leads to decreased heart rate, contractility, and ultimately a decrease in BP
   4. Decreased blood pressure causes:
      a) Sympathetic stimulation
      b) Which leads to an increase in heart rate and an increase in myocardial contractility, increased systemic vascular resistance.
f. Chemoreceptors
   1. Located in carotid body and aortic arch
   2. Monitor blood levels of:
      a) Oxygen
      b) Carbon dioxide
      c) Hydrogen ions (ph)
   3. Send impulses to medulla

       a) Stimulates vasomotor center

       b) Make necessary changes in heart rate and blood pressure

  g. Angiotensin II

    1. Result of renin production by kidneys in response to a low blood pressure

    2. Causes vasoconstriction throughout body

    3. Stimulates production of aldosterone by the adrenal cortex

       a) Causes sodium and water retention

       b) Increase circulating blood volume

  h. Antidiuretic hormone (ADH or vasopressin)

    1. Secreted by pituitary gland in response to a decrease BP

    2. Causes water retention

    3. Causes vasoconstriction

References

Alspach J. Core Curriculum for Critical Care Nursing. 4th Ed. Philadelphia: WB Saunders Co., 1991.

Bullock B. Pathophysiology: Adaptations and Alterations in Function. 2nd ed. Illinois: Scott, Foresman and Co., 1988.

Daily E and Schroeder J. Techniques in Bedside Hemodynamic Monitoring. 4th Ed. St. Louis: CV Mosby Book, 1989.

Headley J. Invasive Hemodynamic Monitoring: Physiological Principles and Clinical Applications. Edwards Critical-Care Division, Baxter, 1989.

Guyton A. Textbook of Medical Physiology. 8th Ed. Philadelphia: WB Saunders Co., 1991.

Hudak C. Critical Care Nursing: A holistic approach. 5th Ed. Philadelphia: JB Lippincott Co., 1989.

Suggested Readings

Sitzer V. Physiologic Framework of Extrinsic Controls. The J Cardiovasc Nurs. 5.4.1–9. 1991.

Barden C. Muscle Dysfunction in the Failing Heart. Nurse Review Series. Springhouse: Spring House Corporation, 1988.

CHAPTER 2.C

Cardiac Anatomy and Physiology
Basic Electrophysiology

Joni Baxter

Subsection:
A–G. Conduction System Topics

An understanding of the basic anatomy and physiology of the heart's conduction system is essential to professionals working in the areas of pacing and electrophysiology. This chapter reviews the anatomy and physiology of the conduction system. Included are the path of normal impulse conduction, cellular behavior, and electrical properties of cardiac cells. Factors influencing conduction, abnormalities that can occur and the locations of conduction delay are discussed.

It is also important to be aware of the methods of evaluating the conduction system. A basic understanding of intracardiac signals is useful whether you are a pacemaker specialist reviewing telemetered signals from a pacemaker or an EP specialist evaluating a patient's electrograms during an electrophysiology study. In this chapter, we will present an overview of the characteristics of both spontaneous and paced electrogram signals. A more in-depth discussion on this topic can be found in the pacing and/or electrophysiology curriculum chapters to follow.

From: Schurig L. *Educational Guidelines: Pacing and Electrophysiology*. Armonk, NY: Futura Publishing Co, Inc, © 1994.

Objectives

1. Describe the normal conduction sequence in the heart.
2. List four properties of cardiac conductive tissue.
3. State two mechanisms of conduction abnormalities.
4. Describe locations in the heart where abnormal conduction delays can occur.
5. List two methods of recording cardiac electrical activity.
6. Describe the common locations of intracardiac catheters used to record cardiac electrical activity.
7. Identify surface electrocardiogram morphology during right ventricular pacing.

Glossary and Abbreviations

Accessory pathway: An extra conduction pathway that travels outside the normal route.

Action potential: The depolarization and repolarization of a cell.

Atrioventricular (AV) node: Area located between the ostium of the coronary sinus and the tricuspid valve annulus through which impulses from the atria pass before continuing into the bundle of His.

Bundle branch: Pathways on both the left and right sides of the heart that conduct impulses from the bundle of His to the ventricles.

Bundle of His: A band of parallel Purkinge fibers that travel from the AV node, conducting impulses through the interventricular septum to the bundle branches.

Electrogram: Recording of cardiac electrical activity.

Refractory period: Period that starts at the onset of the action potential during which a subsequent impulse cannot stimulate the cell.

Sinus (sinoatrial or SA) node: A strip of specialized cardiac tissue located high in the right atrium that under normal conditions is the pacemaker of the heart.

Education Content

A. Anatomy of the Conduction System

   1. Sinus (or SA) node

      a. Located near the junction of the right atrium and superior vena cava

      b. Primary pacemaker of the heart

   2. AV (atrioventricular) node

      a. Located superior to tricuspid valve, anterior to coronary sinus

      b. Impulses travel from the atria through the AV node before continuing into the bundle of His

      c. Secondary pacemaker of the heart

   3. Bundle of His

      a. A band of parallel Purkinje fibers continuous with the distal AV node

      b. Conducts impulses through the interventricular septum to the bundle branches

      c. Normally the sole electrical connection between the atria and ventricles

   4. Bundle branches

      a. Pathways of conductive cells

      b. Transmit impulses from the bundle of His to both ventricles

      c. Bifurcates to right and left bundle

      d. Left branch fans out to anterior and posterior divisions

   5. Purkinje fibers

      a. Specialized cells of electrical conduction throughout the ventricles

      b. Tertiary pacemaker of the heart

B. Physiology of the Conduction System

   1. Cellular electrophysiology

      a. Membrane potentials

         1. Resting potential

           a) The electrical potential difference between intracellular and extracellular fluid

           b) Example: Purkinge cell – 90 mV

         2. Action potential

           a) Depolarization and repolarization of cell

           b) Created as a result of ion currents crossing the cell membrane

              1) Working muscle cells

                • In response to a stimulus

     2) Automatic cells
- Cells which have the ability to initiate an action potential without external stimulation
- Cells with the most automaticity
  — Found in the conductive tissues of the heart
  — SA nodal cells normally have the highest degree of automaticity (dominant pacemaker of the heart)

b. Ion channels

  1. Activity of ion channels during phases of action potential

    a) Phase 0 = depolarization
1) Cell permeability to sodium increases
2) Sodium rushes into cell
3) Rapid upstroke of action potential

    b) Phase 1 = initial rapid repolarization
1) Sodium channels close
2) K^+ and Cl^- leaving cell

    c) Phase 2 = plateau
1) Slow repolarization
2) Slow calcium and sodium inward currents
3) Potassium moving out of cell

    d) Phase 3 = rapid repolarization
1) Potassium levels fall down in concentration gradient

    e) Phase 4 = electrical diastole
1) Potassium leaks out of cell

  2. Electrical properties of cardiac conductive tissue

    a) Excitability
1) Ability to depolarize and create an action potential in response to a stimulus of sufficient magnitude

    b) Automaticity
1) Ability to reach threshold and generate an impulse without an external stimulus
2) Result of spontaneous depolarization during phase 4

    c) Conductivity
1) The ability of a cell to propagate an electrical impulse to a neighboring cell

    d) Refractoriness
1) The temporary inability of a cell to respond to an electrical stimulus and form another action potential.
2) This varies from absolute (unable to respond) to relative (ability to respond depends on timing and strength of stimulus) in different phases of the action potential.

C. Normal Path of Impulse Conduction

	Intrinsic rate
1. Sinus node-pacemaker	70–80 bpm
2 Atria	
3. AV node	40–60 bpm
4. Bundle of His	
5. Bundle branches	
6. Purkinge fibers	20–40 bpm
7. Ventricles	

D. Influences on Conduction
  1. Autonomic nervous system
     a. Sympathetic
        1. Adrenergic – increase rate
     b. Parasympathetic
        1. Vagal – decrease rate
  2. Pathological
     a. Ischemia
     b. Cardiomyopathy
     c. Metabolic
     d. Myocarditis
     e. Calcification
     f. Congenital
     g. Fibrosis
     h. Neurologic
     i. Connective tissue disorders
     j. Tumors
     k. Other
  3. Medication
     a. Cardioactive
        1. Examples: digoxin, antiarrhythmics
  4. Aging

E. Abnormalities of the Conduction System (also refer to Part Three, Chapter 22 for definitions of mechanisms of arrhythmias.)
  1. Mechanisms of arrhythmias
     a. Disorders of impulse formation
        1. Enhanced normal automaticity
        2. Abnormal automaticity
        3. Triggered activity

    b. Disorders of impulse conduction
       1. Reentry
       2. Conduction delay and block
       3. Reflection
    c. Combined disorders of impulse formation and impulse conduction
  2. Locations of conduction delay
    a. May occur in any portion of the conduction system
       1. Sinus node
       2. Atria
       3. AV node
       4. His bundle
       5. Bundle branches
    b. See characteristics of electrograms and normal intracardiac conduction times below

F. Methods of Recording and Characteristics of His Bundle, Atrial, Coronary Sinus and Ventricular Electrograms
  1. Methods of recording
    a. Unipolar vs. bipolar
       1. Unipolar – one electrode inside of the heart and one external to the heart.
       2. Bipolar – two electrodes are at the tip of the catheter inside the heart.
    b. Electrode locations
       1. Surface electrocardiogram
       2. Esophageal – atrial activity enhanced
       3. Myocardial electrogram
         a) Epicardial
           1) Atrial
           2) Ventricular
         b) Endocardial
           1) Atrial – high right atrial
           2) His bundle – tricuspid valve area
           3) Coronary sinus – left sided atrial activity
           4) Ventricular
             • Right ventricular apex
             • Right ventricular outflow tract
             • Left ventricular
      4. Cellular
        a) MAP = monophasic action potential

   c. Filtered
      1. Signal averaged electrocardiogram (SAECG) – Refer to Part Three, Chapter 31.
2. Characteristics of electrograms
   a. Definitions
      1. A represents atrial activation on intracardiac electrograms
      2. H represents His bundle activation on intracardiac electrograms
      3. V represents ventricular activation on intracardiac electrograms
   b. Electrogram interpretation from various electrophysiology catheter locations
      1. High right atrial
         a) A wave on corresponds to P wave on the surface ECG.
      2. His bundle – has atrial (A), His (H) and ventricular (V) electrical activity
         a) PA interval
            1) Normal = 5–40 msec
            2) Intra-atrial conduction time
            3) Time measured from the P wave on a surface ECG or the A wave on the high right atrial catheter to the first rapid deflection of the A wave on the His bundle electrogram
         b) AH interval
            1) Normal = 50–130 msec
            2) AV nodal conduction time
            3) Time measured from the A to the H on the His bundle electrogram
         c) HV interval
            1) Normal = 30–55 msec
            2) Conduction time through the His-Purkinge system
            3) The time measured from the H (His bundle potential on the His bundle electrogram) to the earliest activation of the ventricles
      3. Coronary sinus
         a) Left atrial activity
         b) Left ventricular activity
      4. Ventricular
         a) V wave (right ventricular catheter) corresponds to QRS wave on the surface ECG.
   c. Electrogram characteristics from pacemaker catheters
      1. During device implantation
         a) Atrial lead activity
            1) A wave on corresponds to P wave on the surface ECG
            2) Pacemaker artifact preceeds each evoked A wave

       b) Ventricular activity

          1) V wave (right ventricular catheter) corresponds to QRS wave on the surface ECG

          2) Pacemaker artifact preceeds each evoked V wave

    2. Telemetered intracardiac signals

       a) Intracardiac electrical activity transmitted via pulse generator through device programmer

          1) Unipolar

          2) Bipolar

       b) Waveforms similar to electrograms seen at implant (described above)

G. ECG Morphology During Pacing

    1. Pacemaker artifact preceeds each complex

       a. P wave with atrial pacing

       b. QRS with ventricular pacing

       c. P and QRS with dual chamber pacing

       d. Variations occur depending on

          1. Implanted device

          2. Pacemaker settings

          3. Intrinsic rhythm

    2. Right Ventricular pacing

       a. Surface ECG with catheter in the RV apex

          1. LBBB morphology

          2. Superior left axis deviation (-30 to -90)

       b. Surface ECG with catheter in the RV outflow tract (RVOT)

          1. LBBB morphology

          2. Normal inferior axis (rarely right axis deviation)

    3. Left ventricular pacing

       a. RBBB morphology

    4. ST-T wave changes

    5. Fusion/pseudofusion beats

References

Fogoros R. Electrophysiologic Testing. Boston: Blackwell Scientific Publications, 1991.

Saksena S, Goldschlager N. Electrical Therapy for Cardiac Arrhythmias. Philadelphia: WB Saunders Co., 1990.

Zipes DP, Jalife J. Cardiac Electrophysiology and Arrhythmias. Orlando: Grune & Stratton, Inc., 1985.

Zipes DP, Jalife J. Cardiac Electrophysiology From Cell to Bedside. Philadelphia: WB Saunders Co., 1990.

CHAPTER 3

Assessment

Melanie T. Gura

Subsection:
A. Assessment of History
B. Cardiac Physical Examination
C. Diagnostic Evaluation

Obtaining a health history and physical examination are important aspects of patient care. The history consists of subjective data obtained from the patient and family, whereas the physical examination furnishes objective data through inspection, percussion, palpation and auscultation of the patient.

The cardiac examination usually starts from the head and proceeds downwards. It includes a general patient survey, examination of the heart, the great vessels, the peripheral pulses, and the blood pressure.

In addition to the physical examination, objective data is also obtained from other sources such as diagnostic procedures, which include electrocardiograms, echocardiograms, myocardial perfusion imaging, exercise testing, ambulatory electrocardiogram, head-up tilt table testing, cardiac catheterization/coronary angiography, and electrophysiology studies.

These diagnostic studies, along with the history and physical examination, formulate the patient data base. The data base is then analyzed and synthesized into a problem list which identifies actual, potential, and high-risk problems.

From: Schurig L. *Educational Guidelines: Pacing and Electrophysiology*. Armonk, NY: Futura Publishing Co, Inc, © 1994.

Objectives

1. List the four techniques used in the physical examination to obtain objective data.
2. Demonstrate the proper technique for determining CVP non-invasively.
3. Demonstrate auscultation of the five areas of the heart.
4. Discuss the most commonly utilized method of grading murmurs.
5. Describe a systematic approach to interpret the radiography components of a chest X-ray.
6. List four complications that may occur after invasive diagnostic testing.
7. Describe the diagnostic significance of a right and left cardiac catheterization.
8. Describe the diagnostic significance of cardiac nuclear scanning.
9. Describe the diagnostic significance of the head-up-tilt test (HUT).
10. Describe the diagnostic significance of exercise testing.

Glossary and Abbreviations

Aortic area: Second right intercostal space close to sternum.

Auscultation: The act of listening with our ear or a stethoscope for sounds produced by cardiac activity and any other sounds.

Bell: Used to accentuate low-frequency sounds such as diastolic murmurs and the third (S_3) and fourth (S_4) heart sounds. Should be applied lightly to body surface.

Bruit: An adventitious sound of arterial or venous origin heard on auscultation.

Diaphragm: Used to auscultate high-frequency sound such as systolic murmurs, the first (S_1) and second (S_2) heart sounds. Should be applied firmly against the skin.

Erbs' point: Third left intercostal space close to sternum.

Inspection: Involves objective observation, encompasses our senses of sight, hearing, touch, and smell.

Mitral area: Fifth left intercostal space, medial to midclavicular line.

Palpation: Incorporates our sense of touch. With the examiner's hands, temperature, moisture, texture, vibration, masses, edema, and crepitus are felt.

Paradoxical splitting of S_2: The splitting of S_2 occurs on expiration with P_2 preceding A_2 which is the reverse of normal. This is the rule with RV pacing or left bundle branch block.

Pectus carinatum: Abnormal prominence of the sternum (pigeon breast).

Pectus excavatum: Abnormal congenital depression of sternum (funnel breast).

Percussion: Involves tapping the body surface with a sharp, quick motion to elicit sounds that will assist in determining the location, size, density, and position of the underlying structures.

Physiologic splitting: Pulmonic sound occurs slightly later than aortic closure during inspiration.

Pulmonic area: Second left intercostal space close to sternum.

Stethoscope: Preferred instrument for auscultation. Tubing should be short, 12–14 inches, with an $\frac{1}{8}$ diameter. The ear piece should fit snugly and the diaphragm and bell should be free of cracks.

Tricuspid area: Fifth intercostal space, lower left sternal border.

Xanthoma palpebrarum: Flat, elevated, rounded, chamois-covered plaque affecting the eyelids.

RV: Right ventricle

LV: Left ventricle

Education Content

A. Assessment

    1. History

        a. Chief complaint

            1. Chest pain

                a) Onset, duration

                b) Location, radiation

                c) Severity and character

                d) Aggravating factors

                e) Alleviating factors

                f) Associated symptoms

            2. Dyspnea

            3. Orthopnea

            4. Paroxysmal nocturnal dyspnea

            5. Cyanosis

            6. Palpitations

            7. Fatigue

            8. Cough

            9. Nausea or vomiting

            10. Diaphoresis

            11. Pallor

            12. Fever

            13. Pre-syncope

            14. Syncope

            15. Edema

            16. Cramping

            17. Claudication

            18. Effort intolerance

    2. Past medical history

        a. Previous cardiac problems and procedures

        b. Medication

        c. Allergies

    3. Family history

        a. Coronary artery disease (CAD)

        b. Diabetes mellitus

        c. Cerebrovascular accident (CVA)

        d. Hypertension (HTN)

       e. Heart problems

       f. Sudden death (SCD)

       g. Syncope

       h. Cardiomyopathy (CM)

   4. Social history

       a. Smoking pattern

       b. Dietary pattern

       c. Alcohol consumption

       d. Exercise pattern

       e. Recreation drugs (ex: Cocaine)

   5. Environmental history

   6. Occupational history

B. Cardiac physical examination

   1. Inspection

       a. Skin and mucous membranes

          1. Color

          2. Turgor

          3. Temperature

          4. Eyes

             a) Xanthoma palpebrarum

       b. Neck veins

          1. Internal jugular pulsation waves reflects right atrial pressure

          2. Establish jugular venous pressure (JVP)

             a) Patient supine or 45° angle

             b) Measure in centimeters (cm) the height between the sternal angle (which is 5 cm) and the highest point of oscillation of the internal or external jugular veins

             c) Greater than 2 cm may indicate right-sided heart failure or SVC obstruction

       c. Precordium

          1. Chest shape and contour

             a) Normal

             b) Barrel

             c) Pectus carinatum

             d) Pectus excavatum

             e) Kyphoscoliosis

          2. Visible pulsations

             a) Heaves

             b) Thrills

d. Extremities
   1. Color
   2. Turgor
   3. Nailbeds (160° angle)
      a) Clubbing
      b) Capillary refill
   4. Hair distribution
   5. Edema
      a) Pitting edema grading scale

$$0–1/4'' = +1$$
$$1/4–1/2'' = +2$$
$$1/2–1'' = +3$$
$$>1'' = +4$$

2. Palpation
   a. Pulses
      1. Assess the following bilaterally and simultaneously except carotids:
         a) Rate
         b) Rhythm
         c) Volume
            1) Carotid (upstroke)
            2) Radial
            3) Brachial
            4) Femoral
            5) Popliteal
            6) Posterior tibial
            7) Dorsalis pedis .
      2. Characterize pulse volume on scale of 0–4

$$0 = Absent$$
$$+1 = Weak, thready$$
$$+2 = Normal$$
$$+3 = Full$$
$$+4 = Full and bounding$$

   a) Example: $+2/+4$ would indicate a normal finding on a $+4$ scale
   b. Precordium
      1. Palpate seven fields with ball of hand:

a) Sternoclavicular area

b) Aortic area – base right

c) Pulmonic area

d) Third left intercostal space (ICS) and left lateral sternal border (RV area)

e) LV apical area (PMI area)

f) Epigastric area

g) Ectopic areas – site other than the areas expected based on cardiac anatomy

2. Palpate for:

a) Thrills

b) Heaves

c) Lifts

d) Tenderness

e) Apical impulse location

1) Point of maximal intensity (PMI)

2) Normally fifth intercostal space midclavicular line, 1–2 cm in diameter

3) May be displaced with the following:

- Left ventricular enlargement
- Pleural effusion
- Tension pneumothorax
- Pregnancy
- Tumor, RV or LV
- Chronic obstructive pulmonary disease
- Ascites
- Right ventricular hypertrophy secondary to pulmonary hypertension

3. Percussion

a. Inaccurate to determine heart size, not recommended for use

b. Diagnostic tests replaced percussion secondary to accuracy

1. Chest radiography

2. Echocardiography

4. Auscultation

a. Carotid arteries

1. Sequence with bell

a) Normal

1) Smooth

2) Regular

b) Abnormal turbulent flow

        1) Bruits
- Soft
- Loud

b. Heart (five areas – apex, pulmonic, Erb's point, tricuspid, mitral)

    1. First sequence with diaphragm

        a) Identify S_1 (closing of mitral and tricuspid valves) and S_2 (closing of aortic and pulmonic valves)

        b) Note intensity of S_1 at mitral area

            1) S_1 coincides with upstroke of carotid artery

        c) Note possible splitting of S_1 at tricuspid area

        d) Note intensity of S_2 at aortic area

        e) Note possible splitting of S_2 at pulmonic area

            1) Physiologic splitting
- Normal
- Accentuated by inspiration

            2) Pathological splitting
- Wide split
  - — Audible throughout respiration
  - — Associated with the following:

                Right bundle branch block
                Pulmonic stenosis
                Mitral regurgitation
                Pulmonary hypertension
                Ventricular septal defect

- Paradoxical split
  - — Heard on expiration
  - — Associated with the following:

                Left bundle branch block
                Aortic stenosis
                Patent ductus arteriosus
                Right ventricular pacing
                Left ventricular failure or disease
                Cardiomyopathy
                WPW right accessory pathway
                Ischemia or acute MI

- Fixed split
  - — Atrial septal defect (ASD) with volume overload

    2. Second sequence with bell

        a) S_3 (ventricular gallop) at apex

            1) Occurs in early diastole after S_2

    2) Rhythm sounds like when you say the word "Kentuck'y." The y is the S_3.

    3) Normal in children and young adults

    4) Abnormal in adults >30 years of age
- Ventricular failure
- Chronic mitral insufficiency
- Decreased cardiac output, if due to ventricular failure
- Aortic insufficiency
- Constrictive pericarditis

    5) May occur in last trimester of pregnancy

  b) S_4 (atrial gallop)

    1) Occurs presystolic phase just before S_1

    2) Rhythm sounds like when you say "Ten-ne-see"

    3) May have right and left ventricular origin

    4) Associated with the following:
- Left ventricular hypertrophy
- Coronary artery disease
- Acute, severe mitral insufficiency
- Pulmonary hypertension
- Congestive heart failure
- Hyperthyroidism

  c) Summation gallop

    1) Simultaneous atrial (S_4) and ventricular gallop (S_3)

    2) S_1 and S_2 not as loud as summation

    3) Associated with advanced heart failure

    4) Tachycardia

3. Extra heart sounds in systole

  a) Ejection click

    1) Originate in either the great vessels or their valves

    2) Characteristics
- Shortly after S_1
- Clicking quality
- High pitched

  b) Aortic systolic ejection sound

    1) Heard at apex and base
- Dilated ascending aorta
- Aortic valve disease, post-stenotic dilation

  c) Pulmonic systolic ejection sound

    1) Heard at second and third left interspaces

    2) Dilated pulmonary artery

        3) Pulmonary hypertension

        4) Pulmonary stenosis, post-stenotic dilitation

    d) Mid to late systolic click

        1) Heard at left lower sternal border with the patient in the left lateral decubitus position

        2) Mitral valve prolapse

4. Extra heart sounds in diastole

    a) Opening snap

        1) Heard medial to apex and along left lower sternal border

        2) Heard with the bell and patient positioned on the left side

        3) Stenotic mitral valve

        4) Mitral valve prolapse (MVP)

    b) S_3

    c) S_4

5. Friction rub

    a) Heard fourth and fifth intercostal space at sternal border or anywhere

    b) Single or multicomponent

        1) Inflamed pericardium

        2) Transmural MI

        3) Uremia

6. Murmurs

    a) Turbulent blood flow

        1) Systolic murmurs

- Mitral insufficiency (regurgitation)
- Tricuspid insufficiency (regurgitation)
- Aortic stenosis
    — Valvular stenosis
    — Subvalvular aortic stenosis
    — Supravalvular aortic stenosis
- Pulmonary stenosis
- Interventricular septal defect
- Coarctation of aorta

        2) Diastolic murmurs

- Mitral stenosis
- Tricuspid stenosis
- Aortic insufficiency (regurgitation)
- Pulmonary insufficiency (regurgitation)

- Patent ductus arteriosus (systolic and diastolic components to PDA)
b) Location
  1) Describe in terms of intercostal space and cm from midsternal, midclavicular, or axillary lines
  2) Apex or base
c) Timing
  1) Systole
     - Pansystolic
       — Heard throught systole
     - Mid systolic ejection murmur
       — Heard after S_1
       — Ending before S_2
  2) Diastole
     - Diastolic rumbling murmurs
       — Heard after S_2, can be quite late
       — Bell
     - Semilunar valve incompetence
       — Heard immediately after S_2
       — Diaphragm
     - Intensity
       — Grade on a scale of I to VI
       — Numerator is grade of murmur
       — Denominator shows scale of 6

         Grade I/VI: barely audible; difficult to detect
         Grade II/VI: audible but quiet
         Grade III/VI: moderately loud without thrill
         Grade IV/VI: loud without thrill
         Grade V/VI: very loud, requires the use of a stethoscope to hear; associated with a thrill
         Grade VI/VI: very loud, can be heard with stethoscope off chest; associated with a thrill

     - Radiation
     - Pattern
       — Crescendo
       — Decrescendo
       — Crescendo-decrescendo
     - Quality
       — Musical
       — Blowing

- — Harsh
- — Rumbling
- Pitch
  - — Low
  - — Medium
  - — High
- Flow murmurs
  - — Normal in 50% of children
  - — Anemia
  - — Pregnancy
  - — Change in blood velocity
  - — Hyperthyroidism
  - — Sclerotic valvular disease in the elderly

C. Diagnostic Evaluation
  1. Electrocardiogram ECG
     a. Definition: recording of myocardial electrical activity and conduction throughout the heart from the body surface
     b. Indications: to diagnose the following:
        1. Myocardial infarction (MI)
        2. Myocardial ischemia
        3. Cardiac arrhythmias
        4. Conduction defects
        5. Electrolyte imbalance
        6. Drug toxicity
        7. Chamber enlargement, dilation and hypertrophy
     c. Diagnostic significance: refer to Part One, section IIID
     d. Complications: none
  2. Chest radiography
     a. Definition: x-ray used to visualize silhouette of the heart and great vessels (anatomical assessment)
     b. Indications: to evaluate
        1. Cardiac silhouette, size and position
        2. Pulmonary abnormalities
           a) Effusion
           b) Edema
        3. Ventricular aneurysm (low sensitivity)
        4. Lead and pulse generator placement
        5. ICD patches
     c. Structure, identification:

1. Bony structures
   a) Clavicles
   b) Ribs
2. Trachea
3. Aorta
4. Cardiac shadow
5. Diaphragm
6. Lung
7. Pulse generator
8. Ventricular lead, define unipolar vs. bipolar
9. Atrial lead, define unipolar vs. bipolar
10. ICD patches
   d. Complication: none
3. Echocardiogram
   a. Definition: high-frequency sound waves transmitted transthoracically into the heart and reflected to a transducer
      1. Types
         a) M-mode
         b) 2-dimensional (2D)
         c) Doppler
         d) Color flow
   b. Indications: displays cardiac function and spatial anatomy
   c. Diagnostic significance:
      1. Valvular function
      2. Wall motion of the heart
      3. Pericardial effusion/tamponade
      4. Chamber size
      5. Tumors
      6. Thrombi
      7. RV and LV function
      8. Location of pacemaker leads
      9. Lead perforation
      10. Wall thickness
      11. Congenital malformations
   d. Complications: long-term effect of acoustic radiation is unknown
4. Transesophageal echocardiography
   a. Refer to Part Three, Chapter 27 – Mapping Techniques
5. Myocardial perfusion imaging
   a. Definition: radiopharmaceutical injection into peripheral vein to

determine myocardial perfusion and/or injection of an intravascular agent for ventricular function.

b. Indications:

1. Evaluation of myocardial perfusion during stress and rest
2. Evaluation of ventricular function (requires an intravascular agent injected to complete)
   a) Analysis of ejection fraction (EF)
   b) Analysis of ventricular wall motion
3. Shunt analysis

c. Diagnostic significance:

1. Used to rule out myocardial infarction
2. To indicate areas of ischemia when combined with exercise stress testing or chemical challenge

d. Complications: none, patient is exposed to 0.4–0.6 rads

6. Exercise electrocardiography (stress testing)

a. Definition: evaluate the response of the cardiovascular system to increased physical work levels.

b. Indications: evaluation of the following:

1. Suspected coronary artery disease
2. Cardiovascular functional capacity
3. Arrhythmias
4. Evaluate patient response to medical or surgical therapy
5. Evaluate chronotropic response to exercise
6. Evaluate function of rate adaptive pacemaker
7. Used to determine implantable defibrillator high-rate detection criterion
8. Effect of pacemaker therapy, Ex: device or mode selected
9. Response to antiarrhythmic therapy

c. Diagnostic significance:

1. Routine exercise stress
   a) ECG changes
   b) Blood pressure responses
   c) Symptoms
   d) Arrhythmias
   e) Conduction abnormalities
2. Thallium/Technetium-99m/Sestamibi
   a) Same as routine stress
   b) Nuclear scanning for myocardial perfusion
3. IV dipyridamole-Thallium/Tc99m/Sestamibi
   a) Given in place of exercise to create stress/rest perfusion changes

        b) Used for patients unable to exercise secondary to PVD, arthritis, COPD, orthopedic problems

   4. Chronotropic exercise stress test

        a) Assess appropriate heart rate response to increasing workloads

        b) Indications

           1) Evaluate rate adaptive pacemaker recipients

           2) Evaluate patients with known or suspected autonomic dysfunction

           3) Evaluate patients who cannot achieve a more aggressive exercise protocol

           4) Assess exercise tolerance

           5) Diagnose silent ischemia

 d. Complications:

   1. Chest pain

   2. Dyspnea

   3. Cardiac arrest (rare)

   4. Myocardial infarction (rare)

   5. Exercise induced arrhythmias

        a) Ventricular tachycardia

        b) Complete heart block

        c) Supraventricular tachycardia

   6. Hypotension

   7. Congestive heart failure

   8. Acute CNS events

        a) Syncope

        b) Stroke

   9. Accidental physical trauma, Ex: falls

7. Ambulatory electrocardiogram (AECG, Holter)

 a. Definition: ambulatory ECG monitoring of the patient for 12, 24, or 48 hours

 b. Indications:

   1. Arrhythmia

   2. Symptoms/correlation with arrhythmia

   3. Drug efficacy

   4. Pacemaker function

 c. Diagnostic significance: ECG analyzed and symptoms correlated with ECG changes (need a good historian for accuracy)

 d. Complications: none

8. Transtelephonic monitoring (TTM) and event monitoring

 a. Definition: use of a device capable of recording an electrocardiographic rhythm strip which is transmitted (real time or from memory) via the telephone to a receiving center.

 b. Indications:

1. Arrhythmia/symptom correlation
2. Drug efficacy
3. Pacemaker surveillance
   a) Single and dual chamber pacemakers
   b) Antitachycardia pacemakers
   c) Implantable defibrillator
4. Detection of ischemia episodes

c. Diagnostic significance:
1. ECG rhythm strip analyzed and symptom correlated with ECG changes
2. Pacemaker function
   a) Normal
   b) Malfunction
   c) End-of-service (EOS)

d. Complications: none

9. Head-Up-Tilt (HUT) – Also refer to Part Three, Chapter 32, subsection A.

   a. Definition: a motorized tilting of patient involving a period of supine rest followed by head-up-tilting at different degrees for a specific time concurrent with cardiovascular monitoring
   b. Indications:
      1. Patients with syncope/near syncope of undetermined etiology
      2. To diagnose neurally mediated bradycardia/hypotension
   c. Diagnostic significance:
      1. Absent chronotropic response
      2. Exaggerated chronotropic response
      3. Responses to autonomic dysfunction
      4. Cardioinhibitory response
         a) Vasovagal syncope
         b) Vasodepressor syncope
      5. Pacemaker syndrome
   d. Abnormal findings:
      1. AV block
      2. Bradycardia
      3. Hypotension
      4. Asystole
      5. Syncope

10. Cardiac catheterization/coronary arteriography
    a. Definition: an invasive procedure utilizing several types of catheters to evaluate the anatomical status of the heart and of the coro-

nary arteries. Chamber pressures are recorded and the arteries are filmed following injection of a contrast media.

1. Right heart cath: a catheter is placed into the femoral vein, antecubital vein, subclavian, or internal jugular vein and advanced into the right heart via the right atrium-right ventricle-pulmonary artery
2. Left heart cath: a catheter is placed in either the femoral, brachial, or axilliary artery and advanced into the left heart. A cineangiogram is recorded after injection of contrast media.

b. Indications:
   1. Right heart cath
      a) To evaluate valvular disorders
      b) To assess physiology and pathophysiology of the right heart
      c) To obtain heart pressures, cardiac output, and blood gas content
      d) Evaluate congenital defects
      e) To perform myocardial biopsies
   2. Left heart cath/angiography
      a) To visualize coronary anatomy and presence of coronary disease
      b) To evaluate valvular disorders
      c) To infuse fibrinolytic agents via the intracoronary route
      d) To evaluate LV wall motion, LV function, and ventricular aneurysms
      e) To evaluate CHD

c. Diagnostic significance:
   1. Pressure tracings reviewed for congenital or valvular disorders
   2. Cine coronary angiograms reviewed to determine coronary anatomy and left ventricular function

d. Complications:
   1. Arrhythmias including VT/VF
   2. Infection
      a) Systemic
      b) Insertion site
   3. Hematoma
      a) Insertion site
   4. Conduction disturbances
   5. Perforation of atria or ventricles
   6. Catheter embolism
   7. Catheter knotting
   8. Systemic or pulmonary embolism

9. Arterial thrombus
10. Allergic reaction to contrast media
11. Renal shutdown
12. AV fistula
13. Pseudoaneurysm
14. Tamponade
15. Acute MI
16. Pulmonary edema
17. Respiratory failure
18. Death

11. Electrophysiology studies (EPS)
   a. Refer to Part Three
12. Special Procedures
   a. Plethysmography
      1. Non-invasive
      2. Screening for thrombophlebitis for deep vein thrombus
      3. To evaluate venous blood flow from extremities
   b. Aortography
      1. Invasive
      2. Injection of radiopaque medium and cineangiography (cut film)
      3. Evaluate aortic valve and major vessels
   c. Pericardiocentesis
      1. Invasive
      2. Fluid withdrawn from pericardial sac via needle inserted in the subxiphoid region
      3. Identify pericardial effusion, pressure of pus, blood, pathogens, and malignancy
      4. Treatment of cardiac tamponade

References

Abi-Samra F, Maloney J, Fouad-Tarozi F, Castle L. The usefulness of head-up-tilt testing and hemodynamic investigations in the work-up of syncope of unknown origin. PACE. 11:1202–1214. 1988.

Alspach J, Williams S. Core curriculum for Critical Care Nursing. Philadelphia: WB Saunders Co., 1985.

Anardi D. Assessment of right heart function. J Cardiovasc Nurs 6(1):12–33. 1991.

Andreoli K, et al. Comprehensive Cardiac Care. 6th ed. St. Louis: CV Mosby Co., 1987.

Bates B. A guide to Physical Assessment. 4th ed. Philadelphia; LB Lippincott Co., 1987.

Bier A, Harvey F, Kessle J. Using echocardiography effectively. Patient Care. February. 18–28. 1988.

Blank C, Irvin G. Peripheral vascular disorders: assessment and intervention. Nurs Clin North Am. 25(4):777–794. 1990.

Corbett J. Laboratory Tests and Diagnostic Procedure with Nursing Diagnoses. 2nd ed. Norwalk: Appleton and Lang, 1987.

Fitzpatrick A, Theodorokis G, Verdas P, Sutton R. Methodology of head-up-tilt testing in patients with unexplained syncope. J Am Coll Cardiol. 17(1): 125–130. 1991.

Fuller J, Schaller-Ayers J. Health Assessment: A Nursing Approach. Philadelphia: JB Lippincott, 1990.

Furman S, Hayes D, Holmes D. A practice of Cardiac Pacing. 2nd ed. New York: Futura Publishing Co., Inc., 1991.

Hurst JW, Schlant R. The Heart. 7th ed. New York: McGraw-Hill Book Co., 1990.

Kain C, Reilly N, Schultz E, The older adult: a comparative assessment. Nurs Clin North Am. 25(4):833–848. 1990.

Kay G, Bubien R. Clinical Management of Cardiac Arrhythmias. Maryland: Aspen Publishers, 1992.

Leppo J. Dipyridamole-Thallium: The lazy man's stress test. J Nuclear Med. 30:281–287. 1989.

Malasanos L, et al. Health Assessment. 3rd ed. St. Louis: CV Mosby Co., 1987.

Miracle V. Anatomy of a murmur. Nursing 86:16.7.26. 1986.

Rudy E, Gray VR. Handbook of Health Assessment. 2nd ed. Norwalk: Appleton-Century-Crofts, 1986.

Sokolow M, McIlroy M, Chertlin M. Clinical Cardiology. 5th ed. San Mateo: Appleton and Lang, 1990.

Talbot L, Marquardt M. Pocket Guide to Critical Care Assessment. St. Louis: CV Mosby Co., 1989.

Taber C. Taber's Cyclopedic Medical Dictionary. Philadelphia: FA Davis Co., 1987.

Weber J. Nurses's Handbook for Health Assessment. Philadelphia: JB Lippincott, 1988.

Weed L. Medical records, medical education and patient care. Cleveland: The press of Case Western Reserve, 273. 1969.

Williams E. Essential features of the cardiac history and physical examination. In: Kelley W, (Ed.). Textbook of Internal Medicine, I. Philadelphia: Lippincott, 1989.

Suggested Readings

Alspach J, Williams S. Core Curriculum for Critical Care Nursing. Philadelphia: WB Saunders Co., 1985.

Bates B. A guide to physical Assessment. 4th ed. Philadelphia: JB Lippincott Co., 1987.

Hurst JW, Schlant R. The Heart. 7th ed. New York: McGraw-Hill Book Co., 1990.

Talbo L, Marquardt M. Pocket Guide to Critical Care Assessment. St. Louis: CV Mosby Co., 1989.

Sokolow M, McIlroy M, Chertlin, M. Clinical Cardiology. 5th ed. San Mateo: Appleton and Lang, 1990.

CHAPTER 4

Electrocardiography

Marleen E. Irwin

Subsection:
A. Normal Electrocardiogram
B. Recognition and Diagnosis of Bradycardia/Tachycardia
C. Electrocardiogram of Paced ECG and Timing Cycles

This section introduces principles of electrocardiography for the evaluation of cardiac rhythms. The electrocardiogram (ECG) is a graphic recording of the electrical potentials occurring during cardiac contraction. The electrical impulses emanate from the sinus node and traverse the conduction system of the heart resulting in excitation of the cardiac cells and myocardial contraction. Impulse formation and conduction produce weak electrical current that spread through the body.

The ECG is recorded by applying electrodes to various designated points on the body. The electrical activity is picked up via the electrodes and transmitted to an electrocardiographic device. The recorded presentation graphically presents 12 vectors of the electrical potentials of each contraction of the heart muscle. In conjunction with the assessment of the patients clinical presentation, the ECG provides vital information in the diagnosis of cardiac conditions.

This section deals with the various disturbances of the normal impulse formation and conduction that can occur throughout the cellular structure of the heart responsible for electrical conduction.

It also covers the critical knowledge necessary for gaining competence in understanding and interpreting the paced electrocardiogram and the timing cycles associated with normal single and dual chamber pacing system function. In order to problem solve the paced rhythm, one must have critical knowledge in:

From: Schurig L. *Educational Guidelines: Pacing and Electrophysiology*. Armonk, NY: Futura Publishing Co, Inc, © 1994.

The relationship of interval (time) to rate per minute.

The timing cycles and intervals of the single chamber pacing system.

The timing cycles and intervals of the dual chamber pacing system.

Analysis of the paced cycle and the characteristics of the pulse generators timing intervals.

The pacemaker refractory periods, blanking periods, and pacing intervals and their importance related to the intrinsic cardiac rhythms.

Objectives

1. Describe the usefulness of the electrocardiogram.
2. Demonstrate an understanding of the application of the ECG apparatus.
3. Define the normal electrical events of the cardiac cycle.
4. Describe the characteristics of the normal 12 lead ECG including timing and sequence of recorded leads.
5. Identify normal electrical axis and polarity.
6. Recognize the technical limitations and difficulties associated with the 12 lead ECG.
7. Identify rhythms of normal conduction.
8. Identify the monitoring devices used to detect arrhythmias.
9. Explain the mechanisms of arrhythmias.
10. Recognize and interpret arrhythmias related to abnormal impulse formation and explain the clinical significance of each.
11. Describe the relationship of interval (time) to rate per minute.
12. Identify the timing cycles and intervals of the single chamber pacing system.
13. Identify the timing cycles and intervals of the dual chamber pacing system.
14. Analyze the paced cycle and the characteristics of the pulse generator timing intervals.
15. Describe pacemaker refractory periods, blanking periods, and pacing intervals and their importance related to intrinsic cardiac rhythms.

Glossary and Abbreviations

Automaticity: The property inherent in all pacemaking cells that enables them to form new impulses spontaneously.

Axis: The orientation of the heart's electrical activity in the frontal plane is expressed in terms of axis.

Block: Pathological delay or interruption of impulse conduction.

Cardiac vector: Designates all of the electromotive forces of the heart cycle. It has known magnitude, direction, and polarity.

Depolarization: The initial spread of the stimulus through the muscle.

Downward deflection: The deflection will be negative (below) in relation to the baseline if the stimulus spreads away from the electrode that is at the negative.

Duration: Electrical activation expressed in units of time (seconds, milliseconds).

Einthoven's law: States that a complex in lead II is equal to the sum of the corresponding complexes in leads I and III, (II = I + III)

Electrocardiographic grid: Electrocardiographic paper is a graph in which horizontal and vertical lines are present at 1 mm intervals.

Intrinsicoid deflection: The time required for the spread of the impulse from the stimulated end to the opposite end of the muscle strip, the ventricular activation time (VAT). Measured from the onset of the R wave on the surface ECG to the peak of the R in that lead.

P wave: The deflection produced by right and left atrial depolarization.

P-P interval: This interval is the distance between 2 successive P waves expressed in a unit of time.

P-R interval: This measures the AV conduction time. It includes the time required for: atrial depolarization, normal conduction delay in the AV node, and passage of the impulse through the bundle of His and bundle branches to the onset of ventricular depolarization.

Q wave: The initial negative deflection resulting from ventricular depolarization.

QRS interval: This is the measurement of total ventricular depolarization time.

Q-T interval: This measures the duration of electrical systole.

Q-U interval: This measures total ventricular repolarization including Purkinje fibers.

Repolarization: The return of the stimulated muscle to the resting state.

R wave: The first positive deflection during ventricular depolarization.

R' wave: The second positive deflection.

R-R interval: This interval is the distance between 2 successive R waves expressed in a unit of time (seconds, milliseconds).

S wave: The first negative deflection of ventricular depolarization that follows the first positive deflection.

S-T interval: The duration of the RS-T segment.

T wave: The deflection produced by ventricular repolarization.

Ta wave: The result of atrial repolarization.

U wave: A deflection seen following the T wave and preceding the next P wave.

Upward deflection: The deflection will be positive (above) in relation to the baseline if the stimulus spreads toward the electrode that is at the positive.

Ventricular activation time (VAT): The time it takes an impulse to traverse the myocardium from the endocardial to the epicardial surface, the beginning of the Q wave to the peak of the R wave.

Sinus rhythms:

Sinus arrhythmia: Sinus rhythm with cyclic variations in rate.

Sinus bradycardia: Sinus rhythm, rate less than 60.

Sinus rhythm: Regular and equal atrial and ventricular rates; with normal P waves originating from the sinus node; normal P-R interval.

Sinus tachycardia: Sinus rhythm, rate greater than 100.

AV blocks:

AV block; first degree: Sinus rhythm, P-R interval greater than 0.21 s.

AV block; second degree: At regular or irregular intervals, a P wave is not followed by a QRS complex. The P-P interval is constant.

AV block; second degree; Mobitz I: Cyclically there is progressive lengthening of the P-R interval from beat to beat until a P wave is not followed by a QRS.

AV block; second degree; Mobitz II: In a regular sequence 2:1, 3:1 or in an irregular sequence 3:2, 4:3, a P wave is not followed by a QRS. The P-R interval for the conducted beats is constant or has sinus arrhythmia.

AV block; third degree: Complete dissociation between atrial and ventricular rhythms. The atrial rhythm may be normal sinus or any atrial arrhythmia but the atrial impulse does not capture the ventricle. Ventricular depolarization is initiated by a secondary pacemaker either in the AV junction, or in the ventricle (idioventricular).

Atrial arrhythmias:

Atrial ectopic beats: The atrium is depolarized from a different focus than the sinus node. The P wave may occur prematurely and is followed by normal appearing QRS-T complex or intraventricular aberration. The P-

R interval may be same, longer, or shorter than the P-R interval of the sinus conducted beats.

Atrial fibrillation: There is no regular atrial activity; there are a multitude of deflections seen in the base line ECG, the ventricular rhythm is grossly irregular.

Atrial flutter: There is evidence of regular atrial activity; constant P-P interval and an atrial rate of 260–320. The P waves are often sawtooth configuration and inverted in some leads. AV block is present most commonly 2:1 or 4:1 producing slower and regular ventricular rhythm.

Atrial tachycardia: There is regular atrial activity. Each P may be followed by a QRS (1:1 conduction), or there may be AV block; most commonly 2:1 block resulting in ventricular rates one-half the atrial rate. Can show Wenckebach periodicity.

Blocked (nonconducted) atrial beats: A premature P wave occurs shortly after the preceding QRS, and the AV node is still refractory, therefore does not propagate conduction into the ventricles.

SA block: Periods in which there is an absence of P waves and total absence of atrial electrical activity for one or more seconds.

AV Junctional rhythms:

Junctional ectopic beats (PJB): The P wave is inverted in II, III, aVF, the P-R interval is usually shorter than that of sinus beat. P waves may be within or after the QRS, and not visible.

Junctional rhythm: A regular rhythm at a rate of 50–100. P wave as described above in PJB.

Junctional tachycardia: A regular rhythm at a rate of 120–200. P waves as described above in PJB.

Ventricular rhythms:

Idioventricular rhythm: A regular or irregular ventricular rhythm at a rate of 30–40.

Multifocal (multiform or polymorphic): The ectopic ventricular beats vary in configuration and direction in a single lead.

Unifocal (uniform or monomorphic): All the ectopic ventricular QRS complexes have the same appearance in a single lead.

Ventricular asystole: Absence of ventricular complexes for seconds or minutes.

Ventricular ectopic beats (PVC): Is evidenced by a wide, often notched, or slurred QRS which is not preceded by a P wave and may occur prematurely in relation to the dominant R-R interval.

Ventricular fibrillation (VF): A rapid, irregular wavy electrocardiographic presentation.

Ventricular tachycardia (VT): A run of three or more consecutive ectopic beats. Rate usually 140–200, may be irregular, no P waves seen or if seen, may be dissociated from the ventricular rhythm.

Pacemaker Terminology:

Atrial escape (VA) interval (AEI): The interval from a ventricular output stimulus or sensed ventricular signal to the following atrial output stimulus.

Atrial refractory period (ARP): The period after an atrial sensed or paced event during which the atrial timing circuit ignores any incoming signals.

AV interval (AVI): The programmed interval from the atrial output stimulus to the ventricular output stimulus.

Blanking period/interval: A brief period during which the sensing amplifier in one channel is disabled to avoid its being overdriven by a stimulus produced by the other channel.

Cross-talk: The detection by one channel of a dual chamber pacemaker of the afterpotential associated with the stimulation by the other channel. (The inappropriate detection of atrial output stimulus by the ventricular channel.)

Cross-talk inhibition: The inhibition of the ventricular output when the ventricular channel detects atrial output stimuli as a result of cross-talk. This is a design feature (because of sensing) of the device overcome by the blanking period.

Low rate (base rate) interval (LRI): The programmed lower rate. The longest interval between consecutive ventricular output stimuli without intervening sensed P wave in AAI, DDD, etc., type systems, or from sensed R wave to succeeding ventricular output stimulus.

Maximum sensor driven upper rate: This applies to the upper rate limit determined by the sensor. The maximum sensor rate permits the patient to exceed the upper rate limit.

Post-ventricular atrial refractory interval/period (PVARP): The pulse generator atrial refractory period occurring after the emission of a ventricular output stimulus or a sensed ventricular signal.

Total atrial refractory interval/period (TARP): Consists of two intervals; the AV interval and the post-ventricular atrial refractory interval and is the duration of time that the atrial amplifier is refractory to atrial signals.

Upper rate interval (limit) (URI): This applies to the ventricular channel of a dual chamber system and is the shortest interval between two consecutive ventricular output stimuli or from a sensed ventricular event to the succeeding ventricular output stimulus while maintaining and providing 1:1 AV synchrony with sensed atrial events.

Ventricular refractory interval/period (VRP): The period during which the lower rate interval cannot be reset by any signal.

Abbreviations

ABI: Atrial blanking interval
ABP: Atrial blanking period

AECG: Ambulatory Electrocardiogram/Holter
AEI: Atrial escape interval
AF: Atrial fibrillation
APB: Atrial premature beat
ARI/ARP: Atrial refractory interval/period
AVB: Atrioventricular Block
AVD: Atrioventricular dissociation
AVI: AV interval
BCL: Basic cycle length
CHB: Complete heart block
ECG: Electrocardiogram
EPS: Electrophysiological studies
LAHB: Left anterior hemiblock
LBBB: Left bundle branch block
LGL: Lown-Ganong-Levine
LPHB: Left posterior hemiblock
LRL: Lower rate limit
MCL: Minimum cycle length
PAT: Paroxysmal atrial tachycardia
PCL: Pacing cycle length
PG: Pulse generator
P-P interval
PVARI/PVARP: Post ventricular refractory interval/period
RBBB: Right bundle branch block
SSS: Sick sinus syndrome
SVT: Supraventricular tachycardia
TARI/TARP: Total atrial refractory interval/period
URL: Upper rate limit
VA: Ventriculoatrial
VAC: Ventriculoatrial conduction (VAC)
VAI: VA interval
VAT: Ventricular activation time
VBI: Ventricular blanking interval
VBP: Ventricular blanking period
VF: Ventricular fibrillation
VPB: Ventricular premature beat
VRI: Ventricular refractory interval
VT: Ventricular tachycardia
VTP: Ventricular triggering period
V-V interval
WPW: Wolff-Parkinson-White pattern

Education Content

A. Normal Electrocardiography (ECG)

   1. Usefulness of the 12 Lead electrocardiogram

     a. Application of ECG recordings:

       1. Baseline documentation

       2. Data tracking

       3. Localize infarctions

       4. Differentiate ischemia, injury, or infarction

       5. Evaluate drug administration

       6. Evaluate electrolyte status and administration of supplements, Ex: potassium

       7. Evaluate treatment for MI

       8. Evaluate pacemaker function

       9. Regionalize VT focus

      10. Dx

         a) Cardiac abnormalities

         b) Chamber enlargements

         c) Pre-excitation syndromes

         d) Conduction abnormalities

      11. Arrhythmia analysis

      12. Differentiate wide complex tachycardias

     b. Clinical conditions indicating recording the ECG:

       1. Onset of chest pain

       2. Continuation of chest pain

       3. Severe right upper quadrant pain

       4. Sudden onset of dyspnea

       5. Onset of an arrhythmia

       6. Changes in P-QRS-T configurations on a single lead monitor

       7. Shock state

       8. Syncope

       9. Postoperative hypotension

      10. Coma

      11. Murmur develops

      12. Acquired cyanosis

      13. Trauma to the chest

      14. Preoperatively for patients over 50

      15. Diagnosis of hypertension

      16. Routine coronary care admission
      17. Routine component of pacemaker management
  c. Considerations when using the ECG as a tool for diagnosis
      1. Correlation with clinical evaluation
      2. Evaluation/diagnosis made in conjunction with clinical setting
      3. Extrinsic and technical factors altering the ECG pattern
2. Apparatus for ECG recordings
  a. Recording devices
      1. Radio amplifier
      2. String galvanometer
      3. Oscilloscope
      4. Telemetry and transtelephonic
      5. Ambulatory recorders
      6. Computer facilities
      7. Hardwire or telemetry monitor
  b. Standardization
      1. Amplitude, 10 mm per 1 mV
      2. Recording speed/mm per sec, 25 mm/sec
  c. Electrodes and leads
      1. Leads
         a) Bipolar limb leads: I, II, III
         b) Unipolar limb leads: aVR, aVL, aVF
         c) Unipolar chest leads: $V_1, V_2, V_3, V_4, V_5, V_6, V_7, V_8, V_9$
         d) Unipolar chest leads, right side: V_1–V_6
      2. Lead planes
         a) Frontal
         b) Horizontal
3. Electrophysiologic principles
  a. Wave deflections
      1. Polarity interpretation based on relationship of deflection to the tracing baseline. (One can draw an imaginary reference base by connecting the T and P wave carrying the line through the complex.)
      2. Wave deflection polarity
         a) Positive, above the baseline
         b) Negative, below the baseline
         c) Biphasic, positive and negative
         d) Forms, variations of a through c
  b. Sequence
      1. Atrial depolarization and repolarization

    2. Ventricular depolarization
- **a)** Starts left to right across the septum
- **b)** 0.01 sec, left septal surface
- **c)** 0.02 sec, apical portion RV, lateral wall RV and apical and anterior wall LV
- **d)** 0.04 sec, septum completed and most of lateral wall RV, activate remaining portion of LV
- **e)** 0.06 sec, posterolateral, basal wall LV
- **f)** 0.08 sec, depolarization completed

    3. 0–0.15 sec, ventricular repolarization and T wave completed

  c. Action potentials of the normal cell, Refer to Part One, Chapter 2.C for review.
- **1.** Cell permeability
- **2.** Ionic mechanisms
  - **a)** Polarized, repolarized, and depolarized cell
  - **b)** Slow and fast channels of the conduction system

4. The electrocardiogram (ECG)

  a. Rate and rhythm
- **1.** Systematic examination and evaluation of:
  - **a)** Rhythm, P wave, P-R interval, QRS duration, QRS complex, JT interval, ST segment, T wave, U wave, Q-T duration
  - **b)** Measuring rate and conduction intervals

  b. Complexes and intervals
- **1.** Atrial chamber electrical activation = the P wave
  - **a)** Duration .11 sec
  - **b)** Amplitude 2–3 mm
- **2.** Atrioventricular conduction
- **3.** Ventricular chamber electrical activation = the QRS complex
  - **a)** Sequence (above)
  - **b)** Duration .05–.10 sec
  - **c)** Amplitude (dependent on recorded lead)
- **4.** ST segment
  - **a)** Level to baseline
  - **b)** Take off point from QRS called J point
  - **c)** Shape – normally curves gently into the T wave
- **5.** Ventricular recovery = the T wave
  - **a)** Polarity – same as the QRS complex
  - **b)** Shape – slightly rounded and asymmetrical
  - **c)** Height – 5–10 mm depending on the lead
- **6.** Q-T duration or interval

        a) .39 sec; QTC .41 sec

        b) Varies with rate, age and sex

    7. U wave

        a) Prominence – depends on underlying disease process, potassium deficiency, or drugs

        b) Polarity – same as the T wave

        c) Amplitude – low voltage

    8. QT-U interval when the T wave and U wave are not separate in a given lead

  c. Electrical axis and precordial pattern

    1. QRS orientation, frontal plane

        a) Normal axis; 0 to 90

        b) LAD; -30 to -90

        c) RAD; +90 to +180

    2. Precordial pattern

        a) Intrinsicoid deflection

            1) V_1 = .02 sec

            2) V_6 = .04 sec

        b) Clockwise (left) – counterclockwise (right) rotation

  d. Technical difficulties affecting the recorded ECG

    1. Involuntary/voluntary movement

    2. Incorrect lead placement

    3. Incorrect electrode contact

    4. Incorrect skin preparation

    5. Static and alternating current interference

    6. Poor signal

    7. Uncomfortable patient

    8. Defective components of the system

    9. Broken lead wires

    10. Grounding

    11. Cleaning techniques

    12. Marking and mounting of recording

    13. Recording techniques

    14. Improper standardization

    15. Sensor signals from rate adaptive pacemakers, Ex: META

B. Recognition and Diagnosis of Bradycardia/Tachycardia

  1. Arrhythmia detection

    a. Transtelephonic monitoring

    b. Ambulatory electrocardiography (Holter)

   c. Programmed electrical stimulation
   d. Electrophysiologic studies
   e. Event recorders
2. Mechanisms of arrhythmias – Refer to Part Three, Chapter 22 for further explanation
   a. Abnormal impulse formation
      1. Enhanced automaticity
      2. Triggered activity
   b. Abnormal impulse conduction
      1. Reentry
3. Process for analyzing cardiac rhythms
   a. Gather the clinical information
   b. Inspect the ECG
   c. Determine the dominant rhythm
   d. Determine the atrial rhythm
   e. Determine the origin of the QRS complex
   f. Determine origin of the beats occurring prematurely
   g. Measure all intervals
   h. Conclude on the rhythm and if present, the arrhythmia.
4. Normal and abnormal cardiac rhythms – the study of the cardiac rhythm for: etiology, pattern, significance, incidence, mechanism, diagnostic criteria, evaluation techniques, treatment.
   a. Abnormal impulse formation
      1. Abnormal sinus impulse formation
         a) During sinus rhythm
         b) Sinus extrasystole (premature atrial)
         c) Sinus tachycardia
         d) Sinus bradycardia
         e) During sinus arrhythmia
            1) Respiratory phasic
            2) Ventriculophasic
         f) Sinoatrial block
            1) Partial
            2) Complete
         g) Sinus arrest
            1) Pause
            2) Absent P waves
      2. Ectopic impulse formation
         a) Passive escape beats and rhythms
            1) Atrial

        2) AV junctional
        3) Idioventricular
   b) Originating in the atria
        1) Atrial premature beat (PAC)
        2) Atrial tachycardia
          • Paroxysmal
          • Incessant
        3) Atrial fibrillation
        4) Atrial flutter
        5) AV junctional reentrant, may maintain itself without the atrium
        6) Chaotic atrial rhythm
        7) Pre-excitation (WPW)
   c) Originating in the AV junction
        1) Premature nodal beat (PNB)
        2) AV nodal tachycardia
          • Paroxysmal
   d) Originating in the ventricle
        1) Ventricular extrasystole
        2) Ventricular tachycardia
          • Paroxysmal, nonsustained
          • Sustained
          • Monomorphic
          • Polymorphic
        3) Ventricular flutter
        4) Ventricular fibrillation
b. Disturbances of the conduction system
   1. Sinoatrial (SA) block
      a) Type I
      b) Type II
   2. Intra-atrial block
   3. Atrioventricular (AV) block
      a) First degree
      b) Second degree
         1) Type I
         2) Type II
      c) Advanced or high-grade AV block
      d) Complete (third degree) AV block
   4. Intraventricular block
      a) Right bundle branch block

   b) Left bundle branch block
      1) Fascicular blocks (also called hemiblocks. This is misleading as there are four fascicles.)
         • Left anterior hemiblock
         • Left posterior hemiblock
   c) Bilateral bundle branch block
      1) Bifascicular
      2) Trifascicular
c. Disturbances of impulse formation and conduction
   1. Complete and incomplete atrioventricular dissociation
   2. Preexcitation syndrome (e.g., Wolff-Parkinson-White)
   3. Reciprocal rhythms
   4. Parasystole
      a) Atrial
      b) AV junctional
      c) Ventricular
      d) Combined
   5. Atrial dissociation
   6. Electrical alternans
   7. Lown-Ganong-Levine syndrome
      a) Short PR
      b) Reentrant tachyarrhythmia
   8. Concealed conduction
   9. Artificial pacing system rhythm
d. Reentrant arrhythmias
   1. Extrasystoles – bigeminal or trigeminal
   2. Ventricular tachycardia (VT)
   3. Intraventricular reentry
   4. Paroxysmal supraventricular tachycardias (SVT)
      a) AV nodal reentry (dual AV nodal pathways) – most common type
      b) AV reentry with AV node and an accessory pathway (bypass tract mediated)
      c) SA nodal reentry
      d) Intra-atrial reentry
      e) Atrial flutter
      f) Atrial fibrillation

C. Electrocardiogram of Paced ECG and Timing Cycles (Refer to Part One, Chapter 7, Subsection D.)

1. Process for analyzing paced rhythms
   a. Gather the clinical data and pacing system information
   b. Inspect the ECG/rhythm tracing
   c. Determine the mode of pacing
   d. Determine pacing, sensing, and capture
   e. Measure all pacing intervals
2. Assess intrinsic rate, rhythm, and intervals
   a. Intrinsic rate and rhythm
   b. Programmed pacing rate/interval
      1. Pacing cycle length
      2. With and without magnet application (synchronous and asynchronous operation)
   c. Relationship between the intrinsic events and paced events
      1. Stimulus output intervals
      2. Intervals after sensed events
3. Single chamber timing
   a. Programmed pacing intervals
      1. AAI/AAIR
         a) A-A interval – atrial pacing stimulus cycle
         b) Atrial refractory interval
         c) Sensed to paced escape intervals
         d) Hysteresis interval if programmed
         e) Pacing cycle length with rate adaptive operation
      2. VVI/VVIR
         a) V-V interval – ventricular pacing, output cycle
         b) Ventricular refractory interval
         c) Sensed to paced escape intervals
         d) Hysteresis interval if programmed
         e) Pacing cycle length with rate adaptive operation
   b. Intervals
      1. Refractory
      2. Noise sampling
      3. Alert
      4. Hysteresis
   c. Sensing
      1. Sensed interval
      2. Hysteresis interval
4. Dual chamber timing
   a. Programmed pacing intervals
      1. DVI/VDD/DDD/DDDR

        a) A-A interval
        b) V-V interval
        c) AV interval
        d) Safety pacing interval
        e) Atrial/ventricular blanking intervals
        f) Total atrial refractory interval
        g) Post-ventricular atrial refractory interval (PVARP)
        h) Ventricular refractory interval
            1) Noise sampling interval
        i) V-A interval
        j) Minimum cycle length/upper rate limit
        k) Pacing cycle length
        l) Basic pacing interval/lower rate limit
        m) Minimum sensor pacing interval/max sensor rate

  b. Sensing
    1. P sensing with and without inhibition of atrial output
    2. R sensing
    3. Upper rate behavior
    4. Sensor driven pacing

5. Modes
  a. Asynchronous-VOO/AOO
  b. Atrioventricular sequential asynchronous-DOO
  c. Inhibited-VVI/AAI
  d. Triggered-VVT/AAT
  e. Atrioventricular sequential ventricular inhibited-DVI
  f. Atrioventricular sequential atrial, and ventricular inhibited-DDI
  g. Atrial synchronous-VAT
  h. Atrial synchronous ventricular inhibited-VDD
  i. Atrioventricular "universal" - DDD
    1. Atrioventricular interval (AVI)
    2. Ventriculoatrial interval (VAI)
    3. Lower rate interval (LRI)
    4. Upper rate interval (URI)

6. Timing elements of pacing modes
  a. AOO/VOO (asynchronous atrial or ventricular pacing). Sensing does not occur, consistent pacing with consistent pacing cycle intervals.
  b. DOO – AV sequential asynchronous pacing; atrial and ventricular pacing occurs with fixed intervals between the atrial and ventricular stimulus and between the ventricular stimulus and the succeeding atrial stimulus.

c. VVI/AAI – Inhibited atrial or ventricular pacing; pacemaker stimuli occur at the escape interval in the absence of spontaneous sensed events. In the presence of a spontaneous event provided it occurs after the pacemaker refractory period, the pacing stimulus output is inhibited and the next pacing cycle interval begins to time out.

d. VVT/AAT – triggered atrial or ventricular pacing; the timing of this mode is the same as VVI/AAI; however, when a spontaneous event is sensed, a pacing stimulus output is delivered coincident with the sensed event.

e. DVI – dual chamber AV sequential pacing; the atrium is paced followed by ventricular pacing after a present AV interval. Sensing only occurs through the ventricular circuit, ventricular paced or sensed events begin the time out of subsequent intervals.

f. DDI – AV-sequential, atrial, and ventricular inhibited; sensing of intrinsic atrial events inhibits atrial stimulus output, the V-V pacing cycle length remains consistent except only in the presence of a sensed intrinsic event.

g. VAT – atrial synchronous ventricular pacing; in this mode the pacing system senses the atrium and then delivers a pacing stimulus output to the ventricle after a suitable delay; ventricular sensing is not a function of this mode.

h. VDD – atrial synchronous ventricular inhibited ventricular pacing. In this mode, the pacing system sensed the atrium and delivers pacing stimulus output to the ventricle, sensed intrinsic ventricular events inhibit output and begin the time out of the V-V interval.

i. DDD – In this mode the pacing system delivers output to atrium and ventricle, if intrinsic activity is absent, with atrial sensing the AV interval is timed out, with ventricular sensing, the atrial (VA) escape interval is timed out. (Timing differs depending on A-A timing or V-V timing.)

References

Andreoli KG, Zipes DP, Wallace AG, Kinney MR, Fowkes VK, Eds. Comprehensive Cardiac Care. St. Louis: C.V. Mosby Co., 1987.

Aronson RS, Keung EC. Electrophysiologic mechanism of cardiac arrhythmias. Cardiovasc Rev Rep. 1:403. 1980.

Barold SS, Falkoff MD, Ong LS, Heinle RA. In SS Barold (ed). Modern Cardiac Pacing. Mt. Kisco: Futura Publishing Co., Inc., 645. 1985.

Chung EK. Electrocardiography: practical applications with Vectorial Principles. Harper & Row Publishers, Inc., 1980.

Furman S, Hayes DL, Holmes D, Eds. A Practice of Cardiac Pacing. Mt. Kisco: Futura Publishing Co., Inc., 1989.

Goldman MJ, (ed.). Principles of Clinical Electrocardiography. Los Altos: Lange Medical Publications, 1982.

Goldschlager N. Pacemaker rhythms. PACE. 4:317–320. 1981.

Grant RP. Clinical Electrocardiography. New York: McGraw-Hill. 1957.

Hauser RG. The electrocardiography of AV universal DDD pacemakers. PACE. 6:399–409. 1983.

Hoffman BF. The genesis of cardiac arrhythmias. Prog Cardiovasc Dis. 8:319. 1966.

Josephson ME, Wellens HJ, (Eds). Tachycardias: Mechanisms, Diagnosis Treatment. Philadelphia: Lea & Febiger, 1984.

Kennedy HL. Ambulatory Electrocardiography. Philadelphia: Lea & Febiger. 1981.

Marriott HJL. Practical Electrocardiography. 8th edition. Baltimore: The Williams & Williams Co., 1988.

CHAPTER 5

Basic Pharmacology

Katharine Irene Faitel

A. Types of Drugs
  1. Sympathetic
  2. Parasympathetic
  3. Antiarrhythmic
     a. Electrophysiology of antiarrhythmic drugs
     b. Classification of antiarrhythmic drugs
B. Major Cardiovascular Responses

Although the heart will continue to operate without the nervous system, the autonomic nervous system plays an important part in helping to regulate the heart's impulse formation, conduction, and contractility. The heart operates through two different sets of nerves, the sympathetic and parasympathetic.

Sympathetic nerve fibers are located throughout the atria and ventricles. Stimulation of the sympathetic nervous system increases heart rate, speeds conduction through the atrioventricular (AV) node, and increases the force of contraction.

Parasympathetic nerves (chiefly the right and left vagus nerves) are found primarily in the sinoatrial (SA) node, atrioventricular (AV) node, and atrial myocardium. They are present, although much less densely, in the ventricular myocardium. Stimulation of the vagus nerve causes decreased heart rate, decreased speed of conduction through the AV node, and decreased force of contraction.

Drugs that mimic the action of the sympathetic nervous system are called sympathomimetic. Sympathetic nerves have two kinds of adrenergic receptors, α and β.

α-receptors are located in the peripheral arteries. Their stimulation causes

From: Schurig L. *Educational Guidelines: Pacing and Electrophysiology*. Armonk, NY: Futura Publishing Co, Inc, © 1994.

arterial vasoconstriction resulting in increased arterial resistance (increased arterial pressure) and a variable result on venous return to the heart.

β-stimulation produces vasodilation. β-receptors are divided into β_1 and β_2.

β_1-receptors are located in the myocardium. Their stimulation causes increased heart rate, enhanced AV conduction, increased myocardial contractility, and abnormal automaticity.

β_2-receptors are located in the lungs and arterial walls. Their stimulation causes bronchodilation and arterial vasodilation, decreasing peripheral vascular resistance and the return of more blood to the heart.

Sympathomimetic drugs are similarly divided into α and β, according to their action on peripheral nerve receptor sites. Most sympathomimetic drugs have combined α and β action, although one usually predominates.

This section outlines sympathomimetic and antiarrhythmic drugs, and their influence on the cardiac properties of conduction, automaticity, and contractility in the treatment of cardiac disease. Digitalis is included.

Objectives

1. Identify the two kinds of adrenergic nerve receptors of the sympathetic nervous system and explain the actions of each.
2. State the dose related effects of dopamine.
3. State the receptors responsible for the increased vasodilation of renal, mesenteric, coronary, and intra-cerebral stimulation by dopamine at low doses.
4. Based on their stimulation of α-and/or β-receptors, explain the primary actions of isoproterenol, epinephrine, norepinephrine, and dobutamine.
5. State the advantages of cardioselective β-blocking agents.
6. Name the four classes of the Vaughn-Williams classification of antiarrhythmics and give one example of each.
7. Describe the further breakdown of class I antiarrhythmics and give an example of each.
8. State the actions of digitalis and tell why they are important in the treatment of atrial fibrillation with rapid ventricular response.
9. Name the mechanisms responsible for cardiac arrhythmia.
10. Based on the mechanisms responsible for cardiac arrhythmias identify two modes of action of pharmacologic agents useful in restoring and maintaining normal rhythm.
11. Explain the significance of a prolonged QT interval.

Glossary and Abbreviations

Action potential: The precise, rapid sequence of ionic movement across the cell membrane as a result of electrical stimulation described as a 5 phase process (0–4).

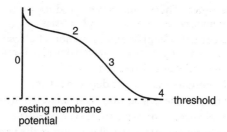

Threshold: Sufficient electrical stimulus to depolarize the cell membrane.

Phase 0: Upstroke; occurs immediately following threshold stimulation; synonymous with the rapid influx of sodium into the cell by way of fast sodium channels causing depolarization.

Phase 1: Closing of sodium channels which inhibits further entry of sodium ions into the cell; the initial phase of repolarization.

Phase 2: Plateau phase; characterized by a balanced influx of calcium into the cell and an outflow of potassium ions. Calcium plays a crucial role in contraction.

Phase 3: Repolarization; continued loss of positive charges as the cell once again reaches equilibrium and resting membrane potential is established (phase 4). Effect is reflected in the QT interval of the surface ECG.

Phase 4: Resting membrane potential; neutral state between electrical stimulations.

α-adrenergic receptors: α-receptors are located in the smooth muscle structure of the blood vessels. Their stimulation causes vasoconstriction.

Automaticity: Property of spontaneous depolarization to threshold during diastole.

β-adrenergic receptors: β-receptors located in the heart are called $β_1$. Their stimulation causes increased heart rate, enhanced AV conduction, and increased myocardial contractility. β-receptors located in the lungs and arterial walls are known as $β_2$. Their stimulation causes bronchodilation and arterial vasodilation.

Cardioselective: Inhibits $β_1$-receptors in the heart, but leaves $β_2$-receptors available to epinephrine stimulation in the lungs and coronary arteries as well as peripheral arteries.

Cell stimulation (all or none law): The ability to stimulate surrounding cells to threshold; (in cardiac cells, by way of a specialized pathway referred to as the conduction system), spreading over the entire atria (resulting in atrial contraction), and then spreading over the ventricle (resulting in ventricular contraction).

Depolarization: Process by which the influx of sodium or other channels such as calcium causes reversal of potential so that the potential of the interior of the cell exceeds that of the exterior; phase 0 of the action potential.

Dopaminergic receptor: Their stimulation produces vasodilation of renal mesenteric, coronary, and intracerebral arteries.

ECG (electrocardiogram): Graphic representation of electrical events associated with the cardiac cycle as obtained from skin (surface) electrodes.

P wave: Represents atrial depolarization.

QRS complex: Represents ventricular depolarization.

QT interval: Represents the period from ventricular stimulation to recovery.

T wave: Represents ventricular repolarization (recovery).

U wave: Thought to represent late repolarization of the ventricular purkinje fibers.

Inotropic action: Effect on cardiac contractility. Agents used to increase contractility have a positive inotropic effect. Those known to decrease contractility have a negative inotropic effect.

Refractory period: Period during which the cell is unable to respond to stimulation with normal depolarization.

Repolarization: Return to resting membrane potential.

Sodium channel blockers: Drugs affecting a decrease in cardiac cells' permeability to sodium during phase 0.

Education Content

A. Types of Drugs
1. Sympathetic
   a. Phenylephrine (Neosynephrine)
      1. Pure α-stimulation
      2. Limited use due to reduced blood flow to the brain and kidneys (coronary blood flow may not be reduced)
   b. Isoproterenol (Isuprel)
      1. Acts on β_1-and β_2-receptors
   c. Adrenalin (Epinephrine)
      1. Smaller doses stimulate β_1-and β_2-receptors
      2. Larger doses stimulate α-receptors
   d. Norepinephrine (Levophed)
      1. Primarily α action
      2. Potent β action (similar to epinephrine)
   e. Dopamine
      1. Effects are dose dependent
         a) Low dose ("renal dose," 1–2 μg/kg per min) stimulates dopaminergic receptors (separate from α and β receptors) produces vasodilation of renal, mesenteric, coronary, and intracerebral arteries. Urine output increased without effecting heart rate or blood pressure
         b) Moderate dose (2–10 μg/kg per min) stimulates β_1 and α-receptors
         c) Doses over 20 μg/kg per min produce primarily α action
   f. Dobutamine (Dobutrex)
      1. Synthesized from the basic chemical structure of isoproterenol
         a) Will not increase heart rate and arrhythmias like Isuprel (except at high doses) or hypovolemia
      2. Causes increased stroke volume
         a) Increases renal and mesenteric blood flow as a result of increased cardiac output and vasodilatation effects
2. Parasympathetic
   a. Atropine
      1. Increases heart rate by blocking parasympathetic effects
         a) Enhances sinoatrial node discharge
         b) Increases the rate of conduction through the AV node
3. Digitalis (Lanoxin)
   a. Increases calcium influx
      1. Increases myocardial contraction

2. Increases cardiac output in the failing heart
3. Causes vasoconstriction of coronary and mesenteric vasculature
4. Increases the rate of atrial conduction by decreasing atrial refractoriness
5. Has effect on sinoatrial and atrioventricular nodes, decreasing the heart rate, making it useful in the treatment of atrial and junctional arrhythmias
   a) Depresses atrioventricular conduction through increased vagal tone
4. Antiarrhythmics
   a. Basic electrophysiology of antiarrhythmic drugs
      1. Mechanisms responsible for cardiac arrhythmias
         a) Alterations in impulse formation (automaticity)
         b) Alterations in impulse conduction (reentry)
         c) Combination of both
      2. Means to restore homogenicity
         a) Suppress ectopic pacemaker sites (automaticity)
            1) Increase threshold (decrease slope of phase 4)
            2) Increase refractory period, phase 3 (making it more difficult to receive an impulse)
         b) Change conduction velocity
            1) Block sodium ion channel, phase 0
   b. Vaughn-Williams classification of antiarrhythmics
      1. Antiarrhythmics classified according to:
         a) Their method of action
         b) Similar ECG effects
         c) May share characteristic side effects
      2. Class I: sodium channel blockers
         a) Ia type – quinidine (Quinidine Sulfate, Quinaglute, Quinidex), procainamide (Procan), disopyramide (Norpace), moricizine (Ethmozine); also has 1c properties (see 1c below)
            1) Decreases automaticity
            2) Decreases conduction velocity
            3) Increases effective refractory period
         b) Ib type – lidocaine, (Xylocaine), mexilitine (Mexitil), tocainide (Tonocard)
            1) Shortening of the action potential
            2) Enhances more normal conduction through ischemic tissue
         c) Ic type – flecainide (Tambocor), encainide (Enkaid), propafenone (Rythmol) n.b. Rythmol also possesses mild β-blocking activity and calcium channel blocking activity

1) Primarily depress conduction velocity, phase O reflected in an increase in the PR and QRS of the surface ECG
2) Patients with sick sinus syndrome and IVC delay should be managed with reduced dosages

d) Class I type drugs (Ia, Ib, Ic) have membrane stabilizing activity present.

3. Class II: β-blockers
   a) Sympathetic stimulation increases O_2 demand; blocking sympathetic stimulation would decrease O_2 demand on the ischemic heart, reducing angina
      1) Used to treat arrhythmias aggravated by increased catacholamine release during exercise or stress
      2) Decreases sinus node automaticity
      3) Reduces sinus rates
      4) Prolongs conduction in the AV node
      5) Pharmacologic effects reflected in an increase in the PR and AH interval
   b) Prototype: propranolol (Inderal)
   c) Cardioselective drugs
      1) Inhibit β_1-receptors stimulation in the heart, leaving β_2-receptors to the lungs and peripheral arteries receptive to β-adrenergic stimulation
      2) Atenolol (Tenormin), metoprolol (Lopressor & Toprol), acebutolol (Sectral)
   d) Non-cardioselective
      1) Propranolol (Inderal), labadolol (Normodyne), timolol (Blocadren), pindolol (Visken), nadolol (Corgard)
   e) Class II type drugs have membrane stabilizing activity present.

4. Class III: drugs that prolong repolarization
   a) Amiodarone (Cordarone), prolongs refractoriness in all cardiac tissue; also possesses noncompetative α-and β-adrenergic inhibition
   b) Bretylium (Bretylol)
   c) Sotalol (Betapace) possess non-cardioselective β-adrenergic blocking properties

5. Class IV: calcium channel blockers
   a) Nifedipine (Procardia) does not possess antiarrhythmic effect
   b) Verapamil (Calan, Isoptin) has the most antiarrhythmic effect
   c) Diltiazem (Cardizem)
   d) Verapamil and Diltizem can inhibit the influence of calcium on smooth muscle

       1) The main focus is in the SA node, AV node, and vascular smooth muscle

       2) Dominant effect is on slowing AV conduction and prolonging the effective refractory period in the AV node, slowing the ventricular response

       3) Antiarrhythmic indications (except nifedipine) include atrial fib, A flutter, and SVT

    e) The effect on smooth muscle causes dilation of peripheral arterioles (reducing afterload) reducing energy requirements and O_2 consumption

       1) Used to treat vasospastic angina and hypertension

    f) Also have negative inotropic effects which are worse with Verapamil.

B. Major Cardiovascular Responses

The presence and severity of cardiac disease has great influence on the response state of the heart, resulting in alterations in conduction, rhythmicity, and contractility. Alterations in impulse formation (automaticity), impulse conduction (reentry), or a combination, are the mechanisms responsible for cardiac arrhythmias. These alterations, complicated by decreased myocardial function, lead to increased risk of morbidity resulting from lethal cardiac arrhythmias. These alterations may be controlled to some degree with pharmacologic treatment.

1. Conductivity

    a. Cardiac muscle is composed of branching columns of fibers that allow electrical energy (stimulus) to flow across the cellular membranes in the form of ions. By propagation, the stimulus travels in an organized manner through conduction pathways which lead to sequential, regular contraction (depolarization).

    b. Following depolarization cardiac tissue requires a recovery period.

       1. The T wave represents repolarization (recovery) of the ventricles

       2. This is a vulnerable period (stimulation can result in ventricular arrhythmias) during the conduction cycle

       3. The heart is unable to respond in an organized manner to stimulus during this period

    c. Other considerations:

       1. R on T phenomenon

          a) Ventricular premature contractions occurring during the vulnerable period of the conduction cycle may generate VT or VF

          b) Sudden death attributed to ventricular fibrillation in many instances is caused by this phenomenon

       2. Torsades de pointes can result from prolonged QT syndromes

        a) Treatment choices: magnesium, increase the heart rate, pacing, discontinue Digitalis or β-blockers

        b) Treatment for VT (see below)

  d. Conduction can be altered by cardiac disease, especially acute myocardial infarction

    1. Ischemic tissue enhances reentry; propagation of the impulse is depressed through the ischemic focus. The impulse is transmitted retrograde resulting in a rapid ectopic rhythm, such as:

        a) PAT (paroxysmal atrial tachycardia)

        b) Paroxysmal junctional tachycardia

        c) Atrial flutter

        d) Atrial fibrillation

        e) Ventricular tachycardia

    2. Principles of arrhythmic control

        a) Block ectopic pacemaker site

           1) Class Ia, Ic, and class III

        b) Enhance conduction through ischemic focus

           1) class Ib

  e. Enhanced parasympathetic influence in diseased myocardium can lead to conduction abnormalities and asystole.

    1. Blocks in conduction

        a) First degree heart block

        b) Second degree heart block (Wenckebach)

        c) Third degree heart block

    2. Pharmacologic treatments for symptomatic bradycardia and heart block:

        a) Atropine

        b) Isoproterenol (Isuprel)

    3. Pharmacologic treatments of asystole

        a) Epinephrine

        b) Atropine

2. Rhythmicity (automaticity)

  a. Inherent property of heart muscle independent of the nervous system

    1. Highly developed in pacemaker cells

    2. The fastest pacemaker will dominate

        a) Various pacemaker sites have various discharge rates

        b) Automaticity of the pacemaker cells decreases with distance from the SA node

           1) SA node (natural primary pacemaker)

        2) AV node, atria (slower rates than SA node)

        3) ventricles (slowest inherent rate)

b. Blocked SA node

    1. Potential pacemaker discharges automatically at its own intrinsic rate

        a) AV nodal (junctional) escape

        b) Ventricular escape

    2. Pharmacologic treatments

        a) Atropine

        b) Isoproterenol (Isuprel)

c. Enhanced SA node automaticity

    1. Sinus tachycardia

        a) Pharmacologic treatments

            1) Digoxin; slow the heart rate

            2) β-blockers; block catacholamine stimulation

d. Enhanced automaticity of an ectopic focus in the atria

    1. PAC (premature atrial contraction)

    2. Atrial tachycardia

    3. Automatic tachycardia

    4. Junctional tachycardia

        a) Pharmacologic treatment

            1) Digitalis; slow the rate if needed

            2) Class II i.e., propranolol; block possible catacholamine influence

            3) Class Ia antiarrhythmics; suppress the ectopic pacemaker

e. Enhanced automaticity in multiple foci can be responsible for atrial fibrillation or atrial flutter (Afib mechanism can also be multiple reentrant circuits)

    1. In combination with enhanced conduction through the atrioventricular node may lead to increased heart rate

    2. Pharmacologic treatments

        a) Digitalis; slow the rate, stabilize atrioventricular conduction

        b) Class Ia antiarrhythmics; suppress ectopic pacemaker sites

        Note: If arrthythmia is multifocal atrial tachycardia they may need $Ca++$ blockers (verapamil or diltiazem)

3. Contractility

a. Mechanical response to the pressure on the walls of the myocardium as they stretch to accommodate the filling of the atrial and ventricular chambers with blood. Muscle fibers shorten and blood is surged forward by the squeezing motion.

b. Chambers that are unable to empty and retain residual blood have poor contractility.

c. Compromised function of either the atria or ventricles affects the heart's overall hemodynamics and other cardiovascular responses.

d. Pharmacologic agents used to increase cardiac contractility have positive inotropic action
   1. Isoproterenol
   2. Epinephrine
   3. Dopamine
   4. Dobutamine
   5. Digoxin
   6. Amrinone

e. Pharmacologic agents that decrease cardiac contractility have negative inotropic action. Contraindicated for patients found to have decreased myocardial function.
   1. Risks and benefits of treatment with such agents must be carefully considered.
      a) β-blockers block the positive inotropic actions mediated by β-receptor stimulation. Cordarone has mild β blocking effect (Initially came on the market in England in 1967 for angina.)
      b) Calcium channel blockers differ in regard to negative inotropic effects
         1) In the clinical setting verapamil has the greatest negative inotropic effect
         2) Although nifedipine has direct negative inotropic effect, reflex sympathetic stimulation of vasodilation (reducing afterload), reduces the result of its negative inotropic effects in the clinical setting
         3) Diltiazem has intermediate negative inotropic effect (Amiodipine may replace diltiazem in this category)
      c) Antiarrhythmic drugs may have negligible negative inotropic effect on a normally functioning myocardium, but may add significantly to an already depressed myocardium.
         1) Disopyramide (Norpace) has the greatest negative inotropic effect of the Class Ia antiarrhythmics
         2) (Ic's) flecainide (Tambocor) has a strong negative inotropic effect. Moricizine (Ethmozine) has minimal negative inotropic effect.
         3) Cordarone has mild negative inotropic effects following intravenous loading, but not oral therapy.

References

Abrams J. Electrophysiology of Arrhythmias. Pract Cardiol, Special Issue. 4–11.

Benge W. Antiarrhythmic Drugs in the United States. Pract Cardiol Special Issue. 35–38.

Funck-Brentano C. Medical intellegence drug therapy Propafenone. New Eng J Med. 322:8:518–523. 1990.

Harrison DC. Symposium on perspectives on the treatment of ventricular arrhythmias. Am J Cardiol Sept. 22:52:6:1c – 2c. 1983.

Patel JM. Arrhythmias: detection, treatment, and cardiac drugs. WB Saunders Co., 3. 1989.

Podrid P. New and investigational antiarrhythmic drugs. Pract Cardiol. 1985.

Pratt CM. Moricizine HCl: mechanism of action, safety, and effectiveness. Intern Med Specialist. 11:8:82–83.

Rinkenberger RL. New antiarrhythmic agents: Part X: safety and efficacy of encainide in the treatment of ventricular arrhythmias. Pract Cardiol. 2–3: 11–12. 1987.

Salerno DM. Review antiarrhythmic drugs: 1987 Part I: cardiac electrophsiology, drug classification, methodology, and approaches to management of ventricular arrhythmia. J Electrophysiol. 12:3:218–226. 1987.

Scheinman MM. Current concepts in arrhythmia management: proceedings of a round table symposium. Arrhythmia Manage, (Suppl). 1990.

Singh SN. New antiarrhythmic agents: Part IX: pharmacology and clinical use of flecainide acetate. Pract Cardiol. 12:13:81. 1986.

Somberg J. Antiarrhythmic therapy and the prevention of sudden death. Cardiol Pract. June, July, Aug: 110. 1986.

CHAPTER 6

Patient Education (General)

Tomas P. Ozahowski
Charles L. Witherell

Subsection:

A. Basic Assumptions
B. Considerations
C. Hoffman's Twelve Principles of Learning
D. Application of the Principles of Learning

Let us consider the in-patient setting. It is there we conduct many of our patient education efforts. Often we are strangers to our patients, identified as an authority figure because of our uniforms, name badges, titles, or all three. We meet them in their rooms, and there they have none of their usual badges of power—they aren't in their places of work, their knowledge of their jobs has no meaning here, their social standing and even their clothing have been taken from them. The centerpiece of their rooms is the bed, a symbol of weakness and passivity, and they are right in the middle of it. When they are eating, it may be food they have not chosen for themselves. They are bombarded with sounds and smells from beyond the closed door to their rooms which, although familiar to us, have ominous meaning for them. Often their conditions or medications dull their sensorium.

Worst of all, they are with us because they perceive themselves to be in danger. We propose tests and procedures to help toward solution of the problem, but these have elements of pain and danger and although aware of this, patients can't say exactly what or how great that danger is. They can't even be sure that we'll come if they call.

It would be difficult to design an atmosphere more hostile to learning. Low-literacy specialists Doak, Doak, and Root, suggest that all failures to

From: Schurig L. *Educational Guidelines: Pacing and Electrophysiology*. Armonk, NY: Futura Publishing Co, Inc, © 1994.

communicate with patients result from problems with logic, language, experience, or combinations of these variables. That is, the material and the task of learning must seem logical to the patient in light of how they live their lives; the language style (not to mention the language itself) must be close to those patients' own; and their personal experiences must be such that they can imagine value for themselves in what we say.

Patient education for the cardiac patient is a subject that has been scrutinized beyond belief. All one has to do is browse through any medical library to realize that you could spend countless hours updating yourself on the subject matter. Most of the articles and textbooks on patient education do not differentiate cardiac patients and arrhythmia patients because their learning needs are quite similar. However, we do need to realize that 30% – 35% of patients fail to follow their physician's recommendations on discharge and that 31% of prescriptions taken are being misused in a manner that poses a serious threat to the patient's health. When you look at these statistics and relate them to patients with life-threatening problems, our role as patient educators becomes extremely vital. Even if your job responsibilities do not include this duty, anyone who has patient contact should become involved in patient teaching.

This chapter will cover the basics of education in the hope of satisfying the ultimate goal of every adult educator to help learners meet their personal needs and achieve their goals. Specific content for patient education has been included in each core section and in related chapters.

Objectives

1. Evaluate patient's environment and how it affects patient's ability to learn.
2. Analyze basic assumptions regarding learning process.
3. Review list of helpful reminders to consider when applying patient education.
4. Identify Hoffman's twelve principles of learning.
5. Describe the best approaches to apply Hoffman's principles.

Education Content

A. Basic Assumptions Leading to Ineffective Teaching

    1. Learning is a change in behavior based on exposure to information, experience, or both. Our basic assumptions as we attempt to teach our patients are:

        a. That because we have presented patients with information in one form or another, we have exposed them to it

        b. That because the patients have had an experience, for example, an electrophysiology study or pacemaker implantation, they have therefore been fully exposed to what that experience has taught other patients

        c. That we have chosen the most effective methods and media for teaching an individual patient

        d. That the patient is capable of learning about the subject under normal circumstances

        e. That the patients' surrounding and internal environments lend themselves to learning now

        f. That patients wants to learn what we want to teach them and

        g. That possessing information gives us competence as teachers.

    When we make these assumptions, we are often wrong.

B. Considerations as one Implements the Education Program

    1. Patients forget much of what the doctor tells them.

    2. The more a patient is told, the greater the proportion he or she will forget.

    3. Patients will remember:

        a. What they are told *first*.

        b. What they consider most important.

    4. Intelligent patients do not remember more than less intelligent patients.

    5. Older patients remember just as much as younger patients.

    6. Moderately anxious patients recall more of what they are told than highly anxious patients or patients who are not anxious.

    7. If a patient writes down what the doctor says, he or she will remember just as well as if he or she hears it.

C. Hoffman's Twelve Principles of Learning

    1. These views have their basis in principles of learning now so well recognized by educators that no one originator can be credited with any of them. Hoffman cites twelve principles particularly important to us as we work directly with patients, paraphrased below:

    a. Perception is required for learning.

    b. Because it is a change in behavior, learning is a threat, and takes place more easily when other threats are minimized.

    c. Learning is more effective when it results from a need felt by the learner.

    d. It is easier to learn when material is related to what the learner already knows.

    e. Material that is meaningful to the learner facilitates learning.

    f. Learning put into immediate use is retained longer.

    g. The learner's active participation is essential for learning.

    h. Plateaus occur normally in learning.

    i. Learning requires reinforcement.

    j. Learners who are made aware of their progress learn more easily.

    k. Organization promotes retention and application of learning.

    l. It is the teacher's job to teach; it is the learner's job to learn.

D. Application of the Principles of Learning

    1. We suggest the following approaches in applying these principles:

        a. Choose the time and place as carefully as you can. If your time with the patient absolutely must be one in a series of several discussions he or she has that morning, do what you can to at least avoid interruptions while you are together. Assuring that medications and vital signs have already been taken and putting a sign on the patient's door can help assure privacy. Likewise, avoid interrupting patients at mealtimes or when they're talking with family on the phone; ask them when you may return. It costs you time, but improves your chance of good communication and shows your respect.

        b. Read the chart first. Never enter a patient's room until you know details of his or her admission and the reasons for it; the patient cannot afford to lose trust in us because we seem ignorant of the problem.

        c. Establish rapport. Knock before entering and introduce yourself to everyone present; shake hands if this is appropriate. Ask for permission to sit; do not sit on the patient's bed, even if there are no chairs available, unless the patient has specifically indicated that you may sit there. Many people find sitting on the bed a comforting gesture, but others find it strongly suggestive of authority, particularly parental authority.

        d. Explain why you've come, in terms of benefit to the patient. For example,"I've come to give you information about the test you'll have tomorrow. With more information, you'll feel more relaxed and comfortable."

        e. Take advantage of the fact that you are not a physician. Particularly if you are dressed in scrubs, be certain to let the patient and family know your title and that you are not a doctor, since people often hesitate to question physicians.

f. Remain constantly aware of non-verbal signals you send to the patient. Sit, speak in a calm voice, gesture smoothly rather than rapidly, avoid looking at your watch, edging toward the door, or finishing the patient's sentences for him or her. Even if you are extremely hurried, do your best to show the patient and family that this time is just for them.

g. Include family members or significant others in the instruction if they and the patient wish it. They may be as much in need of information as the patient, and may later reinforce what you say or give you insights to help in your teaching.

h. Assess the patient's learning needs. Begin by asking patients what they've already heard about the problem and the proposed solutions. Ask to hear whatever questions they may have already formed. Yes, you may provoke a recitation about the problem and its symptoms, but it will be instructive to listen for clues about a patient's grasp of the difficulty and what it means to him or her. Question the patients who use medical terms but seem unsure of them. For example,"What did the doctor say about the local anesthesia he told you would be used?", or, "What did the nurse mean when she told you that you'd be 'NPO after midnight'?"

i. Relate everything you say to sensory or other experiences the patient may expect. For example, "After you get the pacemaker and we bring you back to your room, you can expect the area where the pacemaker is (touch that area as you speak) to become sore," or "Your back may be stiff in here (touch the lumbosacral area as you speak) during or after the electrophysiology study from lying flat on the table."

j. Define new terms as you introduce them. Assume that the patient has no familiarity with medical terminology, even if he or she has had much hospital experience. Also introduce any abbreviations or synonyms for the new term the patient may encounter.

k. Avoid asking "closed" questions—that is, questions which allow only a very brief answer from the patient. Even though these save you time, they give patients no chance to show you in detail what they need to learn. Instead, ask "open-ended" questions,which allow a fuller response. Rather than, "Did the doctor tell you why he thinks amiodarone would be a good medicine for you?," then, ask, "What did the doctor say about amiodarone and why he thinks it's right for you?"

l. Backtrack. Especially when discussing topics the patient finds complicated, bridge to the next thought by returning very briefly to a more familiar one. For example,"This new medicine, propranolol, is a little like the digoxin that you've been taking, in the sense that they both slow the heartbeat."

m. Observe for signs of incomprehension and fatigue. Your teaching efforts will be wasted otherwise. Look for lack of eye contact, a puzzled expression, one-word answers to your questions. Be wary if, when you ask patients for their impressions of what you've said, they repeat your own words exactly for you.

n. Break up learning sessions if necessary. Although it certainly is more time-consuming at first, it is more effective later and therefore may save you time in repeat instruction later.

o. Reinforce the patient's statements of trust and hope for a good outcome. Often people make such statements just to hear them made, so they can begin to believe them more fully while they are afraid. Be as complimentary about your physician colleagues as you can truthfully be, especially about their knowledge, their attention to detail, and their skill in procedures.

p. Never be the first to tell the patient important clinical information. The patient needs and deserves the physician's time and guidance for such things. Associated professionals may and should reinforce what the physician introduces, but do not introduce major topics (the need for a pacemaker, failure at EPS on a trusted medication, failure of an ablation attempt). If we do raise such topics and the patient then responds with questions or concerns which the physician must address, the patient may at best be anxious while waiting for these answers, and at worst may lose confidence in the physician.

q. The learning process for children is different than for adults. Children usually do not have the previous experience which provides a foundation that facilitates future learning. Also, children are interested in the future application of what is learned. Finally, the goals of a child learner are subject-centered rather than problem-centered.

References

Doak LG, Doak CC. Patient comprehension profiles: recent findings and strategies. Patient Counseling Health Ed. 2:3:103–104. Winter, 1980.

Samora J, et al. Medical vocabulary knowledge among hospital patients. Health Human Behav 2:2:83–92. Summer, 1961.

Shuy RW. The medical interview: problems in communication. Primary Care. 3:365–386. September, 1976.

Tuman MC. A comparative review of reading and listening comprehension. J Read. 23:8:702. May, 1980.

CHAPTER 7

Pacemakers

Jennifer Fraser

Subsection:
A. Pacemaker Theory
B. Pacing Codes
C. Indications for Pacing
D. Pacemaker Timing Cycles
E. Pacemaker Surveillance
F. Pulse Generator Programming

This section will describe basic theory including historical development of pacing and the concepts of electrical stimulation of the bradycardic heart. It covers the rationale for selection of a pacemaker along with the electrical concepts of the pacemaker patient interface. It will define the generally accepted clinical indications for the use of antibradycardia pacemakers from the perspective of etiology and results of conduction disorders, autonomic nervous system dysfunction, and ECG features that may predict intermittent AV block. It will provide a preliminary discussion on pacemaker timing cycles by defining accepted terminology for the description of the most commonly used modes of pacing, the revised pacing mode code, and general principles. The goals and methods of pacemaker follow-up will be discussed.

Objectives

1. Understand the clinical consequences of symptomatic bradycardia.
2. Understand the fundamental principles of artificial electrical stimulation of the heart.

From: Schurig L. *Educational Guidelines: Pacing and Electrophysiology*. Armonk, NY: Futura Publishing Co, Inc, © 1994.

3. Understand the etiology of conduction system disturbance.

4. Discuss the reasons for disruption of the conduction system and the resulting arrhythmias.

5. Define the standards of patient care, the goals of pacemaker follow-up, and the plan to ensure safe and efficacious pacemaker programming.

6. Plan the follow-up management of a pacemaker patient and understand the advantages and disadvantages of the different methods.

7. Explain the code by which pacemaker function is universally described.

8. Understand the timing cycles of the major pacing modes in both single and dual chambered devices.

9. Understand the advantages and disadvantages of different methods of follow-up.

10. Discuss the interface between the pacemaker and the patient.

Glossary and Abbreviations

Atrial refractory period: The interval after an atrial sense or paced event during which the atrial channel of a dual chamber pacemaker is insensitive. It is used to prevent the sensing of a non-physiologic event such as a ventricular pacing stimulus, QRS, T wave, intrinsic atrial depolarization faster than the upper rate limit. (Ventricular sensing and pacing also start the atrial refractory period.)

Automatic interval: (pacing interval) The interval between two consecutive pacing spikes. The interval used to evaluate pacing.

AV interval (AV delay): The interval between an atrial pace or sense event and the succeeding ventricular pace or sense event. It is the electronic PR interval.

Blanking periods: The time during and after a pacemaker stimulus during which the opposite channel of the pacemaker is insensitive. The purpose of this interval is to avoid sensing pacemaker stimuli directed at one chamber, in the opposite chamber.

Escape interval: The interval between a sensed or paced event to the next paced event. The interval used to evaluate sensing.

Fusion beat: A ventricular or atrial depolarization that starts from two foci (one spontaneous and one a pacemaker stimulus) and has characteristics of each.

Hysteresis: A prolongation of the pacemaker escape interval following a sensed event. This increases the opportunity for the patient to remain in an intrinsic rhythm.

Lower rate limit: The longest interval allowed between two pacemaker stimuli or between a sensed ventricular event and a paced ventricular event.

Maximum tracking limit: The theoretic maximum pacemaker rate based on atrial refractoriness (which equal the sum of the AVI and PVARP). It may be further limited by electronic circuit-determined absolute limit. The max rate is the maximum rate at which the atrial rate is tracked 1:1.

Refractory period: A component of the pacemaker timing cycle occurring after a sensed or paced event when the pacemaker does not respond to incoming signals. It may be "sensed" but ignored by the pacemaker.

Total atrial refractory period: The time in which the atrial pacemaker channel is insensitive. Generally it consists of the AV interval plus the post-ventricular (PVARP) atrial refractory interval.

Upper rate interval: The shortest interval between ventricular paced events or a sensed ventricular event followed by a paced ventricular event.

Upper rate limit: This may be the same as the maximum rate limit or may be programmed independently. It is the maximum rate at which the ventricle can be stimulated.

VA conduction: The conduction of a ventricular impulse retrograde to the atrium through the AV node or an accessory pathway.

VA interval: The interval between the sensed or paced ventricular event and the next sensed or paced atrial event.

Ventricular refractory period: The interval after a ventricular paced or sensed event during which the ventricular amplifier does not respond to incoming signals. This interval also contains the noise sampling period, which is a brief interval of time at the end of the refractory period where electrical interference causes the pacemaker to revert to fixed rate pacing for one or more cycles.

Vulnerable period: That portion of the electrical complex, either atrial or ventricular, during which stimulation may induce arrhythmia.

Wenckebach: (In pacemaker terms) PV pacing at progressively greater intervals until one P wave is unsensed. The cycle then restarts.

Education Content

A. Pacemaker Theory

   1. History of cardiac pacing

     a. The first documented attempts to stimulate the heart muscle electrically were performed by Luigi Gabrini in the 1790s.

     b. Major advances were made by various scientists in research on human physiology, throughout the 19th century.

     c. 1932: Dr. Albert Hyman, regarded as the father of artificial pacing, developed the "artificial cardiac pacemaker." It was a hand-cranked device and was used in about 40 patients with varying success. Electrical impulses were transmitted to the heart via a bipolar needle inserted between 2 ribs.

     d. 1952: Dr. Paul Zoll reported the successful support of cardiac rhythm through external transcutaneous pacing for patients with Stokes-Adams attacks.

     e. During the early years of heart surgery for congenital repair, Dr. Wilfred Bigelow of Toronto General Hospital, recognized that patients with surgically induced heart block could be sustained through electrical stimulation.

     f. Lillehei and Bakken developed a temporary pacemaker device for use in patients' post-cardiac surgery.

     g. 1958: Dr. Ruse Lumqvist devised the first fully implantable pacemaker. It was implanted by Dr. Senning at Karolenska Hospital in Solna, Sweden.

     h. Concurrently, Furman and Robinson in New York reported the first use of a temporary transvenous pacemaker. The external pacemaker was connected to a wall socket.

     i. 1962: The first programmable pacemaker was developed.

     j. 1966: Multi-programmability in pacemakers became available.

     k. 1971: AV sequential pacing was available and by 1978, dual demand pacemakers were available.

     l. 1981: The first antitachycardia pacemaker was available for use.

     m. 1985: Adaptive-rate pacing was first clinically used.

     n. As a result of the proliferation of devices for a variety of functions and a plethora of programmers to manage them, the clinical practice of cardiac pacing has become a subspecialty for physicians, engineers, and clinically associated professionals.

   2. General principles

     a. The heart muscle is unique in that depolarization of a small group of cells by an electrical impulse will cause depolarization throughout the myocardium and result in mechanical contraction of the heart muscle (systole). After completion of depolarization, the cells repolarize with relaxation of the myocardium. This corresponds to the phase of cardiac filling called diastole.

b. Pathological bradycardia can result in important clinical consequences including sudden cardiac death, syncope with or without injury, presyncope, fatigue, chamber dilatation and cardiac failure, and loss of mental acuity.

c. Pathological bradycardia can be effectively treated over long periods of time by permanent implantable devices which electrically stimulate the endocardial or epicardial surface of the heart and reliably result in depolarization of the atria, ventricles or both.

d. The decision to implant a pacing device can be made on reasonably rigorous clinical grounds with a reasonably high degree of agreement among well-trained and experienced clinicians.

e. Pacemakers are implanted to compensate for failure of atrioventricular conduction or for failure or disruption of impulse formation. Pacemakers are used increasingly to stabilize erratic rhythms and to thereby reduce associated symptoms and improve cardiac performance.

3. Choosing a pacemaker

    a. A rational choice of a specific pacing device can be made based on:

        1. A thorough knowledge of the clinical history and natural history of the condition requiring pacing therapy.

        2. Knowledge of patient lifestyle requirements and expectations.

        3. Follow-up capability of the implanting center.

        4. Patient ability to comply with follow-up.

        5. Does the patient have access to medical care.

        6. Concomitant clinical conditions and the impact of the bradycardia on these conditions.

        7. Likelihood of developing predictable complications of pacing.

    b. Following implantation of a pacing device:

        1. Patient benefits from pacing can be optimized by a carefully planned schedule of follow-up.

        2. Location should be in a setting staffed with specialists thoroughly versed in the clinical and technical aspects of cardiac pacing.

        3. General cardiology care should be available to address the patient's other clinical conditions.

        4. Pacemaker analysis equipment should be available – programmers, ECG machines, magnets, etc.

4. Electrical concepts of the pacemaker patient interface

    a. Electricity flows in a complete circuit only.

    b. In a pacing system, electricity travels from the power source, or battery, through the lead directly to the heart. The electrode must be in direct contact with the epicardial or endocardial surface of the heart in an area with excitable cells.

c. The pacemaker output is delivered to the heart through the lead and electrode. The return pathway of the current is either through blood and tissue to an indifferent electrode on the same lead (20 mm from the tip of the electrode) as in a bipolar system or to the can of the pacemaker, as in a unipolar system.

d. The relatively low amplitude intracardiac signal seen by the pulse generator is amplified by it for proper detection. To avoid amplification of the unwanted signals, the amplifier has a "bandpass filter" through which all signals pass. It has a maximum sensitivity which corresponds to a frequency of the maximum energy in the electrogram for either a P or QRS complexes. Pacemaker sensitivity is expressed in millivolts.

e. Pacemaker output circuit operation is based on five major factors that must be well understood:

    1. Voltage

    2. Current

    3. Charge

    4. Energy

    5. Impedance

    6. Ohms law $V = (I \times R)$

Note: Refer to Part One, Chapter 1, Fundamentals of Electronics for further explanation of 1 through 6.

5. Components of a cardiac pacing system

a. The pulse generator emits stimulation pulses. The "electrode" transmits the stimulation pulse to body tissue. The pulse generator and electrode are interconnected by an insulated electronic conductor. An electrode plus a conductor are called a lead. A pulse generator and lead(s) together are referred to as a "pacemaker." The pulse generator and lead and the patient are a "pacing system."

b. The pulse generator is made up of:

    1. A battery

    2. Electrical output circuit

    3. Timing control to run the output circuit

c. The pacemaker amplifies intracardiac signals and filters unwanted signals via a "bandpass filter"

d. All currently implanted non-nuclear pulse generators are powered by lithium batteries; their longevity is variable. All currently manufactured pulse generators are powered by lithium-iodine.

6. Stimulation threshold

a. The minimal amount of electrical stimulation that consistently results in cardiac depolarization.

    b. May be expressed in terms of amplitude (milliamperes or volts), pulse duration (milliseconds), charge (microcoulombs) or energy (microjoules).

7. Sensing threshold

    a. The minimal atrial or ventricular intrinsic signal to be consistently sensed by the pulse generator sensing amplifier.

    b. May be expressed in millivolts with the smallest number representing the most sensitive setting.

8. The Strength duration curve is:

    a. Created by measuring the voltage or current thresholds for various pulse durations or vice versa and by plotting them on a graph with voltage or current on the vertical axis and pulse duration on the horizontal axis.

    b. The lowest combination of pulse amplitude and pulse duration that reliably results in effective myocardial stimulation.

    c. For all amplitudes and pulse durations above the strength duration curve, the heart is effectively stimulated, and for points below the curve, stimulation is ineffective.

B. Pacing Codes

1. NASPE Mode Code Committee and the British Pacing and Electrophysiology group, through joint effort, developed the NASPE/BPEG (NBG) Generic Code. It meets two major needs not previously dealt with by the Revised ICHD Code; the denotation of rate modulation mechanism that responds to some physiologic variable and the indication of the presence of one or more antitachyarrhythmic function without identifying them specifically. The previously represented bradycardia functions are retained in this code.

2. NASPE/BPEG (NBG) Generic Pacemaker Code for Antibradyarrhythmia, Adaptive-Rate Pacing and Antitachyarrhythmia Devices (Table 1).

3. Definitions of the NASPE/BPEG (NBG) mode code

    a. Position I through III are used exclusively for the description of antibradyarrhythmia function.

    b. Fourth position describes two different device characteristics: the degree of programmability and the presence or absence of an adaptive rate mechanism.

    c. The symbol "0" (None in Position V) indicates both that the device is non-programmable and that it possesses no rate adaptive features.

    d. Any device with one or two programmable features is considered "simple programmable" (P).

    e. Any device with more than two programmable parameters is deemed "multiprogrammable" (M).

    f. An additional option in Position IV is "R" (Rate Modulation).

Table 1
NASPE/BPEG (NBG) Generic Pacemaker Code for Antibradyarrhythmia, Adaptive-Rate Pacing and Antitachyarrhythmia Devices

| | | Position | | |
| | | | IV | V |
I Chamber Pacer	II Chamber Sensed	III Response to Sensing	Program/ Rate Modulation	Antitach/ Arrhythmia Function
0 = None	0 = None	0 = None	0 = None	0 = None
A = Atrium	A = Atrium	T = Triggered	P = Simple	P = Pacing (ATP)
V = Vent.	V = Vent.	I = Inhibit	programmable	S = Shock
D = Dual	D = Dual	D = Dual	M = Multiprogrammable	D = Dual
(A + V)	(A + V)	(T + I)	C = Communicating	(P + S)
			R = Rate modulation	

Vent = Ventricle
ATP = Antitachycardia pacing
  S = Manufacturer's designation only, S = Single (A or V)

    g. "R" takes precedence over the hierarchy of programmability indicators and does not necessarily imply the presence of either programmability or telemetry.

    h. Position V is used to indicate the presence of one or more antitachyarrhythmia functions.

    i. Note the designation for manufacturers which describes the pacemaker's possible use in either chamber, Ex: SSI for single chamber pacing.

C. Indications for Pacing (Refer to Part Two, Chapter 13, covered by specific diagnoses.)

  1. Etiology of conduction system disorders

    a. Any or all parts of the conduction system may be replaced by fibrous tissue, usually in a patchy manner.

    b. When histologic changes are confined to the conduction system, myocardial function is not adversely affected.

    c. Fibrotic changes of the conduction system are usually associated with aging and may have an auto-immune basis.

  2. Causes of conduction system disorders

    a. Patchy fibrosis of conduction tissue (40%)

    b. Cardiomyopathy in which fibrous replacement occurs throughout the myocardium (15%)

    c. Coronary artery disease with infarction or ischemia of part of the conduction system (15% and significantly higher proportionately in patients > 60 years)

   d. Invasion of the conduction system by the calcification of a heart valve (most frequently aortic stenosis)

   e. Congenital heart block

   f. Surgical damage to the conduction system during the repair of VSD or during aortic valve replacement

   g. Less commonly in rheumatoid arthritis, sarcoidosis and amyloid, Lyme disease, Chagas disease, infective endocarditis, aortic valve (ring abcess formation)

   h. May be a result of drugs

3. Clinical results of specific conduction disorders

   a. When the sinoatrial node is involved, there may be a failure or a delay in impulse formation resulting in one or more of the following:

      1. Sinus bradycardia

      2. Sinoatrial block

      3. Sinus arrest

   b. When no atrial activation by the sinus node occurs, another part of the heart may take over the regulating mechanism in a phenomenon known as escape. Escape rhythms may include:

      1. Junctional bradycardia

      2. Ectopic atrial rhythm

      3. His rhythm

      4. Ventricular escape rhythm

   c. If all escape mechanisms fail in combination with sinoatrial arrest, asystole ensues.

   d. Atrioventricular block is a term used to describe block occurring in both the AV node itself and lower in the conduction pathway to the ventricles. It may include the following rhythms:

      1. First degree AV block

      2. Second degree AV block; Mobitz type I or Mobitz type II

      3. Complete or third degree AV block

   e. The majority of patients present with disease in either the sinus node or the AV node and conduction pathway. There is often an extension of disease to other parts of the conducting system over time.

4. Autonomic nervous dystem dysfunction

   a. May result in electrophysiologic abnormalities such as:

      1. Carotid sinus syncope (syndrome)

      2. Vasovagal syncope

5. ECG features that may predict intermittent AV block

a. Conduction defects can be intermittent in nature and therefore result in intermittent symptoms that may be diagnostically challenging. ECG features that may predict the likelihood of intermittent complete AV block are:

1. Mobitz II AV block
2. First degree AV block with right bundle branch block and left posterior fascicular block
3. First degree AV block with left bundle branch block
4. First degree AV block with right bundle branch block and left anterior fascicular block
5. Right bundle branch block with left posterior fascicular block
6. Left bundle branch block
7. Left posterior fascicular block
8. Mobitz I second degree AV block

D. Pacemaker Timing Cycles

1. General principles

a. All pacemaker timing cycles begin and/or end with a sensed spontaneous intrinsic depolarization or a pacemaker stimulus.

b. All pacemaker ECG analysis is based on the understanding of the various stimulation and sensing intervals of that specific device.

c. In a single chambered device, all timing begins and ends by pacing or sensing in that chamber. That chamber determines all timing events.

d. The escape interval varies at times between any two events, sensed or paced. One interval occurs equal to the pacing interval if the timing cycle is begun by a paced event. The second interval that occurs is longer than the pacing interval if it is begun by a sensed event. This variation is called rate hysteresis and is programmable as off, in rate or in milliseconds. Without hysteresis the escape interval in a single chamber device is equal to the pacing interval.

e. The interval after a paced or sensed event that occurs at the beginning of a timing cycle may be broken into several portions; an unresponsive refractory period, a noise sampling period and an alert period.

f. In dual chambered pacing, both the atrium and the ventricle are sensed and initiate separate but related timing cycles. Each chamber's timing cycle has its own blanking, refractory, noise sampling, and alert periods. The various portions of dual chamber timing cycles are generally programmable and must be known in order to verify proper function.

g. There are two different timing systems for dual chamber modes. These are atrial based and ventricular based. Most literature discusses ventricular based timing. The timing cycle of the device you are dealing with must be recognized.

h. Keep in mind, regardless of the type of pacemaker (single or dual chamber), the underlying rhythm determines operation of the pacemaker.

E. Pacemaker Surveillance

1. Follow-up

   a. Pacemaker follow-up was established in the early 1970s to manage an increasing volume of patients, to centralize ancillary equipment and expertise, and to develop surveillance methods that would optimize patient care and safety.

   b. Pacemakers, over time, have become more reliable and of longer life, the interaction between the pacemaker and the patient has become more complex and follow-up more time consuming.

   c. The follow-up service must define its role and responsibility in the care of the pacemaker patient.

      1. This role must be clearly understood by the patient, his family, and the referring doctors.

      2. It may include total cardiologic care, pacemaker care alone or simple observation of pacemaker function with referral for care and intervention.

2. Goals for follow-up

   a. To optimize pacemaker patient interaction and maximize pacemaker longevity.

   b. To minimize patient fear and anxiety through treatment and education.

   c. To verify proper and appropriate pacemaker function.

   d. To recognize, interpret, and correct pacemaker problems prior to symptoms.

   e. To detect pacemakers' approaching end of battery life and replace them in a timely manner.

   f. To act as a repository of pacemaker hardware, information, and technical expertise.

   g. To record patient location and develop a means of notification of those patients should a recall or advisory occur.

   h. To triage non-pacemaker related health problems to the appropriate place (e.g., family physician, emergency room, cardiologist, social worker, public health nurse, etc.)

   i. Develop statistical data that is specific for one clinic or that is part of a larger data base.

3. Methods of follow-up

   a. Hands-on clinical assessment

       1. Allows full assessment of the pacemaker through programming, pocket manipulation, and observation

       2. It allows a trusting relationship to develop between patient and follow-up staff

       3. It is time consuming, often inconvenient and expensive for staff and patient

    b. Transtelephonic monitoring (TTM)

       1. As part of the pacemaker clinic

       2. Independent commercial agency

       3. Efficient, convenient, economical, and readily accessible

       4. Lacks direct patient contact, and relies on patient for observation of symptoms

       5. Problems with artifact and interference

       6. Less successful outcome with psychological support and teaching

       7. Often most useful in patients who are immobile or infirm or those whose pacemakers require frequent assessment

       8. Allows a link between remote clinics and tertiary centers

    c. Combination of clinic and transtelephonic monitoring:

       1. Combines the benefits of clinical assessment with the convenience of TTM

       2. Cost effective and efficient

F. Pulse Generator Programming

  1. General principles

    a. Is defined as the ability to make non-invasive, stable but reversible changes in pacemaker function. It may be used as a diagnostic procedure or a therapeutic measure.

    b. Programmable options vary widely depending on the design of the pulse generator and whether it is intended for use in two chambers or one.

    c. The full benefit of programmability cannot be achieved without a systematic and careful follow-up system run by well-trained staff.

  2. Usefulness of pulse generator programmability

    a. Pacemaker programming to optimal function ensures patient safety and satisfactory pacemaker patient interface.

    b. It prolongs battery life and in some cases, avoids invasive procedures.

    c. Using a pacemaker "programmer" makes it possible to alter some aspect of pulse generator function within a predetermined range. Example rate 30–110 bpm programmers are specific to each manufacturer and often specific within a single manufacturer to various devices. They are not interchangeable.

    d. Improves follow-up procedures.

    e. Permits evaluation of the patient's underlying rhythm.

    f. Provides communication with the device for diagnostic data, measured data, intracardiac electrograms, marker channels, histograms, and programmed settings.

    g. Manages post-implant malfunctions or complications.

3. Guidelines to safe programming

    a. A programming protocol should consider the following fundamental principles:

        1. Know the pulse generator specifications and capabilities

        2. Understand the programmer and its sequence

        3. Know the value and the operation of "emergency" or "stat set"

        4. Know the patient's cardiovascular status and pacemaker dependency

        5. The patient should be supine and monitored by ECG

        6. Emergency life support must be available and staff must be trained

        7. Back-up programmer should be available when programming critical functions in dependent patients

        8. Verify pacemaker settings at completion of the visit

        9. Establish safety margins based on the thresholds obtained

        10. Document events of the visit for tracking patient/device interactions

    b. Pacemaker clinic is the focal point of programming hardware, programming records, and programming procedure. When programming critical parameters such as output, back-up programmers should be available should there be a primary programmer failure.

References

Bernstein A, Brownlee R, Fletcher R, Gold R, Smyth NPD, Spielman S. Pacing mode codes. In Modern Cardiac Pacing. S Barold, Mount Kisco: Futura Publishing Co, Inc., 307–321 (Eds.). 1985.

Bernstein AD, Camm AJ, Fletcher RD, et al. The NASPE/BPEG generic pacemaker code for antibradyarrhythmia and adaptive-rate pacing and antitachyarrhythmia devices. PACE. 10:794–799. 1987.

Ector H, Witters E, Tanghe K, et al. Measurement of pacing threshold. PACE. 8:66–72. 1985.

Elmqvist R, Senning A. An implantable pacemaker for the heart. Proceedings of the Second International Conference on Medical Electronics. London. Iliffe, Smyth CN, 253. 1959.

Furman S, Hayes D, Holmes DR. Comprehension of Pacemaker Timing Cycles: A Practice of Cardiac Pacing. Mount Kisco: Futura Publishing Co Inc., 159–218. 1989.

Furman S. Pacemaker Follow-up. In A Practice of Cardiac Pacing. 1st ed. S Furman (Ed.). Mount Kisco: Futura Publishing Co, Inc., 379–412. 1986.

Furman S. Glossary. A Practice of Cardiac Pacing. 1st ed. In S Furman, (Ed.). Mount Kisco: Futura Publishing Co, Inc., 463–470. 1986.

Harthorne JW. Programmable pacemakers: Technical features and clinical applications. Cardiovasc Clin. 14:135–147. 1983.

Levine PA. Proceedings of the policy conference of NASPE on programmability and pacemaker follow-up programs. Clin Prog Pacing and Electrophysiol. 2:145–191. 1984.

Parsonnet V, Cuddy T, Escher D, et al. A permanent pacemaker capable of external non-invasive programming. Trans Am Soc Artif Int Organs. 19: 224, 1973.

Suggested Readings

Barold SS. Modern Cardiac Pacing, Mount Kisco: Futura Publishing Co, Inc., Ch 23–25. 1985.

Bernstein A, et al. Policy Conference Report, Antibradycardia-pacemaker follow-up: effectiveness, needs, and resources. NASPE Scientific Sessions. 1993.

Dohrmann M, Goldschlager N. Myocardial stimulation threshold in patients with cardiac pacemakers. Cardiol Clin. 3:4:527–537. 1985.

Furman S. Pacemaker follow-up. In A Practice of Cardiac Pacing. 1st ed. S. Furman, (Ed.). Mount Kisco: Futura Publishing Co, Inc., 379–412. 1986.

Furman S. Basic concepts. A Practice of Cardiac Pacing. 1st ed. In S Furman, (Ed.). Mount Kisco: Futura Publishing Co, Inc., 27–68. 1986.

Furman S. Timing cycles. A Practice of Cardiac Pacing. 1st ed. In S Furman (Ed.). Mount Kisco: Futura Publishing Co, Inc., 157–217. 1986.

Hauser R. Programmability: a clinical approach. Cardiol Clin. 3:4:539–550. 1985.

Levine PA, Mace RC. General Considerations Pacing Therapy—A Guide to Cardiac Pacing for Optimum Hemodynamic Benefit. Mount Kisco: Futura Publishing Co, Inc., 65–69. 1983.

Parsonnet V, Furman S, Smythe N, Bilitch M. Optimal Resources for Implantable Cardiac Pacemakers. Circulation 68:1. 1983.

Sutton R, Bourgeois I. What is a Pacemaker? In the Foundations of Cardiac Pacing Part I. The Bakken Research Center Series. Mount Kisco: Futura Publishing Co, Inc., 45–122. 1991.

Sutton R, Bourgeois I. Hemodynamics and Pacing. In the Foundations of Cardiac Pacing Pt 1. The Bakken Research Center Series. Mount Kisco: Futura Publishing Co, Inc., 123–145. 1991.

Furman S, Hayes D, Holmes DR, Comprehension of Pacemaker Timing Cycles: A Practice of Cardiac Pacing. Mount Kisco: Futura Publishing Co, Inc., 159–218. 1986.

CHAPTER 8

Safety

Nancy H. Fullmer

Subsection:
A.   Infection Control/Sterile Technique
B.   Radiation Safety
C.   Electrical Safety
D–F. Drug Interactions
G.   Device Interactions
H.   Electromagnetic Interference (EMI)

Patients experiencing electrophysiologic (EP) studies, EP interventions, and implanted cardiac device therapies are particularly susceptible to environmental hazards. This chapter covers safety aspects to be considered during care of this patient population.

It begins with a discussion of the principles involved in infection control. Concepts of infection control are vitally important for any patient undergoing surgery, but acquire special significance in those experiencing invasive procedures and receiving implanted devices. To protect these patients appropriately, one must understand and apply considerations of pharmacologic prophylactic therapy, proper sterile technique during the procedure, and aseptic practices during the post-procedural recovery and healing period. Since strict sterile technique is integral to infection control practices, it will be addressed in this section.

In various institutions, pacing systems may be implanted in the surgical suite, the cardiac catheterization laboratory, or an electrophysiology laboratory. The implanter may be a cardiologist or surgeon, or the procedure may involve a team approach between the two. No matter what the accustomed practice in the particular institution, proper infection control practices must be carefully observed in order to minimize the risk of infection at the site of implant and the concomitant possibility of transmission of the infection to the cardiac tissue.

From: Schurig L. *Educational Guidelines: Pacing and Electrophysiology.* Armonk, NY: Futura Publishing Co, Inc, © 1994.

Other safety considerations to be covered include radiation safety, electrical safety, and components of a preventive maintenance program to minimize the potential for accidents in this environment.

Device therapy for treatment of arrhythmias has historically been presented without regard to other therapies and conditions that affect myocardial and device interaction. Drug and chemical interventions may have either short- or long-term, adverse therapeutic, or little effect on device function. Effects of the more commonly used pharmacologic agents on the heart's response to antibradycardia pacing, rate modulated pacing, antitachycardia pacing, cardioversion, and defibrillation will be reviewed.

This chapter also discusses concepts of external sources of electromagnetic interference on the functioning of implanted cardiac devices. In this era of rapidly proliferating electronic and magnetically related devices and equipment, the associated professional should keep abreast of long standing sources of interference as well as newly emerging products which could potentially cause problems for this patient population. Each technological development and product release will continue to expand, change, and challenge us.

Objectives

1. Define terms relating to sterile technique, asepsis, and infection control.
2. Identify the "sterile" areas of the implant/testing field as opposed to unsterile areas.
3. Describe appropriate methods of providing sterile supplies to the field during implant/testing procedures.
4. Discuss rationale for appropriate sterile technique during implant/testing procedures.
5. Identify times for administration of antibiotics in relation to infection control for cardiac pacing.
6. Describe activities appropriate to proper and adequate infection control when caring for a patient with an implanted pacing system.
7. Identify basic concepts for radiation safety.
8. Recognize the potential for electrical accidents during pacing and EP studies.
9. List at least three electrolytes that affect thresholds and discuss the effect of severe electrolyte imbalance on thresholds.
10. Name at least six drugs that can at least temporarily increase capture thresholds.
11. List possible sources of electromagnetic interference (EMI).
12. Describe possible effects and symptoms of possible interference.
13. Discuss precautions appropriate to avoid possible deleterious effects of potential sources of EMI.

Glossary and Abbreviations

Acidosis: Chemical accumulation of acid or decrease in base causing an increase in H+ ion concentration and a decrease in pH that may potentially alter pacing thresholds.

Action potential: A brief change in electrical potential across a cell membrane of nerve or muscle tissue in response to some stimulus, typically depolarization and repolarization of the cell.

Alkalosis: Chemical accumulation of base or decrease in acid causing decrease of H+ ion concentration and an increase in pH that may potentially alter pacing thresholds.

Antiarrhythmic: A drug used in management of irregularities in heart rhythm (arrhythmias).

Depolarization: The reversal of the resting potential across an excitable cell membrane, i.e., a reversing of polarity between the inside and outside of a cell membrane.

DFT: Defibrillation threshold

Dosimetry: Measurement and calculation of a radiation dose.

Electrolyte: A substance which dissociates into ions when placed in solution thereby becoming a conductor of electrical current.

Ionized radiation: The process by which energy from a radiation source caused electrons to be dislodged from the outer shell of atoms. Fluoroscopy is an example of ionized radiation.

Millirem: (mrem) A measurement that is one thousandth of a rem.

Radiation: The emission and propagation of energy through space or through a material medium with the release of subatomic particles or waves of energy from the atoms undergoing nuclear disintegration.

RAD: Radiation absorbed dose

REM: Roentgen equivalent man, a measurement that standardizes radiation effects in man.

Roentgen: A measure indicating the total amount of radiation given off into the air by a source of radiation.

Education Content

A. Infection Control and Sterile Technique
    1. Chain of infection
        a. Infectious agent
            1. Bacteria – anaerobic/aerobic
            2. Fungi
            3. Viruses
        b. Susceptible host
            1. Elderly
            2. Breach of anatomical barrier (incision)
            3. Anesthetic effects on normal defense mechanisms
        c. Means of transmission
            1. Contact
                a) Direct
                b) Indirect
                c) Droplet
            2. Airborne
            3. Vehicle or vector-borne
    2. Methods of interruption of chain of infection
        a. Destruction of infectious agent
            1. Heat sterilization (steam, hot air)
            2. Ethylene oxide gas sterilization
            3. Chemical sterilization (Glutaraldehyde/formaldehyde)
        b. Reduction of host susceptibility
            1. Control of chronic disease processes
            2. Optimization of fluid and nutritional status
            3. Use of prophylactic therapy prior to implantation
                a) IV or PO administration of antibiotic agents
                b) Washing/showering with antimicrobial agents
            4. Irrigation of incision site/pocket with antibiotic solution during implant
            5. Use of local anesthetic agents instead of general agents
            6. Use of antibiotic agents following implant
        c. Interruption of transmission
            1. Handwashing
            2. Strict sterile technique intraprocedure
                a) Antimicrobial skin prep
                b) Masks, sterile gowns and gloves, hair coverings

      c) Sterile, waterproofed drapes to isolate incision site

      d) Properly sterilized instruments and supplies

      e) Proper sterile technique intraprocedure

          1) Sterile supply transfer onto field

          2) Control of traffic flow

          3) Control of conversation

      f) Avoidance of drainage devices

      g) Sterile occlusive dressing

   3. Sterile gloves and supplies for incision care

   4. Isolation of incision site from environment

3. Pre-procedure

   a. If ordered, prophylactic antibiotic therapy

   b. Antimicrobial wash within 8 hours

   c. Resolution of current infectious processes

   d. Hydration/nutritional status

   e. Normalization of blood factors and chemistry

4. Intraprocedure

   a. Environmental control

      1. Temperature

      2. Relative humidity

      3. Air-exchange/filtration system

   b. Decontamination of area, equipment, and furniture

   c. Sterile field includes

      1. Waterproof sterile dress

          a) Completely cover patient, only incision area exposed

          b) Only portions of drape above waist level = sterile

          c) Arranged to provide barrier between patient's face and incision area

      2. Waterproof sterile gowns used by implanter and assistant. Sterile areas:

          a) Front of gown from nipple line to waist

          b) Sleeves from wrist to elbow

          c) Other areas of gown are unsterile

      3. Rubber gloves without any holes or tears, completely covering hands and overlapping cuffs of gown sleeves

      4. All other areas of procedure area are unsterile

      5. Provision of sterile supplies to sterile field

          a) Outer, unsterile protective covering opened by unsterile or "circulating" person without touching inner package or edges of packaging

          b) Inner, sterile package removed from opened package by sterile-garbed or "scrubbed" person without touching outer covering or edges of packaging

    c) Unsterile personnel never reach across any sterile area

  6. Testing equipment/cables are passed from sterile field by the "scrubbed" person without touching unsterile areas or personnel

  d. Maintenance of sterility intraprocedure

    1. Sterile drape integrity

      a) Penetration by instruments

      b) Penetration by fluids

    2. No contamination of sterile field

    3. Traffic control

    4. Control of conversation

  e. Sterile occlusive dressing

5. Post-procedure

  a. Use of sterile gloves, supplies by caregivers

  b. Isolation of incision site from environment

  c. Regular checks/changes of dressing

  d. If ordered, prophylactic antibiotic therapy

6. Education

  a. Nursing unit staff

  b. Procedure area staff

  c. Patient/family

7. Drug therapy options

  a. Pre-procedural administration of antibiotics

  b. Intraprocedural administration of antibiotics IV

  c. Intraprocedural irrigation of incision and pacemaker "pocket" with antibiotic solution

  d. Post-procedural administration of antibiotics

8. Universal precautions

  a. Thorough hand washing technique, also upon removal of gloves during patient care

  b. Use protective barriers during high-risk procedures

  c. Take care to prevent cuts and/or puncture injuries during patient care

  d. Use proper disposal techniques and containers for high-risk items, Ex: needles, surgical blades etc.

  e. Minimize exposure during high-risk procedures, Ex: mouth to mouth resuscitation, line insertions, IV insertions, etc.

  f. Transport high-risk specimens in protective containers

B. Radiation Safety

   1. Equipment safety

      a. Inspected at intervals recommended by state/federal guidelines

      b. Maintain ongoing preventive maintenance as per institutional/governmental requirements

      c. Complete repairs promptly

      d. Use appropirate cords, cables, and grounding

      e. Complete calibration/inspection/certification on new equipment prior to use

      f. Post-appropriate signage in areas where x-ray is used

   2. Personnel safety

      a. Wear lead aprons, preferably encircling

      b. Wear "thyroid" collars

      c. Goggles not usually recommended for fluoroscopy

      d. Shield patient if pregnancy suspected or known

      e. Shield room walls and doors

      f. Avoid placing hands directly in the beam

      g. Alert staff when x-ray is activated

      h. Wear radiation safety badge to monitor your exposure to occupational radiation

         1. Collar badge

         2. Whole body badge

         3. Ring badge

      i. Exposure levels for nonoccupationally exposed workers – workers with the potential to receive greater doses must wear a radiation badge.

         1. 500 mrem/year

         2. 125 mrem/quarter

   3. Radiation field

      a. Minimize time and dose of fluoroscopy used

      b. Decrease time in and around radiation field

      c. Increase distance from radiation field – double the distance to decrease dose by a factor of 4

      d. Increase shielding between you and the radiation source – soft tissue as well as lead attenuates ionizing radiation

   4. Lower room lights during procedure – less fluoroscopy time needed

   5. Operation of the equipment is done by qualified technologist

   6. Tube placement

      a. Lower image intensifier close to patient – reduces irradiated field size and scatter

    b. Raise image intensifier from patient – reduces radiation dose to patient

7. Collimate system to area of interest only – reduces field size and scatter

8. Move monitor close to you – reduces time required for study if you can see what you are doing

9. Always record fluoroscopy time and exam – allows for more accurate dosimetry

10. Use common sense when positioning patient with regards to radiation safety.

C. Electrical Safety

1. Environmental precautions
   a. Minimize use of additional line powered equipment
   b. Turn line operated equipment off prior to disconnecting from an outlet
   c. Do not use remote outlets to service equipment on the patient
   d. Keep the patient and area dry
   e. Do not touch electrical equipment with wet hands
   f. Monitor room humidity – 50% – 60% to decrease static electricity
   g. Report sockets that do not hold plugs securely
   h. Know source of emergency power
   i. Do not use cheaters or extension cords
   j. Do not permit temporary or makeshift equipment repairs

2. Equipment precautions
   a. Test all new equipment prior to use
   b. Check inspection tags on equipment in use
   c. Use only properly grounded equipment – 3 prong plugs
   d. Use only hospital grade power cords
   e. Inspect strain relief on equipment power cords
   f. Do not step on plugs or line cords
   g. Do not unplug equipment by pulling the cord from the outlet
   h. Do not use damaged equipment
   i. Report all complaints of shocks or tingling sensations from equipment
   j. Unplug equipment giving off warning signs
   k. Report all equipment that has been dropped
   l. Do not tolerate any deviations from the expected performance of the equipment

3. Pacemaker precautions
   a. Insert a new battery prior to each use of the pacemaker

    b. Maintain a log of generator use

    c. Keep the faceplate cover over the generator controls

    d. Wear rubber gloves when handling the pacing wire

    e. Discharge stray current on a metal surface prior to approaching the patient

    f. Do not allow contact of both extensions of the pacing wire

    g. Cover all exposed parts of the pacing wire with a rubber glove

    h. Do not simultaneously touch electrical equipment and the pacing wire

4. Defibrillator precautions – report any of the following:

    a. Bent electrode paddles

    b. Meter that does not operate smoothly

    c. Circuit breaker or fuse that opens during rapid repetitive discharges

    d. Failure to operate

    e. Failure to hold a charge

    f. Water damage to the unit

    g. Inability to complete the self test procedure

    h. Maximum depletion of the battery

    i. Any suspected problem

5. Monitor precautions – report any of the following:

    a. Poor tracing on the screen

    b. Rate meter malfunction

    c. Alarm malfunction

    d. Poor quality ECG tracing

    e. Automatic direct writers fail to trigger

    f. Water damage to the unit

    g. Any suspected problem

D. Pharmacologic Basis of Drug and Pulse Generator Interactions

1. Mechanisms affecting intrinsic impulse formation and conduction in appropriate single and dual chamber pulse generator response.

    a. Sodium channel blockade

    b. Sympathetic blockade

    c. Effective refractory period prolongation

    d. Calcium channel blockade

    e. Suppression of ectopy

    f. Drug induced arrhythmias (proarrhythmic effects)

    g. Drug toxicity

    h. Drug synergy

2. Mechanisms affecting sensors in rate modulation
   a. Effects on depolarization gradient
      1. Drug effects altering ion concentrations in resting and action potential states
      2. Drug effects altering phases of repolarization
      3. Drug effects on cell membrane during diastole
      4. Drug effects on cell membrane during systole
   b. Effects on pH sensing
      1. Drugs effects altering acid-base balance
      2. Drugs effects indirectly altering acid-base balance
      3. Electrolytes
      4. Glucose – (hyperglycemia-ketoacidosis)
   c. Effects of Pre-ejection Interval
      1. Chronotropic effects
      2. Sympathetic β-blockade
      3. Sympathomimetic effects
   d. Effects on stroke volume
      1. Chronotropic effect
      2. Sympathetic blockade
      3. Drug alteration of preload and afterload
         a) Diuretics
         b) β-blockers
         c) Antihypertensives
      4. Cardiotonic effect – increase strength of contractility or decrease it (negative inotropy)
      5. Sympathomimetic effects
      6. Calcium antagonists

E. Classification of Antiarrhythmic Agents and Mechanisms of Action with Potential Effect on Implanted Device Function
   1. Class I
      a. Class effects
         1. Sodium (fast channel) blockade
         2. Increased refractory periods
         3. Reduced maximum rate of depolarization
   2. Class IA
      a. Description – moderate depression of depolarization rate
      b. Examples
         1. Quinidine (increases capture threshold)

2. Procainamide (increases capture threshold). Toxicity may cause capture and sensing failure
3. Disopyramide (little effect on capture threshold). May increase threshold when taken with other antiarrhythmic drugs
4. Imipramine (increases capture threshold)

3. Class IB
    a. Description – little effect on rate of depolarization
    b. Examples
        1. Lidocaine (no effect on thresholds)
        2. Tocainide (does not affect thresholds)
        3. Phenytoin (slightly reduces pacing thresholds)
        4. Mexiletine (increases capture threshold)

4. Class IC
    a. Description – depresses depolarization with little effect on repolarization
    b. Examples
        1. Flecainide (increases capture thresholds)
        2. Encainide (strongly increases capture threshold)
        3. Propafenone (prolongs AH, HV intervals, no effect on thresholds)

5. Class II
    a. Class effects
        1. β-blockade
        2. Decrease sympathetic stimulation
        3. Increases refractory period lengths
        4. May increase capture and sensing thresholds
    b. Examples
        1. Propranolol
        2. Acebutolol
        3. Practolol
        4. Nadolol
        5. Pindolol
        6. Atenolol
        7. Alprenolol
        8. Oxyprenolol
        9. Metoprolol

6. Class III
    a. Class effects
        1. Uniformly lengthens refractory period (lengthens repolarization without altering depolarization)
        2. Selectively prolongs action potential by delaying repolarization

  b. Examples
   1. Amiodarone (increases capture threshold)
   2. Bretylium (increases capture threshold)
   3. Sotalol (increases capture threshold)
 7. Class IV
  a. Class effects
   1. Calcium channel blockade (selectively depresses SA and AV nodes)
   2. Increases SA and AV conduction time
  b. Examples
   1. Verapamil (slightly increase in threshold). Synergy to digoxin may cause elevated digoxin levels
   2. Diltiazem (as above)
   3. Nifedipine (no effect on threshold)
 8. Non-classified drugs used as antiarrhythmic
  a. Digoxin (no significant effect on thresholds). Toxicity may cause tachyarrhythmias affecting pulse generator or antitachycardia pacemaker performance
   1. Cardiotonic (increase contractility, increase cardiac output)
   2. Negative chronotropic (affects SA impulse formation and conduction)
   3. Interacts more clinically with quinidine and amiodarone
  b. Atropine (no significant effect on pacing thresholds)
   1. Vagal blockade

F. Non-Antiarrhythmic Drugs that Affect Threshold, Sensing, and Other Device Functions
 1. Diuretics
  a. Potassium depleting: (may increase capture threshold due to diuretic induced hypokalemia)
   1. Furosemide
   2. Hydrochlorothiazide (HCTZ)
   3. Ethacrynic Acid
  b. Potassium sparing (no effect on threshold)
   1. Metolazone (Zaroxolyn) – no effect independently potentiates increased potassium depletion when used with furosemide
 2. Corticosteroids (decrease thresholds)
  a. Decadron
  b. Solu Cortef
  c. Solu Medrol
  d. Prednisone

3. Electrolytes
    a. Sodium (hypertonic (3%) IV can increase threshold 50%–60%)
    b. Potassium chloride with ringers solution can briefly reduce capture threshold up to 20%–40%). When given with insulin can increase threshold by 17–30%
    c. Calcium (as gluconate) (can cause slight decrease in capture thresholds)
4. Insulin (see interaction with potassium. Can relieve acid base and chemical imbalance causing increased thresholds in ketoacidosis or hyperglycemia)
5. Sympathomimetics
    a. Isoproterenol (may cause immediate increase in capture threshold followed by a decrease in threshold)
    b. Epinephrine (decrease capture threshold)
    c. Ephedrine (decrease capture threshold)
    d. Metaproterenol (decrease capture threshold)
6. Glucose (increases capture threshold, ie diabetic crisis, hyperglycemia)
7. Phenothiazine based tranquilizers (major tranquilizers, antipsychotic agents) – largely unknown, may increase capture thresholds.
    a. Thioridazine HCL (mellaril)

G. Device interactions
    1. Surgical electrocautery
        a. Possible effects
            1. Reprogramming
            2. Noise reversion
            3. Component damage
            4. Transient/permanent malfunction
            5. Myocardial damage
        b. Precautions
            1. Distance from site
            2. Ground placement – minimize current path through the body
            3. Monitoring
            4. Energy settings – as low as possible
            5. Bipolar cautery if available
            6. Pacing system evaluation – following the procedure
    2. Countershock/defibrillation/cardioversion
        a. Possible effects
            1. Reprogramming
            2. Noise reversion

      3. Component damage
      4. Transient/permanent malfunction
      5. Myocardial damage
      6. Transient loss of capture
   b. Precautions
      1. Distance
      2. Paddle placement
      3. Energy settings
      4. Pacing system evaluation
3. Magnetic resonance imaging
   a. Possible effects
      1. Transient/permanent malfunction
      2. Runaway pacing
      3. Noise reversion
   b. Precautions
      1. Avoid procedure
      2. Emergency equipment
   c. Absolute contraindication for pacemaker patients
4. Radiofrequency ablation – studies underway
5. Lithotripsy
   a. Possible effects
      1. Transient malfunction
      2. Activity sensor malfunction/damage
   b. Precautions
      1. Distance of beam from pacemaker, 8–10 cm
      2. Reprogram device to asynchronous
      3. Pacing system evaluation
6. Radiation therapy (therapeutic not diagnositic radiation)
   a. Possible effects – therapeutic
      1. Reprogramming
      2. Component damage
      3. Transient/permanent malfunction
      4. Cumulative damage
   b. Precautions
      1. Distance
      2. Shielding
      3. Relocation of device
7. Arc welders
   a. Possible effects

        1. Transient/permanent malfunction

        2. Noise reversion

    b. Precautions

        1. Avoid

        2. Distance

        3. Equipment maintenance

        4. Pacing system evaluation

8. Diathermy

    a. Possible effects

        1. Transient/permanent malfunction

        2. Component damage

    b. Precautions

        1. Distance

        2. Monitoring

        3. Pacing system evaluation

9. Transcutaneous electrical nerve stimulation units

    a. Possible effects

        1. Likely with unipolar systems

            a) Transient malfunction

            b) Inhibition/triggering

        2. Precautions

            a) Distance

            b) Pacing system evaluation

    b. Effects on bipolar systems less likely

10. Electroconvulsive therapy

    a. Effects likely

    b. Precautions

        1. Monitoring

        2. Emergency equipment

11. Internal combustion engines

    a. Possible effects

        1. Transient malfunction

    b. Precautions

        1. Distance

        2. Do not lean directly over running engines

12. Airport metal detectors

    a. Possible effects

        1. Transient malfunction

    b. Precautions

        1. Caution with walk-through detectors

      2. Distance with use of hand-held detectors that generate strong magnetic fields

13. Ham radio

    a. Possible effects

      1. Transient malfunction

      2. Noise reversion

      3. Reprogramming

    b. Precautions

      1. Distance

      2. Power settings

14. Unlikely sources

    a. Household appliances

    b. Microwave ovens

    c. Small shop tools

    d. Dental equipment

    e. Television/radio receivers

    f. Passenger automobile ignition systems

15. Pacemaker/ICD

    a. Sensing pacemaker pulses

    b. Undersensing ventricular arrhythmias

    c. Pacing/sensing or capture alterations post defibrillation

    d. Pacemaker magnet operation (dual chamber) trigger defibrillator firing

    e. Reprogramming with defibrillation discharge

H. Electromagnetic Interference

    1. Pacemaker responses to EMI

      a. None

      b. Inhibition

      c. Triggered

      d. Asynchronous

      e. Non-function

      f. Reprogramming

      g. Back-up pacing mode

    2. Management of EMI

      a. Awareness/recognition

        1. Baseline artifact on ECG

        2. Inappropriate pauses on the ECG – not a multiple of the basic rate

3. Inappropriate rate increases – ex: > preset rate, > MTL, at rate protection limit, rates not available in the pacemaker
4. Intermittent abnormal pacing and sensing operations of the pacemaker
5. Identification on the ECG of back-up pacing modes
6. Tingling sensation on the skin
7. Synocpal episodes
8. Event analysis

b. Technology
  1. Programmability
     a) Mode
     b) Configuration
     c) Sensitivity
     d) Responsiveness
     e) Rate
     f) Magnet mode
  2. Shielding
  3. Electrical filtration systems
  4. FDA compatibility standards for medical devices -MDS 201–0004

References

Bartecchi D. Temporary Cardiac Pacing. Chicago: Precept Press. 1987.

Dohrmann ML, Goldschlager N. metabolic and pharmacologic effects on myocardial stimulation threshold in patients with cardiac pacemakers. In: Modern Cardiac Pacing. SS Barold, (Ed.). Mt Kisco: Futura Publishing Co, Inc., 1985.

Dyriakos L, Paul VE, Demosthenes K, et al. Influence of propranolol on the ventricular depolarization gradient. PACE. 14:5:I:787–791. 1991.

Ellenbogen K. Cardiac Pacing. Boston: Blackwell Scientific, 1992.

Furman S, Hayes D, Holmes D. A Practice of Cardiac Pacing. 2nd ed. Mt. Kisco: Futura Publishing Co, Inc., 1989.

Gillette P, Griffin J. Practical Cardiac Pacing. Baltimore: Williams & Wilkins. 1986.

Gottlieb CD, MD, Horowitz LN. Potential interactions between antiarrhythmic medication and the automatic implantable cardioverter defibrillator. PACE. 14:III:989–903. 1991.

Hakki A-H. Ideal Cardiac Pacing. Philadelphia: WB Saunders Co., 1984.

Henry PD. Comparative pharmacology of calcium antagonist: nifedipine, verapamil, and diltiazem. Am J Cardiol 46:1047. 1980.

Kulick D, Shahbudin HR. Techniques & Applications of Interventional Cardiology. St. Louis: Mosby Year Book, 1991.

Levine P, Mace R. Pacing Therapy: A Guide to Cardiac Pacing for Optimum Hemodynamic Benefit. Mt. Kisco: Futura Publishing Co, Inc., 1983.

Moses H, Taylor G, Schneider J, Dove J. A Practical Guide to Cardiac Pacing. Boston: Little Brown, 1987.

Preston TA, Fletcher RD, Eucchesi BR, et al. Changes in myocardial threshold: physiologic and pharmacologic factors in patients with implanted pacemakers. Am Heart J. 74:235–242. 1967.

Reiffel JA, Coromilas J, Simmermam JM, et al. Effect of antiarrhythmic drugs on defibrillation threshold: case report of an adverse effect of mexiletine and review of the literature. PACE. 11:July. 1988.

Salel AF, Seagren SC, Pool PE. Effects of encainide of the function of implanted pacemakers. PACE. September:1439–1444. 1989.

Siddoway MD, Pharmacologic profiles of antiarrhythmic agents. Choices in cardiol. 4(Suppl 1):15–18. 1990.

Singer I, Brennan F, Steinhause, et al. Effects of stress and β_1-blockade on the ventricular depolarization gradient of the rate modulating pacemaker. PACE. March:460–469. 1991.

Singer I, Guarnier T, Kupersmith J. Implanted automatic defibrillators: effects of drugs and pacemakers. PACE. 11:12:December:2250–2261. 1988.

Smith A. Amiodarone, clinical considerations. Focus Crit Care. 11.5:October: 30–37. 1974.

Smyth NPD, Millette ML. Complications of pacemaker implantation. In Modern Cardiac Pacing. SS Barold, (Ed.). Mt Kisco: Futura Publishing Co, Inc., 1985.

Stokes K. The Electrode-Biointerface: stimulation. In Modern Cardiac Pacing. SS Barold, (Ed.). Mt Kisco: Futura Publishing Co, Inc., 1985.

CHAPTER 9

Regulatory and Cost Issues

Lois Schurig
Susan L. Song

Subsections:
A. Diagnosis-Related Groupings
B. National Cardiac Pacemaker Registry
C. Electrophysiology
D. Implantable Cardioverter Defibrillators
E. United States Health Care System
F. Canadian Health Care System
G. Discharge Planning
H. Update on Regulations
I. Managed Care Highlights

Government health care insurance has been a debated subject over many decades by Presidents, Congress, and health care providers. In 1965, through the Social Security Amendments, a federally funded health care program for the elderly and the poor was established by the enactment of medicare and medicaid. The Medicare Hospital Insurance policy for reimbursement, based on the actual cost of healthcare, was fast approaching bankruptcy by the end of 1970s. In 1982, with the enactment of the Tax Equity and Fiscal Responsibility Act (TEFRA), it mandated the Secretary of the Department of Health, Education and Welfare to develop a prospective payment methodology for reimbursement and to set limits on the reasonable cost paid by Medicare. In response to this, a Prospective Payment System (PPS) was established and the basis for payment is the Diagnosis-related groupings (DRGs). This was passed by Congress and became law on April 20, 1983. All health care reimbursements are based on the PPS and DRGs for Medicare insurance.

From: Schurig L. *Educational Guidelines: Pacing and Electrophysiology*. Armonk, NY: Futura Publishing Co, Inc, © 1994.

Regulatory and cost issues are closely related to discharge planning. Therefore, in later sections of this chapter, we will cover the requirements for effective discharge planning and their relationship to reimbursement. Also, in todays (1993) health care market, trends, regulations, rules, etc., are ever changing. It is beyond the scope of this chapter to cover them all in detail. We have elected to provide a checklist of these items. Utilize additional references on them to support your practice.

Objectives

1. Identify and analyze the effects of the DRGs reimbursement on the health care industry.
2. Discuss the benefits derived from the DRGs system.
3. Define the two components of reimbursement in Medicare.
4. Discuss the benefits and the problems of the Canadian health care system.
5. Compare the differences between the United States and the Canadian health care system.
6. Define intensity and severity of service.
7. Identify significant components of a discharge plan.
8. Identify current regulations impact on reimbursement.

Glossary and Abbreviations

CPT-4: *Current Procedural Terminology, 4th Edition.* Descriptive terms and codes for medical services and procedures performed by physicians.

DRGs: Diagnosis-Related Groups. A classification of groups of patients that are clinically coherent and homogenous with respect to resources used.

DRG cost weight: The number or weight that reflects a DRGs resource utilization. This weight is multiplied by the average cost for a Medicare discharge to arrive at the payment for the particular DRG.

DRG creep: The practice of manipulating patients' medical record data to upgrade to a more profitable DRG.

FDA: Food and Drug Administration

GROUPER: Software program. Classifies each case into a DRG on the basis of diagnosis, procedure codes, age, sex, and discharge status.

HCFA: Health Care Financing Administration

HHS: Department of Health and Human Services

ICD-9-CM: *International Classification of Diseases, 9th Revision, Clinical Modification.* This is used by all hospitals to code diagnostic and surgical procedures.

MCE: Medicare code editor. Automated screens in a claim system which are designed to identify cases that require further review before classification into DRG.

MDCs: Major diagnostic categories. A set of 23 broad diagnostic classifications, mainly according to organ system. DRGs fall under the 23 MDCs.

OIG: Office of Inspector General

Outliers: Cases involving unusually long hospital stays, called day outliers, or unusually costly cases, called cost outliers, gain additional payments to hospital.

PHO: Physician Hospital Organization

PPRC: Physician Payment Review Commission

PPS: Prospective payment system. A fixed payment system per discharge for each diagnosis-related group of diseases.

PROs: Peer Review Organizations. An entity which is composed of a substantial number of licensed physicians of medicine and osteopathy engaged in the practice of medicine or surgery to assure the adequate peer review of the service provided to the various medical specialties and sub-specialties.

PRO PAC: Prospective Payment Assessment Commission. Independent advisory group that suggest changes and recommendations to the DHHS DRG payment rates, cost weights, and classification system.

RBRVS: Resource based relative value scale physician's fee schedule system based on resources needed to perform a service.

Education Content

A. Diagnosis-Related Groupings (DRGs)

    1. Development

        a. Yale University researchers in the 1970s

        b. Based on research data 1.4 million cases in New Jersey and other states.

        c. Enacted into law 1983

    2. Utilization

        a. Reimbursement

        b. Quality control

        c. Cost containment

        d. Budget planning

    3. Cases are classified into DRGs based on:

        a. Principal diagnosis and up to four additional diagnoses

        b. Up to three treatments performed

        c. Age

        d. Sex

        e. Discharge status

    4. Prospective payment system (PPS)

        a. 23 Major diagnostic categories (MDCs)

        b. 477 DRGs

        c. Relative weighing factors

        d. Mean length of stay

B. National Cardiac Pacemaker Registry for U.S. Medicare patients

    1. This was mandated by the Deficit Reduction Act of 1984.

        a. Purpose

            1. Determine appropriate payments for pacemaker procedures

            2. Surveillance of implanted devices

            3. Follow-up studies on pacemakers and leads

            4. Determine necessary inspection of pacemaker devices by manufacturers

        b. Registration forms

            1. Hospitals have 60 days to complete the registration form to claim reimbursement for implant procedures.

C. Electrophysiology Studies

    1. Used primarily to diagnose cardiac arrhythmias and to identify the appropriate therapy to be prescribed for patients.

D. Implantable Cardioverter Defibrillator

    1. Reimbursement based on:

        a. Documentation of life-threatening ventricular tachyarrhythmia episodes or cardiac arrest not associated with acute myocardial infarction.

        b. Documented by electrophysiologic studies to have an inducible tachyarrhythmia that is unresponsive to medication or surgical therapy.

E. United States Health Care System

    1. Medicare

        a. A federally funded health program enacted into law in 1965, Title XVIII of the Social Security Act.

        b. Eligibility

            1. Over 65 years old

            2. Disabled < 65 yrs of age

            3. End-stage renal disease

    2. Two components of Medicare

        a. Part A: Hospital insurance funded by:

            1. Taxes on earnings

            2. Proceeds from railroad retirement

            3. Interests on funds from U.S. Treasury

            4. Annual deductible and co-insurance

        b. Part B: Medical insurance, physicians, and other services: funded by:

            1. Small premium

            2. Annual deductible

            3. 20% reasonable charges

    2. Medicaid (National)

        a. A federally funded welfare program with matching funds from the states. Enacted into law in 1965, Title XIX of the Social Security Act.

    3. Military service

        a. Complete health care to the family

    4. Veterans Administration

    5. Employer-paid health insurance benefits

    6. Health Maintenance Organization (HMO)

    7. Private health insurance

    8. Benefits

        a. Health coverage for the elderly

        b. Health coverage for the poor

        c. Alternate system of medical care

9. Disadvantages
   a. 37 million Americans uninsured and a similar number under-insured
   b. Lack of health care protection for the unemployed
   c. Bankrupted by catastrophic illnesses
   d. Medicaid – unequal benefits in different states
   e. Federal budget deficits

F. Canadian Health Care System
   1. Provincial health insurance was established by the parliament in 1965.
      a. Principles of health insurance
         1. Provincial government pays for medical care with provincial and federal funds.
         2. Universal free coverage to all citizens, including long-term homecare and nursing home care.
         3. There are no bills and no money changes between patient and doctors who will bill provincial government.
         4. Provincial government sets budgets for each hospital and sets doctor's fees through negotiation with medical associations.
         5. Government regulates the purchase of high technology equipment as well as the number of trained specialists
         6. Patients may choose their own primary doctor but must have a referral for a specialist.
   2. Benefits
      a. Universal coverage for all citizens
      b. Equal accessibility for all medical services
      c. Cost containment: government control
   3. Disadvantages
      a. Escalating health care costs to the national and provincial government
      b. Global budget limits research and development in new technology and new disease
      c. Extended waiting period for elective procedures, surgeries, and tests
      d. Absence of alternate system of medical care

G. Discharge Planning
   1. Economic concerns
      a. Safe patient discharge
      b. Avoid complications
      c. Decrease length of stay

    d. Optimize use of resources

    e. Cost containment

2. Generic screens, HCFA

    a. Adequacy of discharge planning

    b. Medical stability of the patient

    c. Hospital deaths

    d. Nosocomial infections

    e. Unscheduled return to surgery

    f. Trauma suffered in the hospital

    g. Medications and treatment changes within 24 hours of discharge without adequate observation

3. Reimbursement issues

    a. Transfer of patients between facilities for implantation

    b. Discharge of the patient when the DRG length of service has been completed

    c. Length of service for patients requiring implanted cardiac devices

    d. Coding and billing procedures

    e. Lack of documentation

    f. Increase in the requirements for documentation

    g. Quality control

4. Reimbursement cardiology discharge screens

    a. Patient controlled for last 3 days

    b. No change type/dose of antiarrhythmic $\times$ 2 days

    c. Pain controlled $\times$ 24 hours

    d. No analgesics/narcotics $\times$ 24 hours

    e. Bleeding controlled $\times$ 24 hours

    f. No cardiac change/damage after 3 days of hospitalization

    g. No ECG changes last 3 days

    h. Abnormal physical/laboratory findings addressed and stabilized

    i. Patient and/or care giver instructed on proper administration of medications

    j. Documented by physician that maximum benefit of hospitalization achieved

    k. Patient and/or care giver able to administer medical gases

    l. Patient signs out AMA, refuses Rx or requests transfer

5. Reimbursement considerations

    a. Severity of illness

        1. Vital signs

        2. Labs/Radiology

    3. ECG

    4. Physical findings

  b. Intensity of service

    1. Monitoring

    2. Medications

    3. Treatments

    4. Procedures

6. Components of discharge plan

  a. Contact risk management to help develop policies and procedures to reduce risk

  b. "Medically ready"

  c. Plan for needs post-discharge

  d. Protect the patient from reasonably, foreseeable harm

  e. Included in review program – Quality improvement (QI)

  f. Daily screening for discharge needs

  g. Consideration for physical, emotional, and mental status

  h. Patient received discharge prescriptions

  i. Home care

    1. Education

    2. Wound care

    3. Assessment of vital functions

    4. Medications

  j. Documentation

    1. Explain plan, ensure understanding, who is present, level of understanding by patient and family, acute care needed

7. Discharge planning documentation

  a. Medical records complete and legible

  b. Past and present diagnosis (Co-morbitity)

  c. Rationale for diagnostic testing

  d. Response to treatment

  e. Non-compliance

  f. Complete signatures for each entry

  g. Intensity of patient's evaluation and treatment

    1. Include clinical pathway

    2. Include complexity of diagnosis

  h. Each admission includes

    1. Date

    2. Rationale

    3. Assessment

    4. Treatment plan

5. History and physical appropriateness for the problem
6. Discharge plan
7. Review of information during admission
   i. Risk factors
   j. Care plan
   k. Coding reflects specificity and complexity of condition, treatment plan, diagnostic plan

H. Update on Regulations (Attached references will provide necessary details)
   1. IRS and Inspector General from HHS in an enforcement partnership, dual enforcement
   2. IRS General Counsel Memorandum – 39862, December 91, Cost shifting
   3. Antitrust laws
   4. Medicare Antifraud and Abuse Law
   5. Joint Ventures
   6. Safe Harbors, July 29, 1991
   7. Medicare Patient and Protection Act, 1987
   8. Safe Medical Device Act of 1990 (HR 3095), effective November 29, 1991 (Refer to Part One, Chapter 10, Medical Jurisprudence)
   9. Terms to be familiar with:
      a. Capitation
      b. Managed care (competition)
      c. Common files
      d. Shared risk

I. Managed Care Highlights
   1. HCFA Pilot Project
      a. Packaged pricing for bypass surgery – DRG 106 and 107
      b. Negotiated fees at a reduced rate
      c. Bundled price – surgeon, anesthetists, cardiologist, other physicians and facility costs
   2. Single priced contracts and capitation arrangements are more favorable
   3. Complete cost analysis on your services
   4. Risks involved with various types of contracts
      a. Price
      b. Intensity
      c. Severity
      d. Frequency
   5. Use your computerized data bases to monitor the following indicators:

a. Contribution margin
b. Ancillary services per day
c. Case mix by volume and type
d. Mix of days
e. Length of stay
f. Admission and discharge rates
g. Out of hospital claims cost

References

Binns GS. The relationship among quality, cost, and market share in hospitals. Topics Health Care Finance 18:2: Winter:21–32. 1991.

Blomquist B. Medicare Health Policy Update. Medtronic News, P. Winter: 13–15. 1988.

Boughton-Barnes G. Cardiovascular coding: It's not just a job. Practice Strategies. Fall 92/Winter 93.

Burda D. Insurance & Liability: effective planning can defuse discharge risks. Hospitals. February:39–40. 1987.

Coile R. Forecast of cardiac care "megatrends" for the 1990s. J Cardiovasc Manage. November/December:25–30. 1990.

Federal Register, Part II, Department of Health and Human Services. 55:90: May:1990.

Iglehart JK. Canada's health care system. N Engl J Med. 315:3:202–208. 1986.

Imperiale TF, Siegal AP, Crede WB, Kames EA. Preadmission screening of medicare patients. JAMA. 259:23:3418–3421. 1988.

Inglehart JK. Canada's health care system faces its problems. N Engl J Med. 322:8:562–568. 1990.

KPMG, Peat Marwick. Summary and analysis of the final Medicare and Medicaid "Safe Harbor" Regulations. Dimens Health Care. 92–1:January:1992.

M.R.L. HHS issues patient-transfer regulations. Hospitals. July:22–23. 1988.

Michigan Peer Review Organization. MPR/213Z. HCFA generic quality screens. Exhibit IX. 1–2 and MPR/215Z. Severity of illness/intensity of service criteria. Exhibit X. 1–4. Revised 4/19/89.

Reepmeyer TH. Market forces can boost quality, lower costs. Healthcare Financ Manage. December:1991.

Shaffer FA. DRGs: Changes and Challenges. National League Nurs. 1984.

Sorian R. The Bitter Pills: Tough Choices in American Health Policy. New York: McGraw-Hill Book Co., 1988.

Veltri EP, Mower MM, Mirowski M. Ambulatory monitoring of the automatic implantable cardioverter–defibrillator: a practical guide. PACE. 11: 315–325. 1988.

CHAPTER 10

Medical Jurisprudence

Mary Neubauer

Subsections:

A. Informed Consent
B. Legal Aspects
C. Policy and Procedures
D. Medical Device Safety Act

Basically, the principles of legal and ethical issues in cardiac procedures are not any different from any other medical procedures.

These are issues which apply across the board for all patients, physicians, and health care workers in any health care delivery setting. These matters emerge from dealing with a litigious society, which requires each of us to stand back and take a look at ourselves and how we are accomplishing our work in the profession of delivering the best care possible to the patient. This, in itself, does not portend to be a bad situation, either for ourselves or for the patient. The care we render must not be overshadowed by the fear of legal issues, but should be done in an atmosphere where the rights of the patients come first, followed by the health care workers also protecting their rights by virtue of education to the facts. Compared to the number of patients you will see in your career, the number of lawsuits is minimal. However, it is best to develop good interpersonal relationships with the patients and document the care in a concise, objective manner in which we can defend ourselves, should an untoward event occur.

As part of the legal and ethical education, such issues as advanced directives, consents, malpractice insurance, legal rights of the patient and health care worker, and documentation will be discussed. This will provide the health care workers the knowledge to be able to protect themselves in the

---

From: Schurig L. *Educational Guidelines: Pacing and Electrophysiology*. Armonk, NY: Futura Publishing Co, Inc, © 1994.

event of a problem. It will also enable individuals to conduct themselves in a more professional manner.

Objectives

1. Distinguish the difference between the roles of the physician and the health care worker in informed consent.
2. Identify the rules of negligence.
3. Describe the various types of potential liability.
4. Define the types of professional liability insurance.
5. Illustrate an example of a well-documented record.
6. Demonstrate an example of an advanced directive.
7. Relate several incidents which require occurrence reporting.
8. Discuss the need for policy and procedure.
9. Explain how standards of care are established.

Glossary and Abbreviations

Informed consent: Consent given only after full notice is given as to that which is being consented to; patient must be apprised of the nature and risks of a medical procedure before the physician can claim exemption from liability for battery. Also provides information on options available to the patient.

Malpractice: Any professional misconduct or unreasonable lack of skill in performing professional duties.

Negligence: Failure to exercise that degree of care which a person of ordinary prudence (a reasonable person) would exercise under the same circumstances.

Proximate cause: That which in natural and continuous sequence unbroken by any new independent cause, produces an event, without which the injury would not have occurred.

Standard of care: Rule or procedure adopted by a professional group which outlines a measure of value and quality.

Education Content

A. Informed Consent
  1. Role of physician
     a. Appropriate patient
     b. Complications of procedure
     c. Risks of non-treatment
     d. Risks of procedure
     e. Choice of appropriate pacemaker
  2. Role of cardiac health care worker
     a. Education of patient
     b. Consent form signature
     c. Assist at procedure
     d. Documentation
  3. Requirements of an informed consent
     a. Nature, duration, and purpose of project or procedure
     b. Risks, inconveniences, and hazards
     c. Methods and means
     d. Effects on health of person or subject
     e. Explanation of benefits
     f. Treatment options
     g. Right to privacy
     h. Confidentiality statement
     i. FDA inspection of records of research
     j. Compensation for injury
     k. Contact with the primary investigator if research
     l. Voluntary participation if research
     m. Termination criteria if research
     n. Costs as a result of the project
     o. Number of subjects in the project
     p. New findings which may affect the subjects are revealed

B. Legal Aspects
  1. Rules of negligence
     a. Duty or professional standard of care
     b. Deviation or breach of duty
     c. Causing or proximate cause of injury
     d. Injury or measurable physical or mental harm.
  2. Professional versus ordinary standard of care

    a. Professional held to a higher standard

    b. Circumstances require professional's higher education, training, and experience

    c. Cardiac health care workers trained in superior methods for cardiac procedures

    d. This is a standard on which one will be judged in event of a law suit

3. Complexity of issues in medical professional liability

    a. Informed consent

    b. Privacy of patient

    c. Right to refuse treatment

    d. Right to privacy of medical record

    e. Maintaining accurate and complete records

4. Various types of liability

    a. Negligent provision of care

    b. Negligent application of treatments

    c. Negligent maintenance of records

    d. Violation of rights to privacy

    e. Informed consent – though physician's responsibility, action must be taken for patient's request for information

    f. Failure to follow-up in event of error

5. Insurance requirements

    a. Professional liability market

    b. Requirements for personal insurance

        1. Does organization provide insurance

        2. The independent practitioner

    c. Types of insurance

        1. Occurrence

        2. Claims-made

6. Documentation

    a. Plan of care

    b. Clear, concise and objective

    c. Vital signs as per procedure

    d. Treatment rendered and patient's responses

    e. Education and reflection of patient's knowledge

    f. Medication and patient's response, when appropriate

    g. Assessment of the patient, prior to, during and post-procedure

    h. Discharge instructions and patient/family response

    i. Discharge note – condition of the patient and in whose company

    j. Use approved abbreviations

7. Incident/occurrence reporting
   a. Document any untoward/unexpected event that occurs
   b. Concise, objective-not subjective
   c. Immediate documentation required, while events are still fresh in memory
   d. Administrative tool used to investigate and provide a defense for health care worker and institution
   e. Never used as punitive, but as a protective measure
   f. Use to document potential areas of injury
   g. Use in equipment failure, malfunction
8. Advanced directives
   a. Education to the OBRA, 1990 bill
   b. Living wills as per state law
   c. Medical durable power of attorney

C. Policy and Procedures
   1. Policy and procedure overview
      a. All procedures should have written policy and details of procedure
      b. The health care worker should have knowledge of same
      c. Standard on which one will be judged
      d. Document according to procedure
      e. Treatment should be rendered as per policy
      f. Reviewed and revised, as necessary, on annual basis
      g. Old procedures should be retained. 1989 cases are judged on 1989 procedures.
   2. Guidelines for writing protocols
      a. Violation of a state or government regulation equals negligence
      b. Violation of industry or accreditation requirement equals negligence
      c. Violation of a hospital's policy can be viewed as negligence
      d. Inadequate policy or failure to have a policy may be evidence of negligence
      e. Do not use the word "standard" in hospital policies
      f. Conform to state and federal laws and other external requirements
      g. Be realistic with the desired goal for the policy
      h. Do not use superlatives or make promises
      i. Do not be too specific, allow room for judgment
      j. Be consistent and understandable
      k. Explain the rationale for and limitations of prescribed conduct
      l. Enforce established policies

D. Medical Device Safety Act

   1. Safe Medical Devices Act of 1990 (HR 3095), effective November 28, 1991

   2. Major provisions

      a. Records and reports. Hospitals and other health care facilities must report deaths and serious injuries and distributors are now subject to reporting requirements. Reports are sent to the Department of Health and Human Services.

      b. Civil penalties. FDA could levy up to $15,000 per violation and up to a total of $1 million for all violations adjudicated at a single proceeding.

      c. Recalls. Manufacturers would have to report recalls where a potential for serious, adverse health consequence or death was involved.

      d. Suspension of PMAs. FDA, after an informal hearing, would be permitted to suspend the approval of a premarket approval application (PMA).

      e. Use of PMA data to support other sponsor's PMAs. One year after the fourth approval of a device having the same principles of operation and the same uses as the device initially approved, FDA could use the safety and efficacy data in the approved PMAs to support other pre-market approval applications.

      f. Imposition of post-market surveillance requirements.

      g. Simplification of standards-setting procedures and the addition of alternative controls to standards.

      h. Codification of FDA present criteria for evaluating 510(k)s and requirements for manufacturers to search for adverse safety and effectiveness information for some "predicate" devices listed in Section 510(k) notifications.

      i. Requirements for FDA to regulate device-drug combinations in one center.

      j. Requirements for FDA to review and perhaps reclassify pre 1976 class III devices and transitional devices.

      k. An Office of International Relations would be created and humanitarian devices would have an easier time getting to market.

      l. Hospitals are now required to report whenever "medical personnel become aware of information that reasonably suggests that there is a probability that a device caused or contributed to the death or serious illness of, or serious injury to, a patient of the facility."

      m. Reports are submitted within 10 days.

      n. Hospitals are required to submit semiannual reports summarizing all medical device incidents.

      o. Device tracking requirements exist for "permanently implantable devices, or life-sustaining or life-supporting devices used outside of the user facility."

p. The tracking system will "ensure that patients who receive devices can be provided the notification required."

References

Avery JK. Prevention case of the month: Not my responsibility. J Tenn Med Assoc. August:523. 1988.

Congress Fraud, waste and abuse in the medicare pacemaker industry. Caring. February:1987.

Curran J, William D, Nader R. The consumer and the hospitals. N Engl J Med. May:1017–1018. 1971.

ECRI. Advisory bulletin: new law requires hospital device reporting. November:1990.

Feinstein RJ. The cardiac pacemaker scandal. Miami Med. November:73–75. 1982.

Feutz Shirley. Nursing and the Law. 4th edition. Professional Education Systems, Inc., 1991.

Gifis S. Law Dictionary. Barron's Educational Series, Inc. 1975.

Greatbatch, W. Pacemaker patients: use and misuse, PACE. January:115–116. 1989.

Heller MB. Of pacing, patents and patients. Am J Emerg Med. January:78–79. 1988.

Knight K. Device incident reporting. AAMI. November/December:34–37. 1990.

McCurdy, Melfi, Perkun, Reiter, Perin, Parsons. Critical Legal and Ethical Issues for Nurses. Professional Educational Systems, Inc., 1988.

Sagal M, Elliot D. Legal aspects of cardiac pacemakers. Med Times. October:44–69. 1977.

Sanbar SS. Implantable cardiovascular devices; medico-legal aspects. Legal Med. 56–94. 1986.

Wagner M. Experts see dangers in rules implementing safe medical device act. Mod Healthcare. February:36–39. 1992.

CHAPTER 11

Cardiac Life Support

Susan L. Song

Subsections:
A. Basic Cardiac Life Support
B. Advanced Cardiac Life Support
C. Advanced Defibrillation and Cardioversion
D. Rescue Pacing

Cardiac life support was first introduced with techniques in external chest compression over 30 years ago. In 1966, a National Academy of Sciences—National Research Council (NAS-NRC) Conference on Cardiopulmonary Resuscitation (CPR) recommended the training of the medical and allied health personnel according to the standards of the American Heart Association (AHA). Since then, there have been four more national conferences on CPR and Emergency Cardiac Care (ECC). The AHA has been responsible for establishing standards, policies, procedures and training programs for certifications in both basic life support (BLS) and advanced cardiac life support (ACLS) in life support units, hospitals, and communities throughout the United States. Based on statistics for the pre-hospital cardiac arrest victims, it has been estimated that CPR followed by ACLS may save between 100,000 to 200,000 lives each year in the United States.

Objectives

1. Discuss the major objective for performing CPR.
2. Identify two key factors for successful CPR.

From: Schurig L. *Educational Guidelines: Pacing and Electrophysiology.* Armonk, NY: Futura Publishing Co, Inc, © 1994.

3. Define standards for CPR.
4. Define Certification in BLS and ACLS.
5. Application of the ABCs and CPR.
6. Discuss how modifications in major risk factors can reduce mortality in cardiovascular disease.
7. Discuss the post-management of pacemaker system after defibrillation.
8. List four major reasons for drug therapy in ACLS.

Glossary and Abbreviations

Advanced cardiac life support (ACLS): 1) consist of BLS; 2) adjunctive equipment to maintain effective ventilation and circulation; 3) electrocardiographic monitoring; 4) IV access and drug and electrical therapies; 5) treatment for myocardial infarction.

Basic life support (BLS): Externally supports the circulation and ventilation of a victim of cardiac or respiratory arrest through CPR.

Cardiac pacemaker: Cardiac stimulating system which consists of a pulse generator (power source battery and electronic circuit) a lead and electrode.

Cardiopulmonary resuscitation (CPR): Technique of resuscitation to restore oxygen to the brain by artificial respiration and restoring heart beat by external chest cardiac massage.

Certification in BLS or ACLS: Successful completion according to cognitive and performance testing of BLS or ACLS.

External cardioverter/defibrillator: An apparatus used to counteract ventricular fibrillation by application of electric impulses to the heart.

Implantable cardioverter/defibrillator: Consists of a sensing device, batteries, and energy storage capacitor. The device will sense arrhythmias on the basis of algorithms in heart rate and will discharge.

Standards: Standards for CPR and emergency cardiac care which identify a body of knowledge and skills recommended for successful CPR.

Education Content

A. Basic Life Support (BLS)

    1. CPR is an emergency technique that combines artificial circulation and artificial respiration to maintain life in cases of cardiac arrest until ACLS is available. The three basic principles of CPR are:

    2. Airway

        a. Establish breathlessness

        b. Call for help

        c. Position the victim

        d. Open the airway

    3. Breathing

        a. Establish breathlessness

        b. Rescue breathing

    4. Circulation

        a. Establish pulselessness

        b. External chest compressions

    5. Techniques: One rescuer

    6. Techniques: Two rescuer

    7. Modify techniques for infant and small children

    8. Management of obstructed airway

        a. Causes

        b. Assessment

        c. Heimlich maneuver

            1. Conscious victim

            2. Unconscious victim

            3. Self-administered

B. Advanced Cardiac Life Support (ACLS)

    1. Basic life support

    2. Adjunctive equipment to support ventilation: Correction of hypoxemia

        a. Supplemental oxygen 100%

        b. Masks

        c. Oxygen-powered mechanical breathing device

        d. Oropharyngeal and nasopharyngeal airways

        e. Esophageal obturator airway and esophageal gastric tube airway

        f. Endotracheal intubation

        g. Transtracheal catheter ventilation and cricothyrotomy

        h. Suction devices

    3. Establish intravenous fluid line

4. Drug administration

    a. IV fluid: expansion of blood volume

    b. Analgesic: morphine sulfate – drug of choice for acute myocardial infarction (MI). Also to treat acute pulmonary edema

    c. Control of heart rhythm and rate

        1. Lidocaine – acute control of ventricular ectopic, ventricular tachycardia (VT), and ventricular fibrillation (VF)

        2. Procainamide – suppress ventricular ectopics and ventricular tachycardia and is recommended when lidocaine is contraindicated or has failed to suppress ventricular ectopy.

        3. Bretylium tosylate – to treat resistant VT and VF unresponsive to defibrillation, epinephrine, and lidocaine.

        4. Atenolol, metaprolol, and propranolol – reduces the incidence of VF in post-MI patients who did not receive thrombolytic agents.

        5. Atropine sulfate – reverses cholinergic mediated decreases in heart rate, systemic vascular resistance, and blood pressure. Treat symptomatic sinus bradycardia, AV block at the nodal level or ventricular asystole.

        6. Isoproterenol hydrochloride – increases cardiac output and myocardial contractility

        7. Verapamil and Diltiazem – calcium channel blocking agents that slow conduction and increase refractoriness in the AV node. May terminate reentrant arrhythmias, control ventricular response rate in atrial fibrillation, flutter, or multifocal atrial tachycardia.

        8. Adenosine – terminates arrhythmias in AV node and sinus node. (Atrial fibrillation, flutter, atrial or ventricular tachycardia)

        9. Magnesium – low magnesium is associated with cardiac arrhythmias, insufficiency, and sudden death. It can precipitate refractory VF and hinder replacement of intracellular potassium.

    d. Improve cardiac output and blood pressure

        1. Epinephrine hydrochloride – increase myocardial and central nervous system blood flow

        2. Norepinephrine – vasoconstrictor

        3. Dopamine hydrochloride – dilates renal and mesenteric blood vessels. Increases cardiac output

        4. Dobutamine hydrochloride – increases myocardial contractility

        5. Amrinone – increases cardiac function and induces vasodilation

        6. Calcium chloride – increases ventricular function

        7. Digitalis preparations – decreases ventricular rate in atrial fibrillation, flutter, PSVT

8. Nitroglycerin – effective in relieving angina
9. Sodium nitroprusside – peripheral vasodilator, treat hypertension and heart failure
10. Sodium bicarbonate – control of acid-base balance
11. Diuretics – furosimide, treats acute pulmonary edema and cerebral edema after cardiac arrest
12. Thrombolytic agents – digest fibrin and dissolve clots (timing critical for effectiveness)

5. Cardiac monitoring
6. Defibrillation – early and rapid defibrillation is a major determinant of survival in cardiac arrest
   a. Energy requirements
   b. Paddle position
7. Control of cardiac arrhythmia
8. Post-resuscitation care
9. Supervision by a physician

C. Advance Defibrillation and Cardioversion
  1. Defibrillation technique with implanted devices
     a. Pacemaker system
        1. Recommendations for defibrillation – cardioversion
           a) Keep paddles as far from pulse generator as possible
           b) Use anterior-posterior paddle position
           c) Titrate energy levels
        2. Adverse effects of defibrillation
           a) Irreversible damage to the pulse generator
           b) Reprogramming
           c) Acute and chronic rise in threshold
           d) Transient undersensing
        3. Management of post-defibrillation
           a) Temporary pacing
           b) Evaluation of pacing system
           c) Surgical replacement of system, if needed
     b. Implantable cardioverter/defibrillator (ICD)
        1. Patient education
           a) Carry I.D. card – wear Medi-Alert band
           b) Arrhythmia monitoring
           c) ICD will detect and shock ventricular arrhythmias
        2. External defibrillation
           a) There has been no reports of damage to the ICD

D. Rescue Pacing
   1. Bradycardias
      a. Temporary VVI pacing system
   2. Tachycardias
      a. Antitachycardiac pacing system
   3. Transcutaneous
      a. Please refer to Part Two, Chapter 15, Emergency and Temporary Pacing

References

Annals of emergency medicine. JACEPSAEM. 22:2:2. February. 1993.

Currents in emergency cardiac care. Newsletter of AHA. 3:4:Winter. 1992.

Cannom D, Winkle R. Implantation of the automatic implantable cardioverter defibrillator (AICD): practical aspects. PACE. 9:793–809. 1986.

Grauer K, Cavallaro D. ACLS: Certification, Preparation and a Comprehensive Review. 2nd ed. St.Louis: CV Mosby Book, 1987.

Guidelines for cardiopulmonary resuscitation (CPR) and emergency cardiac care (ECC). JAMA. 268:16:2171–2302. 1992.

Parmely WW, Chatterjee K. Cardiology, Vol I. Philadelphia: Lippencott. 1988.

Willens J. Strengthen your life-support skills. Nursing. 93:23:4:54–58. 1993.

CHAPTER 12

Other Topics

Rosemary S. Bubien
Jo Ellen Thomson

Subsection:
A. Altered Anatomy and Physiology
B. Altered Electrocardiography
C. Arrhythmias Post-Transplantation
D. Contributing Factors to Arrhythmia Development
E. Pharmacology/Electropharmacology
F. Role of Electrophysiology Testing
G. Pacemaker Therapy

The initial clinical experience with transplantation of a human heart occurred in 1967. It has now evolved to an accepted intervention for patients with end-stage cardiac disease. However, transplantation does not eliminate the patient from the population experiencing arrhythmias.

This chapter provides a synopsis of facts relevant to the care of the orthotopic cardiac transplant patient regarding arrhythmias and their treatment.

Objectives

1. Briefly describe the altered anatomy and electrophysiology of the transplanted heart and its implications on the donor sinus node, atrium, and AV node.

From: Schurig L. *Educational Guidelines: Pacing and Electrophysiology.* Armonk, NY: Futura Publishing Co, Inc, © 1994.

2. Discuss the current role of EP in research involving risk stratification and prevention of sudden death in patients awaiting transplant.
3. Discuss the phenomenon of pseudo AV block in orthotopic cardiac transplants recipients.
4. List three contributing factors to atrial and ventricular arrhythmias post-cardiac transplant.
5. Describe the effect of β-adrenergic receptor active drugs, digoxin, and quinidine on the transplanted heart.
6. Discuss the prevalence of permanent cardiac pacing and pacing indications post-cardiac transplant.
7. Describe three methods of providing rate response and AV synchrony in the post-cardiac transplant patient population.

Education Content

A. Altered Anatomy and Physiology

1. Surgical anastomoses create electrical isolation of the native right and left atria from the donor right and left atria.
2. Donor sinus node is transplanted with the donor heart.
3. Donor heart is decentralized (lacks autonomic neural control)
   a. Sympathetic nervous system – The post-ganglionic nerves are severed, thus sympathetic denervation.
   b. Parasympathetic nervous system – The preganglionic neurons are severed, but post-ganglionic neurons are intact.
   c. Increased resting heart rate due to loss of vagal inhibition.
   d. Donor heart rate at rest exceeds native sinus rate.
   e. Circulating catecholamines primarily control heart rate
   f. Heart rate response to exercise may be delayed in both onset and offset
   g. Subsidiary pacemakers in the donor heart may not provide a reliable escape mechanism due to loss of autonomic input.

B. Altered Electrocardiography

1. Native sinus node generates sinus P wave (the atrial cuff supports atrial flutter/fibrillation) which cannot conduct to the donor heart.
   a. Activates atrial remnants
   b. P waves usually have a small amplitude
2. Donor sinus node generates P wave
   a. Conducts through donor atria to the AV junction
   b. P waves generally of larger amplitude and have a typical morphology
3. Decrease in ECG voltage/amplitude does not usually signal rejection

C. Arrhythmias Post-Transplantation

1. Pseudo AV block (due to atrial dissociation between native P wave and donor QRS)
2. Sinus node dysfunction
   a. Usually temporary, reported in 27% of recipients; pacemaker required in approximately 7% of recipients
   b. May sometimes be treated with theophylline
3. Mobitz I AV block
4. Infra-Hisian conduction defects are rare
5. Atrial (55%) and ventricular (79%) arrhythmias incidence
6. Sudden death – usually due to asystole rather than VT/VF

D. Contributing Factors to Arrhythmia Development
  1. Low ejection fraction
  2. Increased pulmonary wedge pressure
  3. Prolonged donor ischemic time–bradyarrhythmias
  4. Pre-operative amiodarone (relative contraindication to transplant at some centers)
  5. Rejection (conflicting data regarding relationship of arrhythmias to rejection – early pre-cyclosporin from Berke & Schroeder; Yes recent data post-cyclosporin from Little; No)

E. Pharmacology/Electropharmacology and Electrical Therapy Post-Cardiac Transplant
  1. Quinidine
     a. Lengthens AH interval in transplanted hearts (opposite to that of innervated hearts)
     b. Other effects such as HV and QT prolongation are same in transplanted and innervated hearts.
  2. β-adrenergic receptor active drugs (norepinephrine, isoproterenol, and propranolol)
     a. Autonomic denervation does not impair β-receptor function; therefore, effects of these drugs on the transplanted heart are similar to those on the innervated heart
     b. Isoproterenol can be used in lieu of atropine to increase heart rate if needed.
  3. Calcium channel blockers – diltiazem and verapamil
     a. Increase the circulating cyclosporin concentration
     b. Does not appear dose-related
     c. In most reported cases, administration did not result in any clinically significant renal impairment, and may be protective to the kidney
  4. Atropine – donor sinus node does not respond
  5. Digoxin
     a. Action is both direct and mediated by the antonomic nervous system
     b. Acute effects are mediated by vagotonic influences; therefore, there is no acute effect on the donor sinus node and AV node. For example, there is no response to intravenous administration
     c. May observe effect with chronic administration because of direct action
  6. Adenosine
     a. Donor sinus node and AV node are significantly more sensitive than native sinus node
     b. Duration of effect on AV node slowing is significantly longer

7. Pacing for atrial flutter (more common), atrial tachycardia, if early post-transplant via epicardial pacing electrodes to donor cuff

F. Role of Electrophysiology Testing
   1. Pre-cardiac transplant
      a. High incidence of sudden death (± 25%) in patients awaiting donor organs
      b. Risk stratification for sudden cardiac death
         1. SAECG
         2. Programmed ventricular stimulation
      c. Clinical trials in progress regarding the role of amiodarone/defibrillator for patients who have not experienced sudden cardiac death
   2. Post-cardiac transplant
      a. Currently, no EP indicators of acute rejection
      b. Endomyocardial biopsy most dependable
      c. Investigational electrophysiologic predictors of rejection
         1. SAECG
         2. Intramyocardial recording
         3. Intra-atrial/AV conduction times

G. Pacemaker Therapy
   1. Indications
      a. Sinus node dysfunction most common
      b. Mobitz II AV block rare
      c. Permanent pacing is not usually necessary
   2. Pacing modes
      a. Mode selection based on clinical indication
      b. Maintenance of AV synchrony and rate response desirable
      c. Flexibility of the pacing system is desirable because of the prevalence of atrial arrhythmias
   3. Implantation techniques
      a. Typically identical to non-transplant patients
         1. Right internal jugular vein is best preserved for biopsy
         2. Leads are positioned in donor atrium and ventricle
         3. Atrial lead positioned to avoid native P wave sensing
      b. Alternative approaches
         1. Atrial triggered – AAT (case study report)
            a) Bipolar single chamber pulse generator
            b) Unipolar atrial lead in recipient atria
            c) Unipolar atrial lead in donor atrial

      d) Triggered mode senses native sinus node and paces donor atria at appropriate physiologic rate

      e) Prevalence of atrial arrhythmias may be problematic

   2. Dual chamber implanted in atrium

      a) 2 atrial leads implanted

      b) Programmed VDD

      c) Provides native P wave synchronized pacing of donor heart maintaining AV synchrony and rate response

      d) Prevalence of atrial arrhythmias may be problematic

4. Follow-up

   a. Frequent right heart catheterizations and biopsies may be hazardous to tranvenous leads

   b. Follow-up must be adjusted accordingly.

   c. Pacemakers may provide an alternate, non-invasive methodology for monitoring the transplant patient for rejection via the use of telemetered information.

      1. Pirolo et al – unipolar peak to peak amplitude of the QRS on the intracardiac electrogram (ICE) was helpful in early detection of rejection

      2. Grace et al – correlation occurs between rejection and a fall in evoked T wave amplitude

   d. More studies need to be done on the evaluation of parameters appropriate for detection of the pre-clinical indicators of rejection.

References

Avitall B, Payne DD, Connolly RJ, et al. Heterotopic heart transplantation: electrophysiology changes during acute rejection. J Heart Transplant. 7: 176–82. 1988.

Banner NR, Lloyd MH, Hamilton RD, et al. Cardiopulmonary response to dynamic exercise after heart and combined heart-lung transplantation. Br Heart J. 61:215–223. 1989.

Berke DK, Graham AF, Schroeder JS, Harrison DC. Circulation. (suppl. III)48: 112–119. 1973.

Bexton RS, Nathan AW, Hellestrand KJ, et al. Sinoatrial function after cardiac transplantation. JACC. 3:712–23. 1984.

Castejon R, Gamallo C, Cabo J, et al. Electrophysiologic changes during acute rejection of heterotopically transplanted rat hearts. J Heart Lung Transplant. 10:100–105. 1991.

Chou, Te-Chuan. Electrocardiography in Clinical Practice. 3rd ed. Philadelphia: WB Saunders Co., 1991.

Ellenbogen K, Marc TD, DiMarco JP, Sheehan H, Lerman BB. Circulation. 81:821–828. 1990.

Grace AA, et al. Diagnosis of early cardiac transplant rejection by fall in evoked T wave amplitude measured using an externalized QT drive rate responsive pacemaker. PACE. 14:1024. 1991.

Heinz G, Ohner T, Laczkovics A. Sinus node dysfunction after orthotopic heart transplantation: comparison of electrophysiologic and clinical parameters in predicting long-term outcome. PACE. 12:673. 1989.

Kacet S, Molin F, Lacroix D, et al. Bipolar atrial triggered pacing to restore normal chronotropic responsiveness in an orthotopic cardiac transplant patient. PACE. 14:1444–1447. 1991.

Liem LB, DiBiase A, Schroeder JS. Arrhythmias and clinical electrophysiology of the transplanted human heart. Sem Thorac Cardiovasc Surg. 2(3): 271–278. 1990.

Lindsay BD, Osborn JL, Kenzora JL, et al. Prospective detection of vulnerability to sustained ventricular tachycardia in patients awaiting cardiac transplantation. Am J Cardiol. 69(6):619–624. 1992.

Little RE, Kay GN, Epstein AE, et al. Arrhythmias after orthotopic cardiac transplantation: prevalence and determinants during initial hospitalization and late follow-up. Circulation. (suppl III)80(5):140–146. 1989.

Loria K, Salinger M, McDonough T, et al. Activitrax AAIR pacing for sinus node dysfunction after orthotopic heart transplantation: an initial report. J Heart Transplant. 7:380–384. 1988.

McManus RP, O'Hair DR, Beltzinger J, et al. Patients who die awaiting heart transplantation, J Heart Lung Transplant. 11(1):191. 1992.

Mackintosh AF, Carmichael DJ, Wren C, et al. Sinus node function in the first three weeks after cardiac transplantation. Br Heart J. 48:584–588. 1982.

Markewitz A, Kemkes BM, Reble B, et al. Particularities of dual chamber pacemaker therapy in patients after orthotopic heart transplantation. PACE. 10:326–332. 1987.

Markewitz A, Osterholzer G, Weinhold C, et al. Recipient P wave synchronized pacing of the donor atrium in a heart-transplanted patient: a case study. PACE. 11:1402–1404. 1988.

Midel MG, Baughman KL, Achuff SC, et al. Is atrial activation beneficial in heart transplant recipients? J Am Coll Cardiol 16(5):1201–1204. 1990.

Miyamoto Y, Curtiss EI, Kormos RL, et al. Bradyarrhythmias after heart transplantation: Incidence, time course, and outcome. Circulation. (suppl IV)82:(5):313–317. 1990.

Osterholzer G, Markevitz A, Anthuber M, et al. An example of how to pace a patient with a heart transplantation. J Heart Transplant. 7:23–25. 1988.

Pirolo JS, et al. Influence of activation origion, lead number, and lead configuration, on the noninvasive electrophysiologic detection of cardiac allograft rejection. Circulation. 84(5 suppl):III344. 1991.

Redmond JM, Zehr K, Gillinov MA, et al. Use of theophylline for treatment of prolonged sinus node dysfunction in human orthotopic heart transplant. J Heart Lung Transplant. Pt 1:133–138. 1993.

Schroeder JS, Berke DK, Graham AF, Rider AK, Harrison DC. Arrhythmias after cardiac transplantation. Am J Cardiol. 33:604–607. 1974.

Scott CD, Omar I, McComb JM, et al. Long-term pacing in heart transplant recipients is usually unnecessary. PACE. 14:1792–1796. 1991.

Part 2

PACEMAKER CURRICULUM

CHAPTER 13

The Patient and the Pacemaker

Marleen E. Irwin

A. Presentations
B. Indications and Contraindications
C. Early Complications
D. Mode Selection
E. Device Selection

This section covers the clinical indications and contraindications for the insertion of cardiac pacing systems for treatment of bradycardia, as well as the early complications associated with insertion of pacing systems. Device selection is also reviewed.

Due to variations in the therapy and advances in research, the absolute indications for permanent pacing are constantly changing. There is general acceptance of definite indications for pacing in some conduction disturbances and there is general agreement that in other conduction disturbances, the need for permanent pacing is not accepted. The patient must be assessed carefully with regard to clinical status and the presenting rhythm. The technology advances in pacing therapy have increased the options for patients requiring control of bradycardia.

Objectives

1. Describe the disturbances of the conduction system that lead to brady-cardia.

From: Schurig L. *Educational Guidelines: Pacing and Electrophysiology*. Armonk, NY: Futura Publishing Co, Inc, © 1994.

2. Describe the various conduction anomalies with associated symptoms that require the implantation of a pacing system.
3. Describe the various conduction anomalies, symptomatic and asymptomatic that do not require the implantation of a permanent pacing system.
4. Describe the process involved in selecting the most appropriate pacing mode.
5. Describe the early complications of pacing therapy.

Glossary and Abbreviations

Adams-Stokes syndrome: A transient loss of consciousness due to inadequate blood flow to the brain due to cardiac arrhythmia to transient cardiac standstill (typically occurs without warning).

Asystole: Absence of ventricular complexes (depolarization) for seconds or minutes.

Block: Delays in or interruptions of impulse conduction.

AV block; first degree: Sinus rhythm, P-R interval greater than 0.20 sec.

AV block; second degree: At regular or irregular intervals, a P wave is not followed by a QRS complex. The P-P interval is constant.

AV block; second degree; Mobitz type I: Cyclically there is progressive lengthening of the P-R interval from beat to beat until a P wave is not followed by a QRS. Mobitz I is usually physiologic with rate and response catecholamine related. The site of block is usually in the AV node.

AV block; second degree; Mobitz type II: In a regular sequence 2:1, 3:1 or in an irregular sequence 3:2, 4:3, a P wave is not followed by a QRS. The P-R interval for the conducted beats is constant. The site of block is usually infranodal.

AV block; third degree: Dissociation occurs between the atrial and ventricular rhythms. The atrial rhythm may be normal sinus or any atrial arrhythmia, but the atrial impulse does not conduct to the ventricle. Ventricular depolarization is initiated by a secondary pacemaker either in the AV node, or in the ventricle (idioventricular). The site of block can be either in the AV node or infranodal.

SA block incomplete: Infrequent failure of the impulse to emerge from the SA node with the result that occasional beats are dropped.

SA block complete: No impulses emerge from the SA node and therefore P waves are not present.

Sinus bradycardia: Sinus rhythm, rate less than 60 beats per minute.

Sinus rhythm: Atrial followed by ventricular activation; with normal P waves (atrial depolarization), normal P-R interval, followed by QRS (ventricular depolarization).

Syncope: A transient loss of consciousness (could be due to cerebral and/or cardiac events).

Abbreviations

ABI: Atrial blanking interval
ABP: Atrial blanking period
AEI: Atrial escape interval
ARI/ARP: Atrial refractory interval/period
AVI: AV interval
BCL: Basic cycle length
LRL: Lower rate limit
MCL: Minimum cycle length
PCL: Pacing cycle length
PG: Pulse generator
P-P interval: interval between consecutive P waves
PVARI/PVARP: Post-ventricular refractory interval/period
TARI/TARP: Total atrial refractory interval/period
URL: Upper rate limit
VA: Ventriculoatrial
VAC: Ventriculoatrial conduction
VAI: VA interval
VBI: Ventricular blanking interval
VBP: Ventricular blanking period
VRI: Ventricular refractory interval
VTP: Ventricular triggering period
V-V interval: interval between consecutive paced complexes

Education Content

A. Presentations
    1. Electrocardiographic presentation of bradycardia
        a. Abnormal sinus impulse formation
            1. Sinus bradycardia
            2. Sinoatrial block
                a) Partial
                b) Complete
            3. Sinus arrest
                a) Pause
        b. Ectopic impulse formation with associated AV block
            1. Originating in the atria
        c. Disturbance of the conduction system
            1. Sinoatrial (SA) block (first, second, third degree)
                a) Incomplete
                b) Complete
            2. Intra-atrial block/conduction delay
            3. Atrioventricular (AV) block
                a) First degree
                b) Second degree
                    1) Type I
                    2) Type II
                    3) Advanced AV block
                c. Third degree/AV block
            4. Intraventricular block (Intra-Hisian block)
                a) Right bundle branch block
                b) Left bundle branch block
                    1) Fascicle blocks
                        • Left anterior hemiblock
                        • Left posterior hemiblock
                c) Bilateral bundle branch block
                    • Bifascicular
                    • Trifascicular
    2. Pacemaker implantation indication classifications
        a. Class I
            1. Conditions for which there is general agreement for implantation of a device

166

    b. Class II

        1. Conditions for which devices are implanted, but there is a divergence of opinion with respect to need

    c. Class III

        1. General agreement that devices are not indicated

B. Indications and Contraindications

    1. Indications for permanent pacing in acquired atrioventricular block in adults

        a. Class I

            1. Complete heart block with any one of the following complications:

                a) Symptomatic bradycardia

                b) Congestive heart failure

                c) Drug induced bradycardia

                d) Documented asystole ≥ 3.0 sec

                e) Post-AV junction ablation

            2. Second degree AV block with symptomatic bradycardia

            3. Atrial fibrillation, atrial flutter with complete heart block, bradycardia unrelated to digitalis or drugs that impair AV conduction

        b. Class II

            1. Asymptomatic complete heart block with ventricular rates of 40 beats per minute or faster

            2. Asymptomatic type II second degree AV block

            3. Asymptomatic type I second degree AV block

        c. Class III

            1. First degree AV block

            2. Asymptomatic type I second degree AV block

    2. After acute myocardial infarction

        a. Class I

            1. Persistent complete heart block and advanced second degree AV block

            2. Transient AV block associated bundle branch block

        b. Class II

            1. Persistent advanced block at AV node

        c. Class III

            1. Transient AV conduction disturbances without conduction defect

            2. Acquired left anterior hemiblock in the absence of AV block

    3. Bifascicular and trifascicular block (chronic)

        a. Class I

        1. With type II AV block without symptoms attributable to heart block

        2. With complete AV block associated with symptomatic bradycardia

    b. Class II

        1. With prolonged H-V interval

        2. With syncope not proved to be due to complete AV block

    c. Class III

        1. Fascicular block without AV block or "symptoms"

        2. Fascicular block with first degree AV block without symptoms

4. Sinus node dysfunction (sinus bradycardia, sinus arrest, sinoatrial block, paroxysmal ectopic atrial rhythms with associated bradycardia)

    a. Class I

        1. Symptomatic bradycardia documented

        2. Tachycardia-bradycardia syndrome

        3. Therapeutic drug provoked sinus bradycardia

    b. Class II

        1. Sinus node dysfunction with rates less than 40–50 bpm with significant symptoms

    c. Class III

        1. Sinus node, dysfunction in asymptomatic patients

5. Hypersensitive carotid sinus and neurovascular syndrome

    a. Class I

        1. Pre-syncope or syncope associated with greater than 3 second asystole with carotid sinus pressure

    b. Class II

        1. Recurrent syncope without clear provocative events with a hypersensitive cardioinhibitory response

    c. Class III

        1. A hypersensitive cardioinhibitory response to carotid sinus stimulation in the absence of symptoms

C. Early Complications

1. Causes, signs, symptoms, diagnostic evaluations and techniques

    a. Traumatic pneumothorax

        1. Laceration of the lung

    b. Traumatic hemothorax

        1. Laceration of the subclavian vein

        2. Myocardial perforations

    c. Traumatic hemopneumothorax

        1. Laceration of the lung, subclavian vein or artery

a) Cause – subclavian vein puncture

b) Signs, symptoms – aspiration of air during the subclavian puncture

    1) Hypotension (unexplained)

    2) Chest pain

    3) Respiratory compromise

c) Diagnostic techniques – intraoperative visualization with fluoroscopy and postoperative chest radiography, repeat chest x-ray in 24 hours to detect late pneumothorax

d. Lead malposition

  1. Perforation

    a) Chest radiography

    b) Electrocardiography

    c) Two-dimensional echocardiography

    d) Pericardial rub

  2. Dislodgement

    a) Failure to capture

    b) Failure to sense

  3. Unexplained and new extrasystoles

e. Wound complications

  1. Hematoma formation

  2. Infection

    a) Most commonly caused by *Staphylococcus epidermidis*

    b) Aggressive and associated with fever and systemic symptoms

    c) Evidence of pocket infection

f. Arrhythmias

  1. Originating at a focus at the same site as that of the pacing lead tip

  2. Seen during lead positioning

g. Pacing lead trauma

  1. Iatrogenesis

    a) Scalpel, scissor cuts – insulation and conducting coil

    b) Insulation damage due to placement of ligature

    c) Insulation puncture by lead guide wires

  2. Manufacturing deficiency

h. External device interference or interactions

  1. Direct current (DC) countershock

  2. Electrocautery

    a) Reprogramming

    b) Reversion to modes not otherwise programmed

            c) Inhibition of pulse generator

            d) Permanent damage to the pacer unit

   i. Pacing system anomalies

       1. Manufacturing design deficiencies and device malfunctions

   j. Acute rise in threshold above device output settings

   k. Cathodal muscle stimulation

       1. Diaphragmatic stimulation

       2. Phrenic nerve stimulation

   l. Anodal stimulation

       1. Pectoral muscle stimulation

   m. Symptoms related to the loss of AV synchrony

       1. Pacemaker syndrome in VVI cardiac pacing

       2. Loss of atrial capture in an implanted dual chamber system with associated retrograde ventriculoatrial conduction or AV dissociation

D. Mode Selection

  1. Non-medical status

    a. Conduction system disorder

       1. AV conduction; normal, blocked, slowed

       2. Atrial arrhythmias; rare, frequent, fixed

       3. VA conduction; documented, elicited

    b. Drugs producing conduction changes

    c. Cardiac anatomy

    d. Surgical considerations

    e. Hemodynamic considerations

       1. Left ventricular (LV) function

    f. Chronotropic competence

    g. Anticipated level(s) of activity

    h. Progression of conduction disease

    i. Consider rate augmentation; indicated, contraindicated

  2. Recommended pacemaker modes "chart"

E. Device Selection

  1. General considerations

    a. Support services

    b. Hemodynamics of cardiac pacing

    c. Cost-effectiveness

    d. Patient – device interaction

    e. Patient lifestyle and mobility to follow-up center

2. Specific considerations
   a. Function and status of the atrium
   b. Function and status of the AV node
   c. Function and status of the sinus node during exercise
   d. Function and status of the ventricle
   e. Frequency and duration of the arrhythmia
   f. Need for maximum exercise capacity
   g. Compliance to follow-up protocol

Recommended Pacemaker Modes

Diagnosis	Optimal	Alternative	Inappropriate
SND	AAIR	AAI	VVI VDD
AVB	DDD	VDD	AAI DDI
SND&AVB	DDDR DDIR	DDD DDI	AAI VVI
Chronic AF with AVB	VVIR	VVI	AAI DDD VDD
CSS	DDI	DDD VVI*	AAI VDD

* - If VVI is ever chosen for the management of carotid sinus syndrome rate hysteresis is recommended.
AVB, atrioventricular block; AF, atrial fibrillation or flutter; SND,sinoatrial node disease; CSS, carotid sinus syndrome.

Recommendations from the British Pacing & EP Group, FEB 1991

References

Barold SS, Falkoff Ong LS, Heinle RA. Modern Cardiac Pacing. In SS Barold, (Ed). Mt. Kisco: Futura Publishing Co, Inc., 645. 1985.

Bernstein AD, Parsonnet V. Strategies for mode selection in antibradyarrhythmia pacing. Cardiol Clin. 10(4) 719–734. 1992.

Bhandari AK, Rahimtoola SH. Indications for cardiac pacing in patients with bradyarrhythmias. JAMA. 252:1327–1328. 1984.

Dreifus LS, Fisch G, Griffin JO, Gillette PC, Mason JW, Parsonnet V. Guidelines for implantation of cardiac pacemakers and antiarrhythmia devices. Circulation. 84:1: July:P455–467. 1991.

Furman S, Hayes DL, Holmes D. A Practice of Cardiac Pacing. Mt. Kisco: Futura Publishing Co, Inc., 1989.

Harthorne JW. Indications for pacemaker insertion: types and modes of pacing. Prog Cardiovasc Dis. 23:393–400. 1981.

Joint American College of Cardiology/American Heart Association Task Force on Assessment of Cardiovascular Procedures: Guidelines for permanent cardiac pacemaker implantation. 18:1:1–13. 1991.

Parsonnet V, Escher DJ, Furman S, et al. Indications for dual chamber pacing. PACE. 7:318–319. 1984.

Pinsky WW, Gillette PC, Garson A Jr, McNamara DG. Diagnosis, management, and long term results of patients with congenital complete atrioventricular block. Pediatrics. 69:728–733. 1982.

CHAPTER 14

Hardware

Richard Forney
Mark Sweesy

Subsections:
A. Generators
B. Leads
C. Programmers
D. Accessories

One of the most exciting and dynamic aspects of cardiac pacing is the associated hardware. The term "hardware has currently become a misnomer since many pulse generators and programmers have become extensively software based.

Doctors Rune Elmquist and Ake Senning implanted the first pacemaker in Arne Larsson in 1958. The early 1960s provided single chamber, non-programmable, mercury zinc battery powered devices containing transistors, resistors, capacitors, wires and other discrete components. The next 30 years documented the transition to dual chamber, lithium iodide batteries, software based, hybrid-circuitry-containing pulse generators with billions of programmable combinations including multisensor rate modulated devices.

Somewhat less exciting until the last decade has been the advancement of pacing electrodes. The requirement of an epicardial lead fortunately was short-lived thanks to Dr. Seymour Furman's introduction of the transvenous approach in 1958. In recent years, smaller, more stable, low threshold atrial and ventricular leads have been developed. These leads are characterized by such features as porous tips, platinized carbon, retractable active fixation mechanisms and steroid eluting mechanisms.

Pacemaker programmers, devices capable of communicating with and

---

From: Schurig L. *Educational Guidelines: Pacing and Electrophysiology*. Armonk, NY: Futura Publishing Co, Inc, © 1994.

altering or programming features of the pacemaker such as the pacing rate have also gone through a tremendous metamorphosis and have increased in importance as an integral part of the pacing system. As Dr. Neal Kay stated "Once the pacemaker has been implanted, I know that pacemaker only by the programmer." Programmers have quickly evolved from being able to program only the paced rate to programming systems which offer features such as batch programming, programmed and measured data available through telemetry, real time ECGs with simultaneous intracardiac electrograms, histograms, event counters, auto-threshold (sensing and capture) testing and many more options.

Objectives

1. To outline and list resources regarding the knowledge base requirements for understanding and utilizing bradycardia and antitachycardia pulse generators.
2. To outline and list resources regarding the knowledge base requirements for understanding and utilizing implantable cardioverter defibrillators.
3. To outline and list resources regarding the knowledge base requirements for understanding and utilizing cardiac pacing leads.
4. To outline and list resources regarding the knowledge base requirements for understanding and utilizing pulse generator programmers.
5. To provide a reference list of recommended resources concerning cardiac pacing hardware.

Glossary and Abbreviations

AV delay hysteresis: (rate-variable hysteresis) A programmable or automatic feature which permits a shorter AV delay after atrial sensed compared to atrial paced events.

CMOS: Complimentary metal oxide semiconductor—a technology term used for integrated circuitry in which two-channel transistors operate within a wide range of voltages. CMOS circuitry provides the logic function in several different circuits of pacemakers and other programmable devices.

dP/dT: Changes in right ventricular pressure over time, reflecting myocardial contractility. dP/dT increases with exertion.

dV/dT (contractility): Changes in right ventricular volume over time, reflecting myocardial contractility. Increased contractility occurs normally with exercise, therefore, an increased heart rate would be indicated by the rate modulation algorithm.

Event counter: A mechanism in the pacemaker that counts and records paced and non-paced events (intrinsic beats). Accessible through the programmer.

Event marker: A mechanism is a pacemaker that permits visual recording on the ECG through a programmer. This feature facilitates ECG interpretation as events are flagged for sensing, pacing, refractory periods, etc. (Varies in devices).

Evoked response: A measured response of the ventricular electrogram following a paced event. The measured area under the electrogram (depolarization gradient) would decrease during exercise. This is used in sensor based systems to signal an increased pacing rate.

Fallback: A programmable upper rate response in some pacemakers. Fallback occurs when the upper rate is reached in dual chamber or rate modulated pacemakers. The ventricular paced rate decelerates to, and is maintained at, a programmable fallback rate that is lower than the programmed upper rate.

Hermetic seal: A fluid-impermeable seal of the pacer case and/or circuitry that protects the circuitry from fluid invasion.

Hysteresis: An extension of the escape interval following a sensed intrinsic event.

IS-1: The most recent attempt to standardize 3.2 mm in-line leads to an industry International Standard.

Pre-ejection interval (PEI): The time interval from electrical depolarization to mechanical ejection. PEI decreases with exercise. This is used in sensor based systems to increase the heart rate.

Rate hysteresis: Extension of the escape interval following a sensed intrinsic event, therefore, the interval is prolonged compared to the pacing or automatic interval.

Rate smoothing: A functional response of some pacemakers that prevents the paced rate, either atrial or ventricular, from changing by more than a programmed percentage from one cardiac cycle to the next cycle.

Reed switch: A switch that consists of two metal strips sealed in a glass tube. Activated by magnet application, closure of the switch results in asynchronous output.

RS232C: Standard computer interface configuration between computers and/or accessory equipment, e.g., programmers.

"Safety Pacing": The delivery of a ventricular output pulse, following atrial pacing, if ventricular sensing occurs during the initial 110 ms of the programmed AV delay. This interval is programmable in some pacemakers.

Semiconductor: An element of electronic circuitry that conducts electricity better than an insulator but not as well as conductive metal. Semiconductors are power efficient and provide electrical amplification and rectification.

VDD orthogonal lead: Single lead for VDD pacing utilizing orthogonal sensing electrodes in the atrial position combined with pacing/sensing electrodes in the ventricular position.

VS-1: Original attempt to standardize lead connections to an industry Voluntary Standard.

Zener diode: A semiconductor element in pacemaker circuitry designed to prevent electrical circuit damage from cardioversion, defibrillation, or other large electrical currents.

Education Content

A. Generators

   1. Major components

      a. Power sources (battery)

         1. Lithium iodide–used almost exclusively today

         2. Lithium cupric sulfide–used infrequently

         3. Promethium 147–nuclear, outdated

         4. Plutonium 238–nuclear, still used infrequently

         5. Nickel cadmium–rechargeable, outdated

         6. Mercury zinc–early devices, outdated

         7. Lithium silver chromate–European battery, outdated

      b. Integrated circuitry

         1. CMOS–complimentary metal oxide semiconductors

         2. NMOS–N-channel metal oxide semiconductors

         3. Discrete components–outdated as sole circuitry component

         4. Hybrid circuitry–combination of integrated circuits and discrete components

      c. Reed switch

         1. Asynchronous output

         2. Magnet activated

      d. Zener diode

         1. Semiconductor element

         2. Power dissipation

      e. Connector block (header)

         1. Lead attachment

            a) Set screw(s)

            b) Side lock mechanism

         2. X-ray identification (radiopaque symbol)

         3. Millimeter sizes and configurations—Table 1.

            a) 6 mm

            b) 5 mm

            c) 3.2 mm–Cordis or Medtronic type

            d) VS-1, VS-1A, VS-1B

            e) IS-1, Figure 1

            f) Bifurcated bipolar

            g) Unipolar or bipolar

            h) In-line bipolar

Table 1. Compatibility Chart for Pacing Leads and Pulse Generators.*

LEADS	PULSE GENERATORS**				
	3.2 mm low-profile or IS-1 • long cavity • sealing rings	IS-1 • short cavity • no sealing rings	VS-1 • short cavity • no sealing rings	VS-1A • long cavity • no sealing rings	VS-1B • long cavity • sealing rings
IS-1 • short pin • sealing rings	YES	YES	YES	YES	YES
VS-1 • short pin • sealing rings	YES	YES	YES	YES	YES
Medtronic 3.2 mm low-profile bipolar • long pin • no sealing rings	YES	NO	NO	NO	YES
Cordis 3.2 mm low-profile unipolar/bipolar • long pin • sealing rings	YES	NO	NO	YES	YES

* The leads and pulse generators listed are designed to fit together. "Designed to fit" means that according to the available documentation, the indicated leads and pulse generators should mechanically fit together. However, manufacturers are responsible for the safety and reliability of the fit. As such, Medtronic assures the fit only between Medtronic products.

** The IS-1 and VS-1 pulse generator connector configurations allow for unipolar and bipolar lead interchangeability. However, when a bipolar pulse generator is connected to a unipolar lead, it must be programmed to a unipolar configuration.

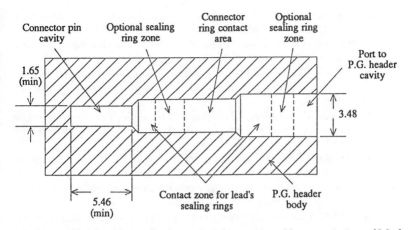

Figure 1. IS-1 Pulse Generator Connector Cavity. Used by permission of Medtronic, Inc.

    f. Case (can)
        1. Titanium
        2. Hermetically sealed
2. Single chamber bradycardia devices
    a. Single lead–atrial or ventricular
    b. Electrode configuration (polarity)–unipolar and/or bipolar
    c. Modes–AOO AAI AAT AAIR VOO VVI VVT VVIR
3. Dual chamber bradycardia devices
    a. Dual leads–atrial and ventricular
    b. Electrode configuration (polarity)–unipolar and/or bipolar with each lead
    c. Modes–DOO DVI VDD DDD DDI DDT DDDR DDIR DVIR VDDR and various modes from single chamber devices
4. Sensors
    a. P-waves–sinus node activity increases with exertion
    b. "Activity"–increased body vibrations are detected by sensor and results in increased paced rate.
        1. Piezoelectric crystal-mounted on pacer can
        2. Accelerometer–piezoelectric crystal or silicon chip mounted on circuit board; also can be mercury ball inside a switch mechanism (gravimetric)
    c. Minute ventilation–product of respiration rate and tidal volume–minute ventilation increases with exertion.
    d. Respiration rate–respiration rate increases with exertion.

    e. Temperature–central venous blood temperature increases with exertion due to heat produced from skeletal muscle.

    f. QT interval–combined duration of ventricular depolarization and repolarization–interval shortens with exertion.

    g. Ventricular depolarization gradient–results from integral derived from ventricular paced beat–as work load increases, integral decreases.

    h. Pre-ejection interval (PEI)–interval from electrical depolarization to mechanical ejection in the ventricle–PEI interval shortens with exertion.

    i. Stroke volume–measurement of amount of blood ejected from the heart during systole–increases with exertion.

    j. dV/dT–changes in ventricular volume over time, reflects contractility–dV/dT increases with exertion.

    k. dP/dT–changes in ventricular pressure over time, reflects contractility–uses piezoelectric crystal in lead–dP/dT increases with exertion

    l. Oxygen saturation–O_2 saturation decreases with exertion.

    m. pH–decreases with exertion due to lactic acid in blood.

5. Multisensor technology

    a. Future sensor combinations

        1. High and low workloads

        2. Slow and rapid responses

            a) Temperature and activity

            b) Minute ventilation and evoked response

            c) dP/dT and activity

            d) Minute ventilation and activity

            e) Oxygen saturation and activity

            f) QT interval and activity

            g) Oxygen saturation and temperature

        3. Physical activity and emotion

6. Multiple modality devices

    a. Automatic mode switching–dual chamber P wave tracking modes to single chamber modes due to atrial arrhythmias

    b. Pacing–cardioversion–defibrillation

    c. Programmable choice of sensor utilized, e.g., pre-ejection interval or stroke volume; oxygen saturation or activity

7. Programmability

    a. Rate–pulses per minute (ppm) or interval (milliseconds)

        1. Base

        2. Upper tracking limit

        3. Upper rate modulated or sensor driven

    4. Interim
    5. Fallback
    6. Rate smoothing
    7. Hysteresis
    8. Circadian response (sleep rate)
b. Sensitivity
    1. P-wave–millivolts
    2. R-wave–millivolts
c. Pulse width (pulse duration)–milliseconds
d. Pulse amplitude–volts, milliamperes
e. AV delay (AV interval)–milliseconds
    1. AV delay hysteresis (differential)
    2. Rate responsive AV delay (rate adaptive AV delay)
f. Refractory periods–milliseconds
    1. Post-ventricular atrial refractory period (PVARP)
    2. Total atrial refractory period (TARP)
    3. Ventricular refractory period
    4. Relative/absolute refractory periods
g. Hysteresis
    1. Rate
    2. AV delay
h. Blanking period
    1. Atrial
    2. Ventricular
i. PVC options–atrial refractory extension
j. Pacemaker mediated tachycardia (PMT) termination algorithms
k. Safety pace–non-physiologic AV delay–ventricular safety standby, programmable on/off
l. Polarity configurations
m. Temporary programming
n. Auto threshold, auto sensing, Vario
o. Emergency, nominal or pre-set parameters
p. Magnet on/off
q. Rate modulated controls
    1. Sensor sensitivity
    2. Slope
    3. Acceleration/deceleration
    4. Onset
    5. Sensor type

8. Telemetry
   a. Type
      1. Magnetic frequency (pulsed magnetic fields)
      2. Radiofrequency transmissions
   b. Programmed data
   c. Measured data
      1. Pulse voltage–volts (V)
      2. Pulse current–milliamperes (mA)
      3. Pulse energy–microjoules (μJ)
      4. Pulse charge–microcoulombs (μC)
      5. Lead impedance–ohms
      6. Battery (cell) voltage–volts
      7. Battery (cell) current–microamperes (μA)
      8. Battery (cell) impedance–Kiloohms (KOhms)
   d. Special features
      1. Standard ECG leads
      2. Intracardiac electrograms
      3. Annotated markers
      4. Event counters
      5. Histograms
      6. Trend analysis
      7. Automatic "patient tailored" sensor parameter selection
9. Antitachycardia pacemakers–see Part Three, Chapter 28.B1
   a. Activation
      1. Automatic
      2. Patient activated
   b. Atrial–used for supraventricular tachycardias
   c. Ventricular–used for ventricular tachycardias, typically used only with implantable defibrillator back-up
   d. Single/dual chamber
   e. Back-up bradycardia pacing
   f. Tachycardia termination algorithms
      1. Burst pacing
      2. Scanning
10. Implantable cardioverter defibrillator (ICD)–see Part Three, Chapter 28.B2
    a. Nonprogrammable–early models now being replaced with programmable ICDs
    b. Programmable
       1. Detection criteria

    2. Energy output–joules, volts
    3. Energy output waveform and sequence
    4. Tachycardia terminating algorithms–tiered therapy
  c. Telemetry
    1. Programmed data
    2. Measured data
    3. Diagnostic data
    4. Event history
  d. Sensing leads
    1. Epicardial
    2. Endocardial
  e. Defibrillation leads
    1. Myocardial patches
    2. Endocardial leads
    3. Subcutaneous patch
    4. SVC spring lead
  f. Antitachycardia features (A9)
  g. Bradycardia pacing
  h. Magnet response

B. Leads
  1. Configuration/electrode location
    a. Configuration (polarity)
      1. Bi-polar
        a) Inline
        b) Bifurcated
      2. Unipolar
    b. Endocardial electrode location
      1. Atrial
        a) J formed
          1) Passive fixation
          2) Active fixation
      2. Ventricular
      3. Coronary sinus
  2. Active and passive fixation
    a. Active fixation
      1. Screw-in
      2. Stab-in
      3. Suture-on

   b. Passive fixation
      1. Tined
      2. Flanged
      3. Finned
3. Epicardial/endocardial
   a. Epicardial
      1. Active fixation
         a) Screw-in
         b) Stab-in
         c) Suture-on
   b. Endocardial
      1. Active fixation
      2. Passive fixation
4. Pacemaker lead materials
   a. Core
      1. Nickel alloy
      2. Elgiloy
      3. Stainless steel
      4. Platinum-iridium
      5. Nickel-silver alloy
      6. Nickel-cobalt alloy
   b. Insulation
      1. Silastic (silicone rubber)
      2. Polyurethane
      3. Polyethylene
   c. Electrodes
      1. Design
         a) Concentric grooves
         b) Porous tip
         c) Polished
         d) Helical coil
         e) Orthogonal
      2. Materials
         a) Elgiloy
         b) Platinum-iridium
         c) Biolite carbon
         d) Platinum
         e) Vitreous carbon
         f) Platinized titanium

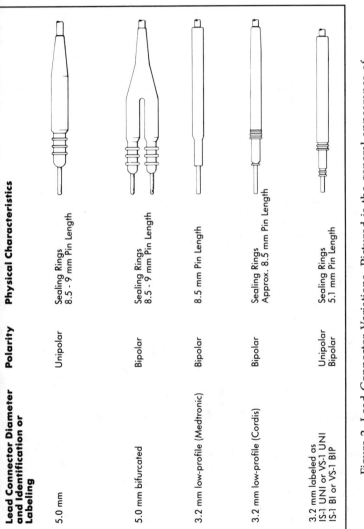

Lead Connector Diameter and Identification or Labeling	Polarity	Physical Characteristics
5.0 mm	Unipolar	Sealing Rings 8.5 - 9 mm Pin Length
5.0 mm bifurcated	Bipolar	Sealing Rings 8.5 - 9 mm Pin Length
3.2 mm low-profile (Medtronic)	Bipolar	8.5 mm Pin Length
3.2 mm low-profile (Cordis)	Bipolar	Sealing Rings Approx. 8.5 mm Pin Length
3.2 mm labeled as IS-1 UNI or VS-1 UNI IS-1 BI or VS-1 BIP	Unipolar Bipolar	Sealing Rings 5.1 mm Pin Length

Figure 2. Lead Connector Variations. Pictured is the general appearance of most currently available leads. Along with connector diameters being different sizes, notice the presence or absence of sealing rings and the connector pin lengths. Used by permission of Medtronic, Inc. (Medtronic News, Winter 1989/90).

      g) Steroid eluting

      h) Iridium oxide

      i) Coated electrodes

         (1) Mannitol

         (2) Polyethylene glycol

  d. Connector systems

     1. Compatibilities

       a) 5 mm

       b) 6 mm

       c) 3.2 mm–Figure 2

          (1) Cordis

          (2) Medtronic

          (3) VS-1

          (4) VS-1A

          (5) VS-1B

          (6) IS-1–Figure 3

 e. Sensors (see A. 4.)

     1. Oxygen saturation

     2. Vibration/motion

     3. pH

     4. Tripolar–stroke volume, PEI, dV/dT

     5. dP/dT

     6. Thermistor

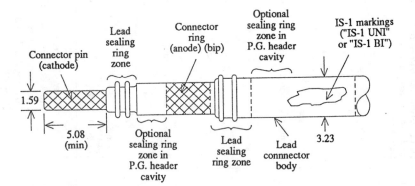

Figure 3. IS-1 Lead Connector—Unipolar/Bipolar. (Used by permission of Medtronic, Inc.)

C. Programmers
   1. Fundamentals
       a. Power source
           1. Battery–AA cells, 9V, C cells, D cells
           2. Line powered
               a) USA–110 to 120 volts AC current
               b) Switchable–for non-USA usage
           3. Both
       b. On/off switch
           1. Automatic power off
       c. Wand or telemetry coil area
           1. Position indicator–may be present
           2. Removable magnet–may be present
           3. Magnetic frequency or radiofrequency telemetry
           4. Battery operated–few devices
           5. On/off switch
           6. Program/interrogate/other function keys
       d. Emergency back-up activation button/switch key
           1. Stat set, emergency VVI, transmit safe program, std prog program user preset values, return to standard, high set, high energy set, safe program, em VVI, emergency, emergency routine
       e. Handheld or desktop size
           1. Display
               a) Liquid crystal
               b) Cathode ray tube
               c) Light emitting diode
               d) None–slide switches
               e) Options–contrast control
           2. Controls
               1. Buttons/keys/switches
               2. Touch sensitive screen
               3. Light pen
               4. Control knob
       f. Software based or dedicated
           1. Software–modules, cartridges, function packs, computer disks
       g. Built-in printer
           1. Print key
           2. Paper feed/advance key
           3. Print type–thermal, dot matrix

       4. Options–print density, stop print, print when interrogated (trace), scroll function

       5. ECG printout

         a) Signal size

         b) Paper speed

         c) Filtered/unfiltered signal

       6. Intracardiac electrogram printout

   h. Accessory hardware

       1. ECG cables

       2. External printer

         a) On/off switch

         b) Power source–battery or line powered

         c) On-line switch

         d) Paper speed

         e) Paper feed/advance switch

       3. RS232C–connection to interface with computer

       4. DC voltage input from wall outlet adapter

       5. External inputs

       6. External outputs

   i. Clock memory

       1. Format selection

         a) Time–24 hour/12 hour clock

         b) Date–selection of order for month, day, year

   j. Training/teaching capabilities

       1. Demo mode, teaching simulator

2. Advanced application of technology

   a. Software based

       1. Help files/screens

       2. Pulse generator specifications

       3. Rate response data collection/display

         a) Histograms

         b) Trend analysis

         c) Auto set features for rate response parameters

       4. Patient information

       5. Non-invasive programmed stimulation (NIPS)

       6. Automatic follow-up algorithms

       7. Holter type capabilities

       8. Event counters

       9. Annotated event markers

      10. Electronic calipers

      11. Retrograde conduction assessment

D. Accessories

1. Adapters
   a. Lead extenders–increase length of lead to relocate pulse generator to new site
   b. Lead caps–used to cover lead pins when lead has been abandoned. Sutured on to prevent erosion and electrically isolate pin.
   c. Lead end pins–to replace or adapt end pin on lead
   d. Lead adapters–rectify connector pin incompatibility
   e. Alligator connectors to specific lead pin size
2. Implantation tools
   a. Vein lifter–used to lift vein(s) for lead introduction
   b. Percutaneous introducer
   c. Lead stylets (guidewires)
   d. Screwdrivers and hex wrenches–tightening/loosening connections in pulse generators connector block
   e. Indifferent electrode–for unipolar devices
   f. Pacing systems analyzer and cables–for testing electrical aspects of implanted lead and pulse generator
   g. Suture sleeves
3. Repair kits
   a. Sleeves–repair "nick" in lead or to upsize lead to connector block
   b. Medical adhesive–for sealing areas that physician does not want fluid intrusion, e.g., connector block
4. Magnets
   a. Shapes–horseshoe, doughnut, bar
5. Lead removal equipment and techniques
   a. Traction–weights attached to lead end, progressively increased until lead pulled from cardiac tissue.
   b. Counter traction sheaths–specialized sheaths are passed over lead bodies, locked in place with locking stylet, lead pulled from cardiac tissue with minor damage.

References

Barold SS, ed. Modern Cardiac Pacing. Mt. Kisco: Futura Publishing Co. Inc., ch 3–6. 1986.

De Belder MA, Malik M, Ward DE, Camm, AJ. Pacing Modalities for Tachycardia Termination. PACE. 13(2):231–248. 1990.

Ellenbogen, KA. Cardiac Pacing. Boston, MA: Blackwell Scientific Publications, 1992. ch 2.

Furman SF, Hayes DL, Holmes DR Jr. A Practice of Cardiac Pacing, 3rd ed. Mt. Kisco: Futura Publishing Co., Inc., 89–134. 1993.

Hayes DL, Maue-Dickson W., Stanton MS. Dictionary of Cardiac Pacing, Electrophysiology and Arrhythmias. Miami Lakes: Peritus Corporation, 1993.

Lau C-P. Rate Adaptive Cardiac Pacing. Single and Dual Chamber. Mt. Kisco: Futura Publishing Co., Inc., 63–237. 1993.

Levine PA, Schuller H, Lindgren A. Pacemaker ECG: Utilization of Pulse Generator Telemetry–A Benefit of Space Age Technology. Solna: Siemens-Elema AB, 1988.

Morse DP, Parsonnet V, Gessman LJ, et al. Durham: Droege Computing Services, Inc., 1991.

Sutton R, Bourgeois I. The Foundations of Cardiac Pacing, Pt. I. An Illustrated Practical Guide to Basic Pacing. Mt Kisco: Futura Publishing Co., Inc., ch 4. 1991.

Physician and technical manuals for every model pulse generator, programmer and software program are available from the manufacturers and should be consulted when utilizing these products. Many manufacturers also print comprehensive booklets concerning battery depletion characteristics, connector sizes, lead compatibility and a wealth of other information concerning all pacing products.

CHAPTER 15

Computer Applications in Pacing

Alan D. Bernstein
Marleen Irwin
Susan L. Song

Subsections:

A. Computer-Based Devices
B. Interfaces with Other Devices and Systems
C. Clinical Practice
D. Data Base Management
E. Signal Acquisition and Processing
F. Research
G. Avoiding Risks with Computerization
H. Rationale for a Computer
I. System Selection

Microprocessor, microcomputer, and mainframe technology play an increasingly prominent role both in pacemaker technology and in clinical pacing practice. These aspects will be considered in the present chapter.

Many pacemaker clinicians are acquainted with computerized data base management applications for maintaining clinical and administrative information and for generating reports, letters, and other documents. Since the early 1980s, however, computers have become increasingly important as integral parts of pacing instrumentation. Today's pacemaker pulse generators, programming devices, pacemaker-systems analyzers, and monitoring systems are largely computer-based, and for good reason. Any function that can be

From: Schurig L. *Educational Guidelines: Pacing and Electrophysiology.* Armonk, NY: Futura Publishing Co, Inc, © 1994.

implemented as a computer program, rather than an electronic circuit, has two important advantages. First, software does not wear out, an important distinction in an application where system reliability is of paramount importance. Second, software is easier to modify than hardware; it is even possible to update the software in some pacemaker pulse generators non-invasively, thus allowing the pulse generator to be redesigned even after it has been implanted.

With the wide proliferation of computer-based pacemaker programming devices and the almost universal presence of data-management computers in clinical facilities, the desirability of allowing devices to communicate with each other, using an agreed upon common language, has become increasingly evident. This matter was addressed by a NASPE policy conference in 1986, and the task of generating a set of standards for such communication has been assigned to the Pacemaker Committee of the Association for Advancement of Medical Instrumentation (AAMI). In the mean time, some pacemaker manufacturers have begun addressing this issue independently, and at least one has made an advanced pacing system available whose programming device consists of a programming head that can be plugged into almost any standard IBM-compatible microcomputer, which then becomes the heart of the programming device, running software provided by the pacemaker manufacturer for that specialized purpose.

Through suitable communication schemes, computers can read the outputs of measurement devices used during pacemaker implantation and follow-up, obviating the need for recording measurement results manually and thus eliminating a major potential source of error. Through analog-to-digital (A/D) conversion, computers can serve as the measurement devices themselves, simplifying the clinical procedures still further. In either case, computer techniques for error trapping can be invoked to identify questionable measurement results as soon as the measurements are made, and (more importantly) can be used to identify and bring to the user's attention any results that indicate the possibility of a pacemaker system problem.

Objectives

1. Identify computer-based devices and systems used in pacing.
2. Describe some of the uses of computer technology during clinical procedures (implantation, clinic follow-up, and transtelephonic monitoring [TTM]).
3. Discuss the role of computer resources in facilitating administrative and research-oriented tasks.
4. Explore the rationale for computer purchases.
5. Identify potential risks in computerization.

Glossary and Abbreviations

Algorithm: A script for performing a task or solving a problem by machine.

Analog signal: A voltage that varies with time. A signal may be generated to represent any time-varying clinical variable, such as pressure or temperature, to allow measurements of that variable to be displayed or processed.

Binary: Number system consisting entirely of ones and zeros.

Bit: A single unit of digital data, i.e., the electrical equivalent of a one or a zero. See Byte.

Byte: A basic unit of computer data storage, consisting of a specified number of bits, each containing a single unit of digital data, i.e., the electrical equivalent of a one or a zero.

Data: Information.

Data base: A table of information organized in records and fields.

Digital: Able to be resolved into a set of basic units, each consisting of the electrical equivalent of a one or a zero.

Error trapping: Identification of erroneous or invalid data by comparison with known or calculated plausible values (e.g., refractory period = 0.4 ms) or stored lists of acceptable values (e.g., mode = VVVR).

Expert system: A computer program that emulates the behavior of a human expert in a strictly limited domain of expertise.

Export: Provision of data for use with another program. Sometimes requires format translation.

Field: A storage area in a record; contains a single data element such as name, pacing mode, or programmed AV interval.

Format: (1) The magnetic "layout" of information storage on a medium such as disk or tape. (2) The conventions by which visible text properties, such as tabulation and typeface size, are represented by codes suitable for computerized manipulation.

Hardware: The electronic circuits and mechanical components that make up the physical form of a computer.

Import: Acquisition of data generated and stored by one program for use by a different program. Sometimes requires format translation.

Interface: A mechanism whereby two computers or computer-based devices can "talk" to each other, using a mutually understood set of symbols and signal voltage conventions.

Macro: A type of program consisting of a sequence of commands each of which could be executed one by one if entered from the keyboard. Used to simplify repetitive tasks.

Memory: Means of storing binary data temporarily or permanently by means of electronic circuits equivalent to on-off switches. See random-access memory and read-only memory.

Microcomputer: A system consisting of a microprocessor, electronic memory, means of data input and output, and (usually) long-term electronic data storage (such as a magnetic disk).

Microprocessor: A specialized integrated electronic circuit able to perform calculations such as addition and subtraction, using binary arithmetic.

Model: A computer program used to emulate the behavior of a mechanical, biological, physiologic, or other system, such as the cardiac conduction system, or a process such as the reasoning by which a pacing mode is selected. See expert system.

Network: A group of computers wired together so that data bases and software programs can be shared by several users.

Program: A set of detailed instructions for executing an algorithm.

Random-access memory (RAM): Computer memory whose contents are lost when the power is turned off. RAM contents can be modified, or "overwritten" during the execution of a computer program.

Read-only memory (ROM): Computer memory whose contents are "burned" into an electronic circuit that retains its properties when the power is turned off. The contents cannot be modified during the execution of a computer program.

Record: A set of fields in a data base, containing information for a single patient, intervention, device, etc.

Software: A combination of instructions (program) and data that controls the operation of a computer.

Education Content

A. Computer-Based Devices
1. Pulse generators
2. Pacemaker systems analyzers
3. Programming and telemetry devices

B. Interfaces With Other Devices and Systems
1. NASPE protocol for computer communications in pacing
2. Local-area networks

C. Clinical Practice
1. Indications for pacing: expert system computer models for application of accepted guidelines for permanent pacing
2. Mode selection: expert system models for pacing-mode selection based on significant clinical criteria
3. Implantation procedure
   a. Measurements
   b. Analog-to-digital conversion for waveform acquisition and analysis
   c. Automatic storage of measurement results
   d. Error trapping: plausibility analysis of measurement results

D. Data Base Management, Implantation, and Follow-up
1. Data acquisition (keyboard, computer-to-computer transfer)
2. Demographic data
3. Administrative data
4. Measurement results
5. Pulse generator and lead specifications
6. Programming choices: patient/pacemaker simulations for parameter choice evaluation
7. Maintenance of programming records
8. Equipment maintenance records
9. Data plausibility assessment, error trapping, and recognition of measurement results that may indicate the presence of clinical or pacing system problems
10. Generation of reports and letters
11. Scheduling (clinic visits, TTM contacts, surgical interventions)
12. Safety advisories: tracking and notifying affected patients

E. Signal Acquisition and Processing
   1. Computer-assisted measurements
   2. Electrocardiogram (ECG), intra-cardiac-electrogram (IEG), and stimulus artifact waveforms
   3. Interface between programming devices and data base management computers
   4. Error trapping: identification of implausible or pathological measurement results
   5. Predictive analysis for follow-up planning (e.g., when will elective replacement time be reached, judging from existing data?)

F. Research
   1. Counting, sorting, and filtering (generating subsets) of data
   2. Statistical calculations
   3. Graphics
   4. Modeling of physiologic systems

G. Avoiding Risks With Computerization
   1. Know what you are getting into
   2. Define what you really want
   3. Look long-term to avoid limitations on the project
   4. Evaluate commitment to the project
   5. Evaluate available resources. Example:
      a. Information system
      b. Computer technology
      c. Programmer
      d. Data entry
      e. Finances
      f. Designer
   6. Evaluate needs for system security
   7. Evaluate environment. Examples:
      a. Ventilation
      b. System service, on site/outside vendor
      c. Space
      d. Location of areas to receive service
      e. Traffic patterns
   8. Have a good manual system prior to the computer system
   9. Determine end point for computer system – prefer options open
   10. Consider what you already have prepared to enter into the system. Examples:
      a. Other functions for import

    b. Data available for import (data bases, word processing, spreadsheets etc.)

    c. Networking

    d. Hardware

    e. Software

  11. Do you have a predetermined deadline for purchase?

  12. Benefits with computerization

    a. Time management

    b. Data tracking

    c. Report generation

    d. Statistics

    e. Management summaries

    f. Performance evaluation

H. Rationale for a Computer Proposal

  1. An organized system promotes the production of revenue.

  2. Computers facilitate effective utilization of existing resources.

  3. The rate of program development permits a gradual need for an increase in resources.

  4. Design of a detailed information system is needed to coordinate services for a patient population such as the pacemaker/ICD patient.

  5. The data base creates a documentation system for reporting/supporting compliance with regulations.

  6. The data base generates reports of significance to the referring physician, efficient and effective marketing.

  7. The computer system maintains the pace with today's technology.

I. System Selection

  1. Review your plan of action before selecting the final product.

  2. Do research and shop around.

  3. Purchase completed program vs. self designed?

    a. Does it meet your needs?

    b. User friendly?

    c. Permit program changes?

    d. Service?

  4. Accessed by a single user or network?

  5. Seek assistance to select

    a. Hardware

    b. Software

    c. Peripherals

d. Communications

e. Network

6. Calculate the amount of space you will need to design or process the amount of data you have

   a. Number of fields to enter

   b. Number of characters for a field

   c. Number of files or data bases to link

   d. Anticipate number of patients

   e. Duration of active storage

References

Benedek ZM, Furman S. The role of the computer in cardiac pacing technology. PACE. 7:1217. 1984.

Bernstein AD, Saksena S, Rathyen W, Parsonnet V. Microcomputer system for serial cardiac potential mapping. Proc. 34th ACEMB. Philadelphia: 258. 1981.

Bernstein AD, Parsonnet V. Computer techniques for pacer artifact waveform analysis. Proc. 35th ACEMB. Philadelphia: September 24, 1982.

Bernstein AD, Parsonnet V. Computer-aided detection of pacemaker system problems. Proc. Seventh Annual Symposium on Computer Applications in Medical Care (SCAMC), IEEE Computer Society. 398–401. 1983.

Bernstein AD, Parsonnet V. Microcomputer and microprocessor applications in cardiac pacing. Med Instrum. 17:329–333. 1983.

Bernstein AD, Parsonnet V. Computer-assisted measurements in pacemaker follow-up. PACE. 9:392–400. 1986.

Bernstein AD, Alexandersson M, Benedek M, et al. Report of the policy conference on computer communications in pacing sponsored by the North American Society of Pacing and Electrophysiology. PACE. 11:784–788, 1988.

Bernstein, AD. Computer assistance in research-protocol evaluation. J Clin Eng. 14:285–288. 1988.

Bernstein AD, Parsonnet V. Computer-assisted mode selection in antibrady-arrhythmia pacing. J Am Coll Cardiol. 15:266A. 1990.

Bernstein AD, Parsonnet V. Strategies for mode selection in antibradyarrhythmia pacing. In Cardiology Clinics. JC Griffin, (Ed.) Philadelphia: WB Saunders, 719–734. 1992.

Byrd CB, Halberg BS, Byrd CL. Computerized pacemaker patient analysis. PACE. 13:1779–1781. 1990.

MacArthur AM, Sampson MR. Screen design of a hospital information system. Nursing Clin North Am. 20:3:471-486. 1985.

Parken P, Saksena S, Bernstein AD, Rodgers TK, Parsonnet V. Computer simulation of complex cardiac arrhythmias: preliminary evaluation of an electrophysiologic model. PACE. 4:242. 1981.

Shepard RB, Blum RI. Cardiology office computer use: primer, pointers, pitfalls. ACC. 8:4:933–940. 1986.

Tao DK. System architecture designed to manage care. Top Health Care Finance. 14:2:52–29. 1987.

CHAPTER 16

Emergency and Temporary Pacing

Robert Audette
Kathleen Strong

Subsections:
A. Temporary
   1. Transvenous
   2. Esophageal Cardiac Pacing
   3. Epicardial (Post-Surgical)
B. Emergency
   1. Transthoracic Cardiac Pacing
   2. Transcutaneous Pacing

Temporary cardiac pacing was first made clinically feasible in the early 1950s by Paul Zoll, MD. Since then, great advances have been made in all areas of temporary pacing, including the development of a faster easier method of transvenous access, in 1958, by Seymour Furman, MD.

Temporary cardiac pacing is used in elective situations as well as in emergencies. It is utilized most often for life-threatening ventricular bradyarrhythmias. It can be used prophylactically while evaluating the need for permanent pacing, after cardiac surgery, or it can be used in emergency situations during CPR or when sinus arrest, symptomatic sinus bradycardias or complete AV block occurs. Temporary pacing may also be used to correct tachyarrhythmias that fail to respond to drug therapy, i.e., paroxysmal supraventricular tachycardia, atrial flutter, and ventricular tachycardias. Each method of temporarily pacing the heart has advantages and disadvantages that must be weighed by the physician to decide the proper method appropriate for each individual

From: Schurig L. *Educational Guidelines: Pacing and Electrophysiology.* Armonk, NY: Futura Publishing Co, Inc, © 1994.

situation. Temporary pacing, in general, is a safe, quick, and effective method of maintaining hemodynamic stability until further treatment can be administered. Many of the indications for the utilization of temporary pacing support are transient, and either resolve spontaneously, can be corrected, or require more permanent pacing methods.

Objectives

1. Identify indications for use of each specific pacing modality.
2. Overview of implantation techniques or application methods for each type of temporary pacing.
3. Understand specific equipment used for each method of temporary pacing.
4. Assess appropriate capture and sensing for each method.
5. Plan for the management of each patient with the specific type of temporary pacing used.
6. Outline complications for each method.
7. Review safety precautions for each type of pacing utilized.
8. Outline the set up and methods of assisting with implementation of each modality.
9. Outline the essential patient education for each modality.
10. Assess long-term needs, if appropriate.

Education Content

A. Temporary

1. Transvenous

   a. Indications for use

      1. Complete AV block
         a) Congenital symptomatic
         b) Acquired symptomatic
         c) Surgical (asymptomatic and symptomatic)

      2. Second degree AV block
         a) Type I – (AV nodal – symptomatic)
         b) Type II – (His Purkinje, symptomatic)

      3. Bundle branch blocks
         a) Pre-existing LBBB in a patient having a right heart catheterization

      4. Atrial fibrillation with slow vent response when presence or increased risk of symptomatic bradycardias exists

      5. Sick sinus syndrome – Brady-tachy syndrome when presence or increased risk of symptomatic bradycardias exists

      6. Hypersensitive carotid sinus syndrome when presence or increased risk of symptomatic bradycardias exists

      7. Tachycardia prevention associated with long QT (torsades de pointes)

      8. Tachycardia termination (after drug failure)
         a) Atrial flutter
         b) AV nodal reentry
         c) Reciprocating tachycardia WPW syndrome
         d) Ventricular tachycardia

      9. Acute MI
         a) Newly acquired bifascicular BBB
         b) Newly acquired BBB plus transient complete AV block
         c) second degree AV block type II
         d) Complete AV block

      10. Diagnostic tool in electrophysiology studies

      11. Emergency treatment of permanent pacemaker malfunction

      12. Support during cardiac surgical procedures

      13. Used for electrolyte imbalance causing extreme bradycardia or blocks, i.e., hyperkalemia

      14. Heart block or bradycardia secondary to drug therapy with β-blockers, lidocaine, etc. (often in patients with previously well tolerated intranodal blocks)

      15. Prophylactically – prior to cardioversion/defibrillation in patients with sick sinus syndrome

      16. To improve hemodynamics in severe CHF

b. Overview of use of transvenous pacing

      1. Offers stable rate support

      2. Is easily tolerated by the patient

      3. It can be utilized to stabilize a clinical situation until the need for permanent pacing is established.

      4. Many situations requiring temporary pacing support are transient or have a correctable cause.

      5. A physician is required to insert a temporary pacing wire.

      6. It can be implemented at the bedside using ECG guidance or under fluoroscopy.

c. Specific equipment

      1. Pacing wire

          a) Balloon tipped or stiff electrode is inserted through one of the venous access routes

          b) Two wires needed if dual chamber pacing is to be utilized

      2. Pulse generator

          a) Battery powered external device

          b) Pace and sense in the atrium, ventricle or both

          c) Has an on/off switch

          d) Ability to pace demand, triggered and asynchronous modes

          e) Controls for rate, output, sensitivity and AV interval in dual chamber models

          f) Some have light indicators for pace/sense/battery (lights flash with each output pulse, detected P or R wave or low battery)

          g) Generator has positive and negative poles, two sets for atrium and ventricle in dual chamber models and one set of poles for single chamber pacing

          h) Extension cable may also be used

      3. Cardiac monitor

          a) Connected to patient with display of intrinsic rhythm and pacing operation

          b) Able to document with rhythm strips

      4. ECG machine

          a) Insertion done at bedside

          b) Connect to patient using limb leads

          c) Connect the V lead via alligator clamp to negative tip of the pacing wire (records changes in the intracardiac electrogram

> (ICE) during passage of pacing wire will guide placement of catheter into right ventricle)

5. Fluoroscopy
   a) Utilized to guide placement of wire into the appropriate chamber(s) to be paced if not utilizing ECG guidance
   b) Always use when a stiff catheter is used
6. Crash cart
   a) Defibrillator
   b) Essential medications
   c) Emergency supplies for codes
   d) Pericardiocentesis tray

d. Setup and procedure
   1. Explain procedure to patient and family when appropriate
   2. Obtain consent if possible from patient or family
   3. Establish patent IV line or venous access
   4. Prepare skin with betadine or follow hospital procedure
   5. Gather equipment
      a) Local anesthetic (lidocaine 1 or 2%)
      b) Pacemaker catheters (stiff wire, preformed J, balloon, etc.) This should be selected by physician
      c) Introducer for pacing catheter
      d) Sterile dressings, gloves, gown, towels, etc.
      e) Cutdown tray if needed
      f) Alligator clamps
      g) Suture material
      h) Generator – insert new battery and check for pacing operation of generator
   6. Attach ECG machine to patient
   7. Patient may be apprehensive and require sedation (check with physician)
   8. Assist physician as needed during insertion
   9. Monitor cardiac rhythm closely, watch for ventricular arrhythmias
   10. Monitor vital signs q 15 minutes or more frequently if patient is symptomatic
   11. After pacing catheter is in place, establish thresholds, establish pacing capture and establish settings for pacemaker (rate, output, sensitivity and mode)
   12. Dry sterile dressing applied after pacing wire is anchored by physician (one or two sutures) (check positive and negative connectors and note pacing capture on cardiac monitor)
   13. Obtain paced ECG for documentation of pacing rhythm

14. Obtain overpenetrated chest x-ray (lateral view if possible) to rule out pneumothorax and assess lead(s) position(s)

15. Bed rest initially, note physicians orders regarding increased activity

16. Record on nurses notes
    a) Time and date of insertion, type of wire used, generator settings including rate, mA, sensitivity and mode (DDD,VVI, etc.)
    b) Record threshold information (sensitivity and stimulation thresholds)
    c) Monitor strips recorded during insertion and every 4 hours post insertion

17. Secure generator to patient – note manufacturers recommendations and site of insertion to determine where generator will be secured to patient

e. Sites for insertion
Consideration must be given to the advantages and disadvantages of each approach and long-term pacing needs.

1. Brachial
    a) Attach BP cuff to upper arm, to make vein more prominent
    b) Basilic or median antecubital vein in antecubital fossa of right arm, usual site
    c) Needle and introducer inserted, needle removed
    d) Pacing catheter electrode advanced through sheath to right ventricle to establish pacing
    e) Immobilize the arm to prevent dislodging the wire
    f) Main advantage
        1) Compressible vessel, use for patients on anticoagulation
    g) Disadvantages
        1) Requires immobilization of the arm
        2) Limits activity
        3) Increased incidence of phlebitis and arterial or nerve injury (especially if cutdown used)

2. Femoral approach
    a) Fast, easy access to the right heart
    b) No cutdown required
    c) Fluoroscopy should be used (may have difficulty advancing pacing wire across the tricuspid valve from the inferior approach)
    d) Advantages
        1) Low incidence of phlebitis
        2) Catheter dislodgement
        3) Thrombus formation

e) Disadvantage
1) Limited movement
2) Usually immobilized or restricted to bed to prevent wire dislodgement or perforation of the myocardium

3. Internal jugular approach
   a) Reasonably easy access, commonly used (may use Trendelenburg to increase venous flow, dilate the vessel, and facilitate access)
   b) More direct access to right ventricle from right internal jugular
   c) Disadvantages
      1) Patient discomfort is greater with this approach
      2) Neck movement is difficult
      3) Pacing wire more easily dislodged
      4) Risks include:
         • air embolism
         • hematoma
         • infection and pneumothorax
         • brachial plexus injury

4. External jugular approach
   a) Easily accessed and compressed
   b) Disadvantages
      1) Tortuous vessel with valves, making advancement difficult (may result in perforation of the vessel)
      2) Intolerance due to position in neck of pacing wire
      3) Increased lead instability due to head movement

5. Subclavian vein approach
   a) Large vessel, can accommodate large or multiple wires (use of percutaneous introducer for venous access without cutdown)
   b) Easy access (can facilitate access with patient in Trendelenburg position)
   c) Advantages
      1) Left subclavian – easier passage and rapid positioning in right ventricular apex
      2) Can use ECG or fluoroscopy for insertion
      3) Stability of lead is good and well tolerated by patient (does not require patient immobilization)
   d) Disadvantages
      1) Risks due to air embolism, pneumothorax or hemothorax, subclavian artery perforation, infection or injury to the brachial nerve plexus

      2) This approach may not be the best choice if the vein will be used for permanent pacing

      *Note: Choice of sites must consider degree of emergency, other medical therapy (i.e., anticoagulation), length of time pacing may be needed, and consideration of need for permanent pacing

f. Troubleshooting problems

    1. Two major areas to consider – pacing and sensing

      a) Non-capture or loss of capture

        1) Due to lead dislodgement or fracture – reposition patient, increase pacing output, lead reposition by physician

        2) Threshold rise due to medications, fibrosis, etc. – increase pacing output, physician reposition wire

        3) Electrolyte imbalance – correct the imbalance

        4) Ischemia or MI at electrode site – increase output, physician may need to reposition pacing wire

        5) Low battery in pacing generator – change battery

      b) No output

        1) Low battery – change battery

        2) Lead not connected to generator – check all connections

        3) Unable to visualize pacing spike in current ECG lead – change ECG lead

        4) Lead fracture – physician replace pacing wire

        5) Pacemaker generator in off position – check all settings, turn pacemaker generator to on position

        6) Output too low – increase output (mA)

        7) Generator may be oversensing – check for muscle interference and EMI

      c) Stimulation of diaphragm

        1) Output too high – decrease output, change position of patient, physician reposition lead wire

        2) Possible perforation – obtain 12 lead ECG and chest x-ray, and if available, tip electrogram

      d) Undersensing – not sensing intrinsic beats

        1) Due to lead dislodgement – obtain chest x-ray, 12 lead ECG. Physician reposition or replace pacing wire

        2) Due to low sensitivity setting of pulse generator – increase sensitivity

        3) Due to low battery – check all connections, replace battery

        4) Due to a lead fracture – obtain 12 lead ECG and chest x-ray, physician replace pacing lead wire

        5) Due to pacemaker refractory period – not sensing APCs or VPCs (too close to be sensed)

    e) Oversensing – pacemaker sensing something other than intrinsic beats (muscle movement – sensing other chamber activity, cross-talk)

        1) Due to sensing of P/T waves – may need to decrease sensitivity

        2) Electromagnetic interference (EMI) – find source of the interference and eliminate

        3) Due to myopotentials – decrease sensitivity

        4) Lead fracture – physician replace lead wire

g. Special considerations

  1. Defibrillation and cardioversion

    a) Most manufacturers do not require disconnection of the pulse generator, up to 400 joules

    b) Disconnecting the generator may prevent diverting current from the heart to the generator

  2. Potential danger for inducing VT/VF

    a) Greatest if there is undersensing in the presence of acute cardiac ischemia, digoxin toxicity, and hypokalemia

  3. Stimulation and sensing thresholds should be assessed daily (thresholds may increase over time)

  4. Temporary transvenous pacing may be contraindicated

    a) In patients who are immune-compromised

    b) In patients with tricuspid valve prosthesis

    c) In patients receiving thrombolytic therapy (if necessary to use transvenous pacing, must use a compressible venous access)

h. Considerations for use with:

  1. Acute myocardial infarction

    a) Inferior wall MI – temporary pacing for sinus node dysfunction, to treat hypotension, heart failure, AV block, ischemia, or arrhythmias, to increase cardiac output and decrease cardiac ischemia due to decreased blood flow from low heart rates

    b) Anterior wall MI – with development of AV block, pacing may be necessary to prevent hemodynamic compromise

    c) Alternating bilateral bundle branch blocks in acute MI requires pacing due to high risk of complete AV block

    d) Some blocks or infarct-related conduction disorders may require temporary pacing

  2. Sick sinus syndrome (SSS), sinus node disease (due to coronary artery disease), sclerodegenerative disorders, cardiomyopathies

      a) Use temporary pacing if cause unknown and patient is symptomatic

      b) When attempting cardioversion in patients with SSS

      c) Use if patient on medications that may worsen SSS, temporarily until condition is resolved due to the medications or until permanent pacing is determined to be necessary

      d) For control of tachyarrhythmias associated with sick sinus syndrome

   3. For control of cardiac rhythms

      a) Can be useful in the diagnosis of rhythms

      b) Can be used for the treatment of suppression of arrhythmias VT (especially torsade) or PAT

      c) Treatment of arrhythmias occurring during cardiac catheterization procedures

      d) Treatment of arrhythmias not responsive to drug therapy

      e) For suspected prolonged bradyrhythms after cardioversion or if DC cardioversion may be dangerous to the patient (digoxin toxicity)

      f) Overdrive pacing (especially useful in torsade de pointes)

      g) Burst pacing – (pacing the ventricle 4–15 extrastimulus, 30 or more beats faster than the tachy rate, or using timed ventricular extrastimulus

 i. Electrical safety precautions – Also refer to Part One, Chapter 8, Safety

   1. Review

      a) All invasive temporary pacing has the potential to deliver a shock directly to the heart along the pacing wire

      b) Electric shock can cause atrial or ventricular fibrillation

      c) Follow all recommended electric safety precautions

2. Esophageal cardiac pacing

 a. Overview of transesophageal pacing – introduced in 1957

   1. It is simple, quick to initiate, and safer than endocardial pacing

   2. Particularly useful in infants and children when venous access is often difficult

   3. Increased interest in transesophageal pacing as a non-invasive diagnostic therapeutic and investigational technique

   4. Uniform success with atrial transesophageal pacing for termination of SVT and atrial flutter due to close proximity of the esophagus to the atrium

   5. Only variable success with ventricular esophageal pacing

 b. Indications for use

   1. Emergency pacing for acute treatment of bradyarrhythmias or sinus arrest in patients with an intact sinus node

2. Induction and termination of SVTs for diagnostic and therapeutic purposes (primary use)
3. Conversion of atrial flutter to RSR or other more hemodynamically stable rhythm in both children and adults
4. Elective induction of atrial fibrillation and flutter in patients with WPW, for assessment of ventricular response and prognosis
5. Assessment of the presence and severity of coronary artery disease
6. Control of heart rate during cardiac imaging studies (echocardiography, radionuclide ventriculography and thallium scintigraphy)
7. Assessment of parameters in the conduction system dealing with AV nodal refractoriness and sinus node recovery times
8. Assessment of the efficacy of antiarrhythmic and antianginal medications
9. Inhibition of VVI pacemakers to analyze the intrinsic cardiac rhythm and assessment of improper electrical outputs of ICD during SVT

c. Specific equipment
   1. Esophageal electrode (bipolar electrode recommended)
      a) Pill electrode
         1) Swallowed by the patient
         2) Technician or nurse gradually releases the wires
         3) Capsule dissolves
         4) Peristalsis lowers the electrode into the esophagus
      b) Balloon electrode (not commercially available at present)
         1) Inserted through nares
         2) Consists of one or more inflatable balloons
         3) Balloons inflated with air in esophagus. This, in theory, decreases the distance between the pacing wire and cardiac muscle, less current is needed for pacing and less discomfort to the patient
   2. Esophageal cardiac stimulator – special stimulator to provide:
      a) Constant current pulses of at least 30 mA, and pulse widths of at least 10 msec, for successful atrial pacing
      b) Stimulator must be capable of output voltages of 60 volts (be sure one is not pacing the ventricle).
      c) Rate control should adjust to 600 ppm (for atrial flutter termination in infants) to 200 ppm for other circumstances.
      d) Standard temporary generator will not work because energy output is not high enough.
   3. ECG machine and monitoring equipment for position assessment of electrode and to assess and document patient's rhythm
   4. Crash cart and defibrillator

d. Set up and procedure
  1. Prepare conscious patient
    a) Explain procedure
    b) Acquaint the patient with the particular sensation experienced with esophageal pacing, pace at low-current levels until the patient experiences the feeling. Stop the pacing to insure the immediate cessation of symptoms (done after electrode is in place)
    c) Prepare the patient for the possibility of diaphragmatic stimulation. Coughing and hiccoughing may occur depending on the position of the electrode
  2. Patient instructions
    a) Patient instructed to swallow capsule containing the electrode, with water

e. Complications and safety precautions
  1. Minimal esophageal damage has been noted in a few cases (epithelial erosion with pacing for long durations)
  2. Atrial fibrillation may be induced by rapid esophageal pacing with the possibility of rapid ventricular response in patients with WPW
  3. Rare phrenic pacing or brachial plexus stimulation has been observed in infants
  4. Patients complain of "pulsatial heartburn" (disappears with termination of pacing)
  5. Esophageal pacing should not be used in patients with esophageal disorders
  6. Patients complain of excessive pain and skeletal muscle stimulation (patient may swallow viscous lidocaine after electrode is positioned). Analgesia or sedation may be appropriate in the conscious patient
  7. With any pacing method, there is a risk for arrhythmias and necessary precautions should be taken (crash cart, emergency medications, and defibrillation should be available)

3. Epicardial cardiac pacing
  a. Overview
    1. Surgery performed on the heart has the potential to cause conduction disturbances both of a temporary or permanent nature
    2. Heart block may be noted intraoperatively or early postoperatively. Ventricular or AV sequential pacing may be needed to maintain hemodynamic stability
    3. Temporary pacing wires (thin stainless steel wires coated with Teflon) are routinely attached during surgery to the epicardial surface of the atrium and one may be placed on the right ventricle

    4. The wires are brought through the chest wall and sutured to the skin.

    5. An easy method of temporary pacing used postoperatively only:

        a) To overdrive and terminate arrhythmias

        b) To increase cardiac output by increasing heart rate

        c) To aid in the diagnosis of arrhythmias, through use of epicardial electrograms

        d) Can be used safely with digoxin related arrhythmias

        e) Used for the postoperative treatment of medication resistant arrhythmias

b. Indications for use

    1. Post-open heart surgery in patients with potential for AV blocks or other arrhythmias that may require temporary pacing

    2. Postoperatively in patients that may require increased cardiac output

    3. In patients post-open heart surgery (corrective or palliative) for congenital heart disease

    4. For back-up pacing

    5. For diagnosis of arrhythmias by epicardial electrograms

c. Specific equipment

    1. Pacing wires – already in place postoperatively (if not in use, should be insulated and protected from microshocks)

    2. AV sequential demand pulse generator or DDD generator with:

        a) Atrial and ventricular positive and negative output terminals

        b) Controls for atrial and ventricular output

        c) Ventricular rate and sensitivity control

        d) AV interval control

        e) DDD has similar control settings as a permanent unit

        f) Off and on switch

    3. Generator used for asynchronous atrial or ventricular pacing, demand ventricular pacing, AV sequential pacing, dual chambered pacing, paired atrial stimulation, and rapid atrial stimulation

    4. Cardiac monitoring equipment

    5. Crash cart and defibrillator

d. Set up and procedure

    1. Small gauge insulated wire with a straight needle or blunt pin at distal end – curved needle at proximal end

        a) If unipolar electrode is used, a surface ground wire or needle implanted in skin is needed (for pacing). Avoid using the other chamber's wire as a ground.

        b) If bipolar electrode is used

1) It provides both unipolar and bipolar electrograms
2) Offers back-up in case of failure of one wire
3) Is more comfortable for the patient

2. Atrial and ventricular electrodes are traditionally located
   a) Atrial – to the right of the sternum
   b) Ventricular – to the left of the sternum
3. Sites are protected from infection with providon-iodine ointment and small dressing
4. Electrodes are individually wrapped in a glove or in barrel of a plastic syringe and covered with gauze taped to the chest wall
5. Site and electrodes must be kept dry at all times
6. To initiate atrial pacing, to diagnose or treat transient arrhythmias:
   a) Atrial electrodes are connected to pulse generator (use gloves to prevent microshocks)
   b) With bipolar electrodes, one wire is connected to positive terminal, the other to negative terminal
   c) With unipolar electrodes, atrial wire is connected to negative terminal and a skin electrode to the positive terminal (with atrial pacing, negative and positive are less relevant than with ventricular pacing)
   d) The output (mA) and rate are set as ordered (stimulation thresholds are usually obtained and usual procedure for initiation of pacing is followed)
7. Rapid atrial pacing – used to overdrive most atrial dysrhythmias (except atrial fibrillation, sinus tachycardia and some types of atrial flutter)
   a) Attach pacing wires as above to pulse generator
   b) Achieve capture at rate higher than intrinsic atrial rate
   c) Maintain higher rate for brief period, then terminate pacing or quickly reduce pacing rate
8. Ventricular pacing – used to treat transient arrhythmias
   a) To initiate ventricular pacing, the ventricular electrode(s) are connected to pulse generator using same procedure as used for atrial pacing
   b) Rapid ventricular pacing can be instituted to overdrive VT by following same procedure used for trial pacing
9. AV Sequential pacing – the most commonly used mode of temporary pacing postoperatively after cardiac surgery
   a) To initiate AV sequential pacing, attach atrial electrodes to appropriate terminals of the pulse generators
   b) Atrial rate, AV interval, and output is set for each chamber.

(Thresholds are obtained and values are set with appropriate safety margins)

   c) Some pulse generators are unable to sense atrial activity and DVI mode must be used (atrial rate must exceed intrinsic rate)

10. Reevaluate patient as patient stabilizes. Intrinsic rate may now exceed the programmed rate and pacing needs and parameters may need to be adjusted

11. Removal of epicardial electrodes
    a) Performed at bedside (usually 4 days postop)
    b) Anchoring sutures are removed
    c) Physician gently pulls wires, expecting minimal resistance
    d) Dry sterile dressing applied as per hospital policy
    e) Patient should be observed for signs and symptoms of cardiac tamponade
    f) Watch for signs and symptoms of infection
    g) Prevent microshocks by insulating terminals from shocks and moisture
    h) Patient to remain on bed rest for 6 hours post-removal

e. Troubleshooting problems
   1. If pacing is required and there is failure to stimulate
      a) No output
         1) Check if pacer is on
         2) Check output dial
         3) Check battery
         4) Check dislodgement of pacing wire
         5) Pacemaker generator may be undersensing or oversensing
   2. If pacing is required and there is failure to capture
      a) May be due to increasing stimulation thresholds – may need to increase output (mA)
      b) Lead may be fractured or dislodged
      c) May be due to perforation – check signs of cardiac tamponade, including pacing of the diaphragm
      d) Check battery status and parameters on pulse generator (have extra pulse generator available)
   3. If pacing is required and there is failure to sense
      a) May be due to EMI (some generators will revert to asyncronous operation)
      b) If utilizing the DDD mode, watch for cross talk possibility, or if unipolar, watch for possibility of myopotential inhibition
      c) May need to reevaluate and adjust sensitivity settings

f. Special considerations

    1. Prevention of electrical shocks from electrical hazards is extremely important with the use of epicardial wires

        a) Wear gloves when handling pacing wires

        b) Keep moisture from wires and skin

        c) Insulate wires and all connections to temporary wires with insulated nonconductive moisture proof material such as a disposable glove

        d) Ground all electrical equipment that comes in contact with the patient (encourage use of battery powered equipment to the patient)

        e) Keep extra pacemaker generator and battery at bedside in case of failure

B. Emergency

    1. Transthoracic cardiac pacing (rarely used)

      a. Overview

        1. Used traditionally as a final desperate measure in emergency situations

        2. It involves puncture of the myocardial wall with a long needle, introduced through the skin

        3. The pacing catheter can be introduced into the ventricular chamber of the heart through the needle

        4. Rapid method of initiating pacing, but generally unsuccessful and difficult to position the pacing wire into the ventricular cavity (reason for unsuccessful statistics has been due to utilization after the patient had failed to respond to chronotropic or inotropic agents)

        5. Not generally utilized today due to improvements in other invasive and noninvasive methods of pacing

      b. Indications for use

        1. Usually in emergency situations for patients with bradyasystolic cardiac arrest

      c. Specific equipment

        1. Pacing wire – includes

           a) Transthoracic pacing catheter

           b) Needle, long enough to penetrate chest wall to myocardium

           c) Connecting cable (all three items usually contained in transthoracic pacing kit)

        2. Battery powered pulse generator with positive and negative pole connections

3. ECG monitor connected to patient to assess intrinsic and pacing rhythms
4. Crash cart and defibrillator

d. Set up and procedure
   1. Explain procedure to patient and family when appropriate
   2. Monitor vital signs and cardiac rhythm
   3. Clean area with appropriate antibacterial agent
   4. Approach to consider for placement of percutaneous transthoracic pacemakers
      a) Fifth intercostal space, 6 cm left of midsternal line
      b) Fifth intercostal space, 4 cm left of midsternal line
      c) Fifth intercostal space, parasternal line
      d) Sub-zyphoid toward left shoulder
      e) Sub-zyphoid toward sternal notch
      (Note that free withdrawal of blood does not guarantee ventricular placement of the pacing wire)
   5. After pacing wire is placed in the ventricle, attach positive and negative terminals to the pacemaker generator.
      a) Adjust rate
      b) Adjust sensitivity
      c) Adjust output to obtain capture
   6. Document capture on ECG and generator settings
   7. Dry sterile dressing applied as per guidelines for your institution

e. Complications
   1. Puncture of lung – liver
   2. Puncture of internal mammary vessel
   3. Lacerations of RCA and LAD
   4. Air embolism
   5. Bacterial endocarditis
   6. Thrombus formation
   7. Myocardial infarction due to coronary artery damage
   8. Pericardial tamponade
   9. Improper position of pacing wire (free withdrawal of blood does not insure proper position in ventricle) pacing wire could be located in inferior vena cava, right atrium or pulmonary artery

2. Transcutaneous pacing
   a. Overview
      1. Introduced in 1981 by Dr. Paul Zoll
      2. Two large electrodes with non-metallic inner surfaces transmit electrical stimulus of low and uniform current across the skin

3. Some units reduce the skeletal muscle contractions by using a pulse duration of 40 msec

4. Provides non-invasive VVI pacing, usually effective, and easily applied (patient tolerance varies and sedation should be available)

5. Physician not necessary for application (nurse or other trained personnel can initiate pacing)

6. Included in ACLS protocol

b. Indications for use

1. Bradycardia or asystole of any origin

2. Stokes Adams disease
   a) Reflex vagal stimulation
   b) Drug induced

3. Overdrive suppression of ventricular ectopic activity and tachycardia

4. Stand-by for patients at risk for AV block during acute myocardial infarction or ischemia (especially if thrombolytics used)

5. Stand-by during anesthesia

6. Stand-by during pacemaker procedures, especially during generator replacements

7. For cardiac arrest (included in ACLS protocol)

c. Specific equipment

1. Non-invasive pacemaker with the ability to adjust rate and mA (output)

2. Cardiac monitor – (adjustment needed to use in-house equipment due to output stimulus that will saturate the bedside equipment and ECG machine when pacing) assessment of rhythm, pacing capture, and documentation strips are most accurate using generator's printout and screen

3. Self adhesive pacing electrodes
   a) Applied to clean dry skin
   b) Position in left anterior/posterior position, or according to manufacturer's recommendations (position to provide the shortest current pathway to the heart)

4. Crash cart – with essential medications, supplies and defibrillators

d. Set up and procedure

1. Explain procedure to patient and family when appropriate

2. Connect patient to monitor and obtain rhythm strip

3. Apply adhesive pacing electrodes (if excessive hair, clip – do not shave the area – tiny nicks in the skin may cause discomfort)

4. Connect pacing cable to non-invasive pacemaker

5. Select demand pacing mode, select pacing rate
6. Select the output (mA) until stimulation is effective. Check for pulses to assess hemodynamic effectiveness (pacing capture is usually evidenced by wide complex QRS and preceded by spike on generator's monitor)
7. Assess patient comfort level (many conscious patients require sedation)
8. Document
   a) Time pacing initiated
   b) Current required to capture
   c) Pacing rate
   d) Evaluation of patient response
   e) Medications used
   f) Date and time pacing terminated
9. Follow electrical safety guidelines for pacemakers to prevent microshocks

e. Troubleshooting problems
   1. No electrical capture
      a) Increase current
      b) Check pacing electrode positions
      c) Correct electrolyte imbalances
      d) Reposition electrodes
      e) Check for skeletal muscle twitching (if none present, check battery status, plug machine into outlet if appropriate, check all connections, if unsuccessful, obtain another generator)
      f) If patient has prolonged cardiac arrest, or extensive myocardial damage, patient may not be viable and no electrical capture will be possible
   2. Electrical capture, but no mechanical cardiac output
      a) Too much time has elapsed and the patient may not be viable
   3. Pacemaker unable to sense
      a) Reposition ECG electrodes, obtain new lead position, if needed to obtain better complexes
      b) If noisy signal, reposition electrodes, check for sources of EMI
   4. Discomfort during pacing
      a) Use sedation or analgesia
      b) Keep output (mA) at level of capture, not above, to minimize patient discomfort from pacing. Verify capture is occurring.

f. Special considerations
   1. Use of temporary transcutaneous pacing in neonates

   a) Check area under electrodes frequently for burns
   b) Use of shin electrodes be kept to a minimum
2. Patients with underlying conditions (pulmonary emphysema and patients with large pectoral muscles) may require high thresholds for stimulation and therefore experience strong painful contractions
3. If ventricular fibrillation occurs, defibrillate promptly (consult manufacturer's recommendations for use during defibrillation)
4. Defibrillation paddles should be placed in the standard apex-sternum position. Do not place on pacing electrodes
5. Care should be taken to wipe off any excess gel that may be on the skin surface to avoid arching and burns. (If unit has both pacing and defibrillation capabilities, the electrodes can be used for both functions, and no paddles are needed.)

References

Bartecchi CE, DE Mann. Temporary Cardiac Pacing. Chicago: Precept Press, Inc., 1990.

Bass L, Meissner J. Cardiovascular care. Illustrated Manual of Nursing Practice. Springhouse: Springhouse. 1991.

Benson WD. Transesophageal electrocardiography and cardiac pacing: state of the art. Circulation. 75: (supl III):4:86–90. 1987.

Benson WD, et al. Transesophageal cardiac pacing: history, Application, technique. Clin Prog Pacing Electrophysiol. 2:4.360–372. 1984.

Benson WD. Transesophageal pacing and electrocardiography in the neonate. Clin Perinatol. 3:619–631. 1988.

Brodine WN. Evaluation of pacemaker function. Hospit Med. October:64–86. 1986.

Clinton JE, et. al. Emergency non-invasive external cardiac pacing. J Emerg Med. 2:155–162. 1985.

Dunn D, JJ Gregory. Non-invasive temporary pacing: experience in a community hospital. Heart Lung. 18:23–28. 1989.

Gallagher JJ. Esophageal pacing: diagnostic and therapeutic uses. In Modern Cardiac Pacing. S. Barold (Ed.). Mt. Kisco: Futura Publishing Co, Inc., 1985.

Gould B, Marshall A. Non-invasive temporary pacemakers. PACE. 11: 1331–1334. 1988.

Grenvik A, Hennesy R. Critical Care Cardiology. New York: Churchhill Livingstone. 1989.

Guarnerio M, et. al. Transesophageal atrial pacing: a first choice technique in atrial flutter therapy. Am Heart J. 117:6.24–52. 1989.

Hakki A-Hadi. Ideal Cardiac Pacing. Philadelphia: WB Saunders Co., 1984.

Hurst J. The Heart. 6th edition. New York: McGraw Hill Book Co. 1986.

Jenkins JM, et al. Use of the pill electrode for transesophageal atrial facing. PACE. 8:512–527. 1985.

Littleford, PO. Physiological temporary pacing: techniques and indications. In modern cardiac pacing. S. Barold, (Ed.). Mt Kisco: Futura Publishing Co, Inc., 231–55. 1985.

Phillips B, et al. TAP-Transesophageal atrial pacing. Med Electron: December. 1987.

Silver M, Goldschlager N. Temporary transvenous cardiac pacing in the critical care setting. Chest. 93:607–613. 1988.

Underhill S et al. Cardiac Nursing. 2nd edition. Philadelphia: Lippencott. 1989.

Warnowicz-Papp, MA. The pacemaker patient and the electromagnetic environment. Clin Prog Pacing Electrophysiol. 1:2:166–176. 1983.

Zoble RG. Cardiac Pacing: Critical Care Cardiology. New York: Churchill Livingstone, 102–126. 1989.

Zoll PM, et al. External non-invasive temporary cardiac pacing: clinical trials. Circulation. 71:5:937–944. 1985.

CHAPTER 17

Pacemaker Implantation

John Gentzel

Subsection:
A. Pre-implantation
B. Implantation

Clinical assessment prior to the implantation of a permanent cardiac pacing system is imperative. Need for device therapy must be clearly documented in order for most insurance companies to reimburse payment. Typically most cardiac pacing is performed for the necessity of back-up bradycardia support. (Refer to Part One, Chapter 9).

Current pulse generator selection is complex, at best. Today's devices are multiprogrammable and add to the confusion in selecting the device which best suits the individual patient. Careful attention must be given to the pacing prescription. Single chamber versus dual chamber; rate modulation versus none, are all important considerations. (Refer to Part Two, Chapter 13).

Cardiac pacemaker implantation has evolved over the years from thoracotomy to simple percutaneous technique. The advancement came due to lead design, placement technique, and overall design of the pulse generator itself. Early models where quite cumbersome, and today's smaller devices can be implanted easily in the region of the pectoral muscle group. Although newer implant techniques are performed, other methods may become necessary to consider based on individual needs.

Objectives

1. Assess patient/device need.
2. Evaluate electrolyte balance and drug toxicity.

From: Schurig L. *Educational Guidelines: Pacing and Electrophysiology*. Armonk, NY: Futura Publishing Co, Inc, © 1994.

3. Proper physician documentation, and supporting documentation, e.g., 12 lead, Holter monitoring report.
4. Identify proper procedure coding (CPT-4), and master diagnosis code (ICD-9-CM)
5. Identify surgical asepsis.
6. Understand the meaning and importance of threshold measurement and intracardiac electrograms.
7. Identify possible complications associated with pacemaker implantation, and the need for emergent procedures.

Education Content

A. Pre-Implantation
   1. Clinical assessment
      a. Patient
         1. Age
         2. Size
         3. Evaluate activities of daily living
         4. Underlying cardiac rhythm
         5. Underlying medical/health state
         6. Future needs of the patient
      b. Diagnostic evaluation
         1. 12 lead ECG
         2. 24 hour Holtor monitor
         3. Cardiac event recorder/monitor
         4. Electrolyte balance
            a) Potassium
            b) Magnesium
         5. Concurrent drug levels
            a) Anti-arrhythmics
         6. Electrophysiologic evaluation
      c. Device selection
         1. Single chamber (SSI)
            a) Atrial (AAI/AAT)
            b) Ventricular (VVI/VVT)
         2. Dual chamber (DDD,DDI,VDD)
         3. Rate modulated
            a) Single chamber (SSIR)
               1) atrial (AAIR)
               2) ventricular (VVIR)
            b) Dual chamber (DDDR, DDIR)
   2. Patient education pre-implant
      a. Informed consent
         1. Explain need for device
         2. Explain operative site
         3. Describe procedure
            a) Location
               1) OR
               2) Cath lab

           3) EP lab

           4) Special procedure room

       b) Duration

       c) Anesthesia

           1) local

           2) general

       d) Recovery immediate post-implant

   4. Follow-up requirements

3. Documentation of indications for pacing

   a. Written indication of need

      1. Patient symptoms

       a) Syncope/near syncope

       b) Congestive heart failure

       c) Chronotropic incompetence

      2. ECG findings

       a) 12 lead

       b) Holtor monitor

       c) Cardiac event recordings

       d) Telemetry strips

      3. Laboratory findings

       a) Electrolyte balance

       b) Drug levels

      4. Documentation recorded

       a) Physicians' progress notes

       b) History and physical

       c) Laboratory reports

       d) Nurses' notes

       e) Graphic charts

   b. Documentation/correlation for billing purposes (concept of a common file between hospital and physician bills)

      1. CPT-4 coding

       a) Relationship to physician billing

       b) Relationship to outpatient charges

      2. ICD-9-CM coding

       a) Relationship to in-hospital charges

      3. DRG coding

       a) Relationship to in-hospital charges

B. Implantation

   1. Instrumentation

a. Environmental considerations
   1. Area lends itself to aseptic environment
   2. Emergency code cart
   3. Defibrillator
   4. Cardiac monitors
   5. High-grade fluoroscopy
   6. Electrocautery
b. Procedure area
   1. Surgical suite
   2. Cardiac cath lab
   3. Electrophysiology lab
   4. Special procedures lab
c. Instrumentation
   1. Drapes
   2. Surgical instruments
      a) Stainless steel back table (1)
      b) Basin 250 cc (1)
      c) Basin 100 cc (2)
      d) Hemostats (6)
      e) Mosquito clamp (4)
      f) Right angles (2)
      g) Needle holders (3)
      h) Retractors
         1) Army/Navy (2)
         2) Medium rakes (2)
         3) Senn retractor (2)
         4) Self retaining retractor
            • Gelpi (1)
            • Weitlander (1)
      i) Suture scissors (1)
      j) Metz (1)
      k) Vein lifter/pick (1)
      l) Knife handle(s) (2)
      m) Radiographic 4 × 4s (20)
      n) Lap sponges (10)
      o) Appropriate suture
      p) Appropriate size introducer(s)
2. Patient preparation
   a. Monitoring
      1. ECG

     a) Multiple monitors (> = 2)

     b) Lead configuration

       1) limb leads (easiest access)

     c) Cables for electrograms

  2. Blood pressure monitor (automatic)

  3. Pulse oximetry

  4. Oxygen administration

  5. Patients' level of comfort

     a) Anesthesia

     b) Sedation

       1) Evaluate level of consciousness

b. Site preparation

  1. In accordance with surgical asepsis

3. Implantation techniques (See also pediatric implantation)

  a. Indications for site choice

    1. Age of patient

    2. Concurrent surgery

    3. Physician preference

    4. Concurrent devices (i.e., prior ICD)

    5. Prior pacemaker implant

  b. Endocardial

    1. Cutdown method

    2. Percutaneous (transvenous)

      a) Retained guide wire technique

        1) 1 French size larger introducer than lead being used

    3. Epicardial

      a) Thoracic

        1) General anesthesia

        2) Performed in OR suite

        3) Concurrent surgery

      b) Epigastric (subxiphoid)

        1) General anesthesia

        2) Performed in OR suite

        3) Concurrent surgery

4. Implantation analysis

  a. Pacing system analyzer (PSA)

    1. Sterile cables

      a) Lead cables

      b) Pacemaker cables

  b. Threshold measurements

1. Atrial
    a) Sensing determination
        1) P wave amplitude
        2) Slew rate (optional)
    b) Capture threshold
        1) Set PSA to > = 10 ppm over intrinsic rate
        2) Set pulse duration to match pacemaker
        3) Decrement voltage
    c) Impedance measurement
        1) Know lead characteristics
            • Low-impedance leads
            • High-impedance leads
c. Ventricular threshold measurements
    1. Sensing determination
        a) R wave amplitude
        b) Slew rate (optional)
    2. Capture threshold
        a) Set PSA to > = 10 ppm over intrinsic rate
        b) Set pulse duration to match pacemaker
        c) Decrement voltage
    3. Impedance measurement
        a) Know lead characteristics
            1) Low-impedance leads
            2) High-impedance leads
d. Strength duration curves
    1. Pulse width
    2. Pulse amplitude
e. Special considerations
    1. Pacemaker syndrome
        a) Pace ventricle and note change in blood pressure
        b) Decreased blood pressure indicates pacemaker syndrome
    2. V-A conduction
        a) Pace ventricle, note activation in atrium
    3. Replacement/revision
        a) Follow basic steps outlined above
        b) Have appropriate wrenches available for pacemaker removal or lead revision
5. Complications
    a. Immediate to 24 hours
        1. Hematoma

   2. Pneumothorax
   3. Subclavian vein tear
   4. Cardiac tamponade
      a) Lead perforation
   5. Lead dislodgement
      a) Failure to capture
   6. Induced arrhythmias
   7. Pectoral or diaphragmatic twitching
   8. Failure to sense
   9. Air embolus
   b. >24 hours to discharge
      1. Same as 1–9
      2. Infection
6. Troubleshooting
   a. Insure proper connections
      1. On PSA to leads
      2. On leads to pacemaker
   b. Proper battery voltage on PSA
7. Documentation of implant data
   a. Patient demographics per hospital protocol
      1. Indications
      2. Access
      3. Complications
      4. Date of procedure
   b. Lead data
      1. Manufacturer
      2. Model number
      3. Serial number
      4. Mode of fixation
         a) Active
         b) Passive
      5. Endocardial
      6. Epicardial
      7. Polarity
         a) Unipolar
         b) Bipolar
   c. Pacemaker generator data
      1. Manufacturer
      2. Model number
      3. Serial number

4. Polarity
   a) Unipolar
   b) Bipolar
   c) Unipolar/bipolar programmable
5. Pacemaker settings at implant

d. Previous pacemaker
   1. Date of implant
   2. Model number
   3. Serial number
   4. Indication for removal
   5. Disposition of the removed device

e. Staff present
   1. Implanting physician
   2. Assistant
   3. Scrub nurse/technologist
   4. Circulator
   5. Analysis performed by
   6. Following or referring physician

8. Emergency procedures
   a. Bradycardia support
      1. Pharmacologic support
         a) Atropine
         b) Isuproterenol
      2. Temporary pacing
         a) Non-invasive (transcutaneous)
         b) Invasive

   b. Chest tube
      1. Pneumothorax
      2. Hemothorax

   c. Cardiac tamponade
      1. Pericardiocentesis

References

Barold SS, Mugica J. New Perspectives in Cardiac Pacing. 2nd edition. Mt. Kisco: Futura Publishing Co, Inc. 1991.

Barold SS. Modern Cardiac Pacing. Mt. Kisco: Futura Publishing Co, Inc. 1985.

Furman S, Hayes D, Holmes D. A Practice of Cardiac Pacing. 2nd edition. New York: Futura Publishing Co, Inc. 1989.

CPT 1992. American Medical Association. Chicago, Il.

International Classification of Diseases, 9th Revision, 4th Edition Clinical Modification. 1,2: 1992. Los Angeles: Practice Management Information Corporation. 1992

Suggested Readings

Higano ST, Hayes DL, Spittell PC. Facilitation of subclavian-introducer technique with contrast venography. PACE. 13(5):681–684. 1990.

Moak E. Perioperative implications of pacemaker implantation. Today's OR Nurse. 12(5):19–23. 1990.

Molina JE. New technique for pacemaker implantation in the upper chest of children and women. Ann Thorac Surg 51:(6):992–995. 1991.

Samet P, el-Sherif N. Cardiac Pacing and Electrophysiology. 3rd edition. Philadelphia: WB Saunders, Co. 1991.

CHAPTER 18

Pacemaker Follow-up

Jennifer Fraser

Subsection:
A. Rationale, Goals, and Methods of Pacemaker Follow-up
B. Logistics of a Clinical Follow-up Center
C. Specific Follow-up Protocols
D. Pacemaker Programming
E. Identification and Management of Pacemaker Malfunction
F. Management of Recalls Advisories

Centralization of pacemaker patient follow-up allows clinical centers to take advantage of dedicated resources, including the expertise of associated professionals and pacing physicians. This section will describe the reasons, methods, and usefulness of organized pacemaker follow-up. The reader will be provided with the necessary information to develop policies and procedures, specific for their institution, for pacemaker follow-up.

Objectives

1. Understand the reasons for an organized approach to pacemaker follow-up.
2. Plan the follow-up management for a population of pacemaker patients.
3. Assign appropriate equipment, personnel, and resources for the operation of pacemaker follow-up.

From: Schurig L. *Educational Guidelines: Pacing and Electrophysiology.* Armonk, NY: Futura Publishing Co, Inc, © 1994.

4. Institute safe, effective, and efficient protocols for the assessment of all types of pacemakers and patients.

5. Develop a patient education plan that incorporates all aspects of pacemaker function and care.

6. Develop an appropriate schedule of follow-up for all pacemaker types and for all stages of pacemaker longevity.

7. Understand the importance of an accurate, complete, and easily accessed method of pacemaker follow-up documentation.

8. Describe the complications of cardiac pacing and how they can best be diagnosed and treated.

9. Understand the sequence of actions and the responsibilities relating to the recall or advisory of a pacemaker or a lead.

10. Understand the uses and the safe implementation of diagnostic and therapeutic pacemaker programming.

Education Content

A. Rationale, Goals, and Methods of Pacemaker Follow-up

1. Reasons for organized pacemaker follow-up

  a. Routine follow-up allows pacemaker battery EOS (end-of-service) to be predicted and thereby allows elective and non-urgent replacement.

  b. Effective follow-up identifies pacemaker system abnormalities and allows prompt treatment of the abnormalities.

  c. Effective follow-up allows the non-invasive adjustment of the pacemaker to maximize longevity and to optimize patient function. The paced electrocardiogram is analyzed, sensing and pacing thresholds are determined and a pacemaker prescription is developed utilizing the full range of programmable options.

  d. Continual observation of pacemaker function reduces the incidence of sudden and unpredicted pacemaker system failure and allows detection of suboptimal performance.

  e. Follow-up clinics allow the accumulation of a data bank on individual patients, on various models of leads and pacemakers (to monitor reliability) and on the investigation of new devices.

  f. A pacemaker clinic may provide a site for the training of medical and para-medical personnel.

2. Goals of pacemaker follow-up are to:

  a. Optimize device function consistent with the patient's clinical requirements

  b. Maximize pacemaker longevity while maintaining patient safety

  c. Minimize patient fear and anxiety through emotional support and education

  d. Verify proper and appropriate pacemaker function.

  e. Recognize, interpret and correct pacemaker problems prior to symptoms

  f. Detect pacemakers approaching end of battery service and replace them in a timely manner

  g. Act as a repository of pacemaker hardware, information, and technical expertise

  h. Record patient location and develop a means of notification of those patients should a recall or advisory occur

  i. Triage non-pacemaker related health problems to the appropriate place (e.g., family physician, emergency room, cardiologist, social worker, public health nurse, etc.)

  j. Develop statistical data that is specific for one clinic or that is part of a larger data base

3. Methods of pacemaker follow-up

   a. Direct evaluation and clinical examination

      1. Allows full assessment of the pacemaker through programming, patient questioning, observation and provocative testing

      2. Allows corrective action of the pacemaker through programming

      3. Allows a trusting relationship to develop between a patient and their family and follow-up staff

      4. Is time consuming, often inconvenient and expensive for staff and patient

   b. Transtelephonic monitoring (TTM)

      1. May be done as part of a pacemaker clinic or may be done through a commercial agency

      2. Efficient, convenient, economical and, readily accessible

      3. Lacks direct patient contact and relies on patient for the observation of symptoms

      4. May have problems with artifact and interference

      5. Patient must be seen for confirmation or correction of any problem

      6. Often most useful in patients who are immobile, infirmed or living in remote areas

      7. Allows a link between tertiary follow-up centers and remote clinics or physician offices

   c. Combined direct evaluation follow-up and transtelephonic monitoring

      1. Combines the benefits of clinical assessment with the convenience of TTM

B. Logistics of a Clinical Follow-up Center

  1. Human resources

   a. There is no standard training or common background for associated professionals (AP) involved in pacemaker follow-up. A number of sub-specialty health care providers are often involved in the implantation and the follow-up of pacemakers. These sub-specialties include: nurses, cardiovascular technologists, exercise physiologists, physician assistants, and others.

   b. Education of both associated professionals (AP) and physicians is frequently done by the manufacturers of pacemakers. The appropriateness of this, for other than specific product information, has been the subject of debate.

   c. Whatever the AP's educational background, she/he must have an understanding of cardiac physiology and be able to interpret patient symptoms. They must also be skilled in ECG rhythm interpretation and in cardiac emergency procedures. It is a further advantage for the AP to have a working knowledge of computer based technology.

    d. Many procedures related to the assessment of pacemaker function are delegated to the associated professional by the supervising physician. The scope and limitations of these acts, must be clearly defined in the procedure and policies of the institution.

2. Physical plant

    a. Pacemaker follow-up centers can be located in a department of their own or as part of a department with space shared for other activities.

    b. Adequate space must be provided for the following:

        1. Chart filing

        2. Patient reception and waiting

        3. Programmer storage (may be a significant amount of space)

        4. Private patient examination area

        5. Patient exercise area (corridor or flight of stairs)

        6. Patient and family teaching (video and written materials)

3. Equipment resources

    a. Minimal recommended equipment and clinical tools

        1. ECG strip chart recorder with real-time rhythm strip

        2. ECG display monitor

        3. Electronic measurement device for pulse duration and interval (digital interval timer)

        4. Magnets

        5. Programmers for all pacemakers implanted in the region and access to others through manufacturer's representative

        6. Technical information on the behavior of all implantable pacemakers whether implanted in that institution or not

    b. Recommended optional equipment

        1. 12 lead ECG recorder

        2. External pacemaker with skin electrodes and cables

        3. Oscilloscope to visualize pulse waveform (This is optional)

        4. Resuscitation equipment including defibrillator and transcutaneous pacemaker

        5. Solutions and sterile trays for the treatment of pacemaker wounds

    c. Support resources

        1. Transtelephonic receiving center

        2. Fluoroscopy and x-ray

        3. Ambulatory monitoring (event recorders)

        4. Exercise treadmill

        5. Tilt test laboratory

6. Echo-Doppler facility
7. Electrophysiology lab
8. Operating room
9. Computerized data base

4. Documentation
    a. Documentation of all aspects of pacemaker patient's care should be accessible 24 hours a day to health care workers
    b. Ideally, it should be computerized and used to:
        1. Store manufacturers' specifications and recommendations
        2. Store patient follow-up records
        3. Generate reports
        4. As an instrument of follow-up for analysis and programming
    c. Pacemaker follow-up records (computerized or manual) should include:
        1. Patient demographic information
        2. Location and contact of the referring physician
        3. Complete history and physical findings leading to implantation
        4. Operative notes and details of implantation
        5. Model and serial numbers of all previously and currently implanted hardware
        6. Specifications, warranty and technical information on all hardware
        7. Technical notes, advisories and recall information on any implanted hardware
        8. Patient notification of device recall or advisory
        9. Current programmed settings and any program changes, including the reason for programmed change
    d. Patients must be provided with identification and programmed settings of their pacemakers to provide sufficient information for any physician consulted.

C. Specific Follow-up Protocols

1. Determinants of follow-up schedule
    a. Health care economy and environment
    b. Patient distance from follow-up
    c. Duration of implant for both lead and pulse generator
    d. Reliability of implanted hardware
    e. Complexity of the pacemaker
    f. Patient dependency and general cardiovascular status
    g. Availability and utility of transtelephonic monitoring
    h. Recommended schedule and protocol

1. Predischarge; within the first week
   a) 12 lead ECG; free running and magnet
   b) Wound and pocket assessment
   c) Chest x-ray; PA and lateral
   d) Intracardiac electrogram (ICE) and/or marker channels; if available
   e) Diagnostic stimulation and sensing threshold determination
   f) Programming based on patient's status, on thresholds at implantation and on most current stimulation threshold, and on lead type
   g) Patient and family support and education
2. First outpatient visit; 4–8 weeks post-implant
   a) History and physical
   b) Rhythm strip with and without magnet
   c) Stimulation and sensing thresholds
   d) Dependency assessment
   e) Telemetry, event counts and electrograms
   f) Provocative maneuvers for muscle potential
   g) VA conduction tests
   h) Cross-talk testing
   i) Therapeutic programming of all parameters
   j) Patient and family education and support
3. Maintenance period (approximately 5 months)
   a) Full direct evaluation (as described above)
   b) May initiate TTM at 3 month intervals
   c) Perform direct evaluation at 1 year intervals for single chamber devices
   d) Perform direct evaluation at 6 month to 1 year interval for dual chamber and adaptive rate systems
4. Intensified follow-up
   a) TTM or direct evaluation at up to 1 month intervals

2. Components of direct clinical evaluation
   a. Review of patient's clinical history and device history:
      1. The pathophysiology of conduction disorder and the pre-implantation symptoms
      2. The number and age of the pacemaker and the lead
      3. Previous pacemaker complications
   b. Brief history, specific to cardiovascular system:
      1. Changes in cardiovascular status as revealed through change in symptoms

 2. Specific questions about symptoms reflecting decreased cerebral perfusion or cardiac output

 3. A return of pre-implantation symptoms may suggest malfunction or inappropriate mode selection

c. General health inquiry and medication review:
 1. Medications that directly affect pacemaker thresholds should be understood

 2. Patient medication errors may be noticed during routine inquiry

 3. Non-pacemaker health problems may be revealed and must be triaged in an appropriate manner

d. Physical assessment:
 1. Evaluation of the pocket for signs of infection or erosion (pain, swelling, erythema or tightly stretched skin)

 2. Evaluation of neck veins for evidence of distention or cannon waves

 3. Skin color and clinical signs of cardiac compensation

e. All available telemetry and diagnostic data:
 1. Available telemetry features of the pacemaker must be known

 2. Pacemaker memory contents may be: data placed in memory or data derived during pacemaker operation

 3. ECG interpretation channel is displayed with a surface ECG and may mark the pacing and sensing function of the pulse generator

 4. Programmed setting may be confirmed through telemetry

 5. Hardware identification including: battery status, battery voltage and impedance, the model and serial number

 6. Electrogram transmission indicates the quality of the signal the pacemaker senses and responds to

f. 12 lead ECG:
 1. Three simultaneous channels will optimize detection of the stimulus artifact and the atrial and ventricular depolarization

 2. Is useful to monitor axis shift and diagnose lead dislodgement

g. Free running ECG with electronic measurement:
 1. Allows visualization of the interaction of the pacemaker and the intrinsic rhythm at rest

 2. Allows precise measurement of rate, pulse duration and AV interval

 3. Generally provides sufficient information to determine capture and sensing

 4. Should be done while isometric exercise is performed to uncover myopotential inhibition or myopotential triggering

 5. Should be done continuously during threshold determination

    6. Programmer screen and printout can be used as an alternative to ECG in some models

h. Magnet application:

    1. A reed switch is activated to shut off demand function and cause asynchronous output

    2. Asynchronous output allows demonstration of the paced rhythm, even when the intrinsic rate exceeds the paced rate

    3. The magnet rate, pulse duration and mode are often indicators of battery status (ERI – Elective replacement, EOS – end-of-service)

    4. Applying a magnet over a pacemaker opens the telemetry link

    5. In some pacemakers, the initial magnet sequence is a crude threshold assessment

    6. Some devices reduce output in a cyclical fashion for threshold determination

    7. Some aspects of pacemaker behavior in the magnet mode are used to verify proper receipt of programming

    8. The application of a magnet to a pacemaker is generally accepted as a safe practice that may be performed by trained personnel

    9. There have been rare reports of magnet application inducing atrial fibrillation, ventricular tachycardia, and pacemaker mediated tachycardias (should be avoided in acute ischemia or infarction setting)

    10. Appropriate magnet response of the specific device being assessed must be understood from technical information provided

    11. Possible responses to magnet application include:

        a) Asynchronous pacing in single chamber devices

        b) Asynchronous pacing in both chambers in dual devices (usually)

        c) Asynchronous pacing for a specific number of beats following magnet removal (may do so at more than one rate)

        d) Asynchronous rate may be the same as programmed rate

        e) Asynchronous rate may be independent of programmed rate (usually faster)

        f) Some single and dual devices require that magnet response be programmed "on" before any response is seen

        g) The same device may respond with a different magnet rate dependent on the programmed mode

        h) Magnet application may begin an output threshold assessment (output decreases over a specified number of beats)

        i) Magnet rate may decrease as EOS approaches

      j) Use the reference manual for the device to understand the expected response to magnet application

i. Exercise or other maneuvers to alter rate or rhythm:

    1. Exercise will often raise the sinus rate to demonstrate pacemaker sensing or P wave tracking

    2. Valsalva or carotid sinus massage (CSM) will allow the observation of pacing when the pacemaker is inhibited

j. End-of-service (EOS)

    1. Most manufacturers' pacemakers monitor battery voltage to indicate battery depletion

    2. When battery voltage reaches a fixed minimal level, a signal of impending end-of-service is given

    3. EOS indicators may include

        a) Increase in escape interval (rate slowing)

        b) Change in magnet rate

        c) Increase in pulse width

        d) Mode changes

        e) Changes in threshold margin test

        f) Loss of rate responsive mode or antitachycardia mode

        g) Real-time telemetry

            1) Increasing battery impedance

            2) Decline in battery voltage

k. Dependency assessment:

    1. Threshold determination should begin with an assessment of pacemaker dependency

    2. Knowledge of pacemaker dependency influences patient management

        a) Who may program (e.g., physician or AP)

        b) Need for emergency equipment

        c) Management of recall

        d) Clinical management of patient during pulse generator or lead replacement

    3. Suggested scoring of dependency: (Cameron, DA Fraser JA – Toronto General Hospital 1984)

        1+ Intrinsic rhythm exceeds paced rate (>50 bpm)

        2+ Intrinsic rhythm visible with rate slowing or competition

        3+ • Fully paced at lowest programmed setting (40 bpm)

           • Intrinsic rate 30–50 bpm

        4+ Pacer inhibition results in no escape ventricular rhythm or one that is < 30 bpm

l. Diagnostic programming:

    1. To determine normal or abnormal pacemaker function and gather data to determine the pacemaker prescription

m. Therapeutic programming to fill pacemaker prescription:

    1. Permanent changes made to the pacemaker based on the findings of diagnostic programming and on clinical need

    2. Must be recorded in the patient record

n. Waveform analysis:

    1. Requires a specialized oscilloscope or specially designed follow-up equipment

    2. Is useful in detecting lead insulation failure or pending lead wire fracture

o. Final interrogation of the pacemaker:

    1. Must be done to ensure the pacemaker program was entered and received by the pacemaker correctly

    2. To provide documentation for the patient and the chart regarding programmed settings

p. Documentation of all findings and report to referring physician.

q. Scheduling of subsequent follow-up visits:

    1. Providing patients with their subsequent follow-up appointment each time they are seen is efficient and results in low lost-to-follow-up rate

r. Patient and family support and education

    1. Must begin prior to implant and extend throughout the patient's life

3. Considerations for rate-adaptive follow-up:

    a. Evaluation of chronotropic response with exercise during ECG monitoring

    b. Rate histograms when available

    c. Evaluation of sensor activity during activities of daily living (telemetry or ambulatory monitoring with diary)

4. Transtelephonic monitoring

    a. A transmitter used by the patient converts an ECG signal into an audible tone by frequency modulation for transmission over phone lines

    b. A receiving device regenerates the ECG signal for analysis

    c. Usefulness of TMM:

        1. To unburden a busy clinic from patient visits

        2. To service remote areas

        3. To monitor infirmed or immobile patients

        4. To institute frequent observation of devices and leads under advisory or those known to have poor reliability

        5. Monitoring on intermittent and symptomatic arrhythmia

      6. To provide technical expertise between follow-up centers or between manufacturer and clinical center

      7. Serves only as a screening method of detection of problems that must be assessed by direct evaluation

  d. Requirements:

      1. Specialized sending and receiving equipment

      2. Patient teaching; written and demonstration

      3. A cooperative patient, family member or patient care giver

      4. Adequate telephone lines

      5. 24 hour access

  e. Abnormalities that may be found by TTM:

      1. Pacing or magnet rate change

      2. Pulse duration widening

      3. Sensing or pacing failures

      4. Pulse generator failure

      5. Arrhythmia (this monitoring may be a primary use of TTM)

      6. Rough estimate of adequacy of output safety margin (in some devices only)

  f. Suggested protocol:

      1. Confirm patient identification and match patient to his records

      2. Question patient regarding any new symptoms or problems

      3. Verbally review instructions to the patient

      4. Record and assess free running ECG

      5. Record and assess magnet mode ECG, repeat 4 (above)

      6. Assure patient or advise patient of need for care or intervention

      7. Establish next assessment time

      8. Document findings and create a report

  g. Limitations of TTM:

      1. Single lead ECG

      2. Definitive tests and corrective measures cannot be undertaken

      3. Susceptible to motion artifact and EMI

      4. Must rely on patient or family for quality of transmission

      5. Problems such as suboptimal cardiac output cannot be detected

      6. High misdiagnosis rate with TTM

D. Pacemaker Programming

  1. During routine clinical visits

    a. Diagnostic programming should be done to:

      1. Assess pacemaker therapeutic efficacy

      2. Determine pacemaker related causes of any symptoms

   3. Document threshold trends
   b. Therapeutic programming should be done to:
      1. Correct malfunction
      2. Improve patient's functional status
      3. Provide output safety margin
2. Diagnostic programming
   a. Suggested guidelines for safe pacemaker programming:
      1. Know the pacemaker specifications
      2. Understand the programmer and its operating sequence
      3. Know the value and the operation of emergency or stat set
      4. The patient should be supine and monitored (real-time)
      5. Emergency life support equipment must be available
      6. Operator must be trained in emergency life support
      7. Back-up programmer should be available
   b. Assessment of stimulation threshold (see section on stimulation threshold for more detail):
      1. Recognize patient's dependency
      2. Evaluate voltage and pulse width threshold and create a strength duration curve
      3. Maintain a four fold voltage safety margin during acute threshold phase
      4. Maintain a two fold voltage safety margin once lead maturation has occurred
      5. Use temporary or automatically decrementing threshold whenever possible
      6. Should be done intraoperatively, at 4–8 weeks, 3 months, 6 months and yearly if stable; and any time the patient has symptoms or changes cardiac medications
   c. Sensitivity threshold assessment:
      1. The R or P wave must have adequate amplitude and slew rate for proper sensing to occur
      2. The atrial electrogram is of lower amplitude than the ventricular and requires an increase in the sensitivity of the pacemaker amplifier
      3. When possible, allow intrinsic rhythm to predominate and decrease sensitivity until sensing is lost by ECG criteria or telemetered criteria (marker channels) – allow a safety margin between this and permanent setting
      4. In high-grade dependency, adjust sensitivity to as low as possible (while still sensing extrasystole) to avoid potential inhibition from far field signals
3. Therapeutic programming

a. The final program should be tailored to clinical needs:
   1. Angina threshold
   2. Patient functional status
   3. Ventricular function
   4. Intrinsic rhythm
   5. ECG and symptomatic indication for pacing
b. Uses of programmability
   1. Mode:
      a) The inhibited mode is most commonly used
      b) The triggered mode is useful to determine normal sensing and in the presence of electromagnetic interference
      c) Asynchronous pacing is seldom used due to the potential for competitive pacing
      d) Dual chambered devices have multiple modes to meet most clinical needs and circumvent problems
      e) Adaptive-rate mode is only available in pacemakers specifically indicated as such (may be one or more sensors)
   2. Rate:
      a) May be increased to optimize cardiac output
      b) May be decreased to allow sinus rhythm to predominate
      c) May be decreased below angina threshold
   3. Output (may be amplitude or pulse duration)
      a) Adjust according to stimulation threshold
      b) Lower to reduce battery current drain and increase longevity
      c) Lower to reduce or eliminate extracardiac stimulation
   4. Sensitivity:
      a) Increase to correct undersensing of low endocardial signals
      b) Decrease to reduce sensing of other far-field intracardiac signals (T waves)
      c) Decrease to reduce the sensing of far-field extracardiac signals (myopotential, environmental)
      d) Higher number = low sensitivity
   5. AV delay:
      a) Increase to allow spontaneous ventricular depolarization
      b) Decrease to allow full ventricular capture
   6. Refractory period:
      a) Increase to reduce the chance of T-wave sensing
      b) Increase in AAI mode, to avoid QRS sensing
      c) In dual chambered pacing, extend the post-ventricular re-

fractory period to prevent VA conduction from being sensed and creating pacemaker mediated tachycardia (PMT)

7. Hysteresis:
   a) Delays the onset of pacing and allows sinus rhythm and AV synchrony to be maintained (available in both single and dual chamber device)

8. Polarity:
   a) Bipolar to unipolar
      1) May amplify a low endocardial signal
      2) May correct function temporarily in a bipolar lead fracture
   b) Unipolar to bipolar
      1) May decrease the ECG distortion of pacemaker artifact
      2) May decrease the chance of electromagnetic or myopotential interference
      3) May correct pectoral muscle stimulation
      4) Requires a bipolar lead and may result in loss of pacing if a unipolar lead is in situ

4. Emergency programming
   a. The operator must always understand the emergency sequence and values of the "emergency" or "stat set" button
   b. When programming critical values such as output, every attempt should be made to use temporary settings that may be restored rapidly once loss of capture is identified
   c. Real-time ECG monitoring is imperative for stimulation threshold assessment
   d. Patients undergoing stimulation threshold assessment must be in a supine position to reduce any neurologic symptoms resulting from loss of capture
   e. When selecting the device for a specific patient, automatic threshold determination features should be available in the pacemaker selected for the dependent patient

E. Identification and Management of Pacemaker Malfunction

1. Recognition of symptoms
   a. Symptomatology related to pacemaker malfunction:
      1. Return of pre-pacing symptoms may be caused by:
         a) Loss of capture for any reason
         b) Incorrect preoperative diagnosis (pacing does not prevent symptoms)
         c) Inappropriate pacemaker inhibition (oversensing)
      2. Pectoral or diaphragmatic stimulation may be caused by:

       a) Lead insulation failure
       b) Connector insulation failure (self sealing grommet failure)
       c) Disruption of silastic coating on unipolar pulse generator
       d) High output of unipolar pulse generator
       e) Electrode perforation
       f) Atrial lead stimulation of phrenic nerve

3. Palpitations may be:
   a) Paroxysmal SVT (not involving the pacer)
   b) Tracking flutter or fibrillation waves with a DDD system
   c) PMT in dual chambered system
   d) Oversensing in the triggered mode (or DDD)
   e) Inappropriate settings of an adaptive-rate pacemaker

4. Fatigue, dyspnea, pre-syncope may be due to:
   a) Low cardiac output
   b) Pacemaker syndrome
   c) Minimum rate too low
   d) Failure to capture

5. Painful pacemaker pocket may be due to:
   a) Infection
   b) Hematoma
   c) Pending erosion
   d) Pocket too small
   e) Pocket too high – pacer rubbing clavicle
   f) Neurinoma

2. Recognition of device indicators of malfunction
   a. Loss of capture with artifact present may be:
      1. Exit block
      2. Lead dislodgement
      3. Insulation failure
      4. Perforation
      5. Air or blood in pocket
      6. Stimuli in the refractory period of the myocardium
   b. Loss of capture with artifact absent may be:
      1. Misinterpretation of normal pacemaker inhibition
      2. Intermittent connection or disconnected pulse generator and lead
      3. Lead conductor failure with intact insulation
      4. Battery exhaustion
      5. Output failure of the pulse generator (component failure)
      6. Lead fracture (may have small spike artifact)

   c. Oversensing may be:
      1. T-wave sensing in VVI
      2. R-wave sensing in AAI (or other far-field sensing)
      3. Partial lead fracture
      4. Two leads touching (eg., temporary and permanent)
      5. Myopotential inhibition
      6. Electromagnetic interference
      7. Concealed conduction (rare)

   d. Undersensing may be:
      1. Inadequate amplitude or slew rate of electrogram signal
      2. Dislodged lead
      3. Conductor failure with intact insulation
      4. Connector failure
      5. Pulse generator failure (sense amplifier)
      6. Misinterpretation of fusion beats
      7. Asynchronous noise mode

   e. Alteration in programmed parameters may be:
      1. Phantom programming
      2. End-of-service
      3. Component failure
      4. Misinterpretation of normal function
      5. Following exposure to electrocautery, defibrillation
      6. Misprogramming

3. Troubleshooting
   a. Early complications
      1. Pneumothorax:
         a) Prompt chest x-ray after subclavian puncture done, also repeat prior to discharge to uncover late pneumothorax
         b) May manifest at time of implant or up to 48 hours later
         c) Symptoms may include: hypotension, chest pain, respiratory distress

      2. Lead perforation
         a) May lead to pericardial tamponade or subacute effusion
         b) Findings may include: rising threshold, RBBB pattern, diaphragmatic stimulation, friction rub or pericarditis
         c) May be diagnosed by x-ray or two-dimensional echocardiography

      3. Pocket hematoma
         a) If there is continued bleeding or the pocket is painful, it should be evacuated

      b) If not expanding or compromising the sutures, observe without intervention

  4. Lead dislodgement

      a) More common in atrial passive fixation than ventricular leads

      b) Use the initial postoperative x-ray as a reference if dislodgement is suspected

  5. Primary pulse generator component failure

      a) Is rare, but may result in unusual paced rates or rhythms

      b) Is usually seen early following implant, but may be anytime

b. Late complications:

  1. Infection

      a) Treatment often requires removal of the entire pacing system

      b) Patients should be instructed to examine their pacemaker pocket routinely for signs of infection

  2. Erosion of lead or pacemaker:

      a) The only treatment is surgical revision

      b) Is often associated with infection

  3. Thrombosis:

      a) Of the superior vena cava, axillary vein or around lead can be serious

      b) Of the cephalic vein is expected and is not associated with problems

  4. Exit block or development of high thresholds:

      a) May be related to administration of threshold elevating drugs

      b) May be due to excessive scar formation at the heart-electrode interference

      c) May be due to myocardial infarction at electrode site

      d) This may be temporary if related to local edema (resolving after the healing process is complete), or permanent if related to the nature of the endocardium

  5. Lead insulation failure:

      a) Is rare, but has been seen in certain batches of polyurethane insulation material (most common at suture tie site)

      b) May involve the outer coil of unipolar leads or the inner coil or bipolar leads

  6. Twiddler's syndrome:

      a) Purposeful or absent-minded manipulation of the pulse generator causing rotation and lead twisting and lead dislodgement

      b) The use of a tight fitting Dacron pouch may prevent the rotation

4. Finding solutions
   a. Approach to pacemaker troubleshooting:
      1. Question the patient regarding symptoms; frequency, duration, onset, secondary features
      2. Review of the patient's medical and pacemaker history
      3. Limited physical examination including the pacemaker pocket
      4. 12 lead ECG
      5. Rhythm strip with provocative maneuvers such as pocket tug, arm resistance or arm stretching (with and without magnet)
      6. Interrogation and telemetry when available
      7. Checking of pacemaker specifications if not known
      8. Overpenetrated chest x-ray
      9. Diagnostic programming
   b. Correction of pacemaker malfunction:
      1. Non-invasively
         a) Programming
         b) Medication
      2. Surgically
         a) Lead reposition, repair or replacement reposition
         b) Pulse generator replacement or reposition
         c) Correction of connector problems
         d) Evacuation of air or hematoma

F. Management of Recalls and Advisories

1. Determining the severity of the problem
   a. Recall may be generated by manufacturer, government agency or by the follow-up physician
   b. The United States FDA has established regulatory definitions for pacemaker recall or "Recall Classes" (they also use the word "Recall" to describe corrective actions, field repairs, labeling changes, hazard warnings and other situations) of the failure mode
   c. Recall/advisory may be inclusive of all models of a given product, or may be limited to those of certain serial numbers, representing a time period of manufacturing
   d. Pacemaker system performance monitoring should include: device performance of both pacemaker and lead, and clinical aspects such as infections, lead dislodgement connector problems
2. Individual patient assessment and decision making
   a. Patient dependency and pre-pacing symptoms are an important factor in the decision management of corrective actions, such as

whether to surgically replace or to monitor (a normally functioning device under recall)

b. In the event of a large recall, the order of scheduling of both assessment and surgical replacement can be guided by patient's known dependency and their implied risk should the device fail

c. It is advisable that an individual's pacemaker dependency be indicated on their record and updated at regular intervals to assist in the management of patients immediately upon notification of recall

3. Management considerations

a. A failure pattern, once identified, must be reported to the manufacturer and to the appropriate government agency

b. The recall or advisory must be classified based on the nature of the malfunction and the patient risk. This may be done by the manufacturer or by the responsible government agency

c. The physician responsible for the patient must be notified by the manufacturer

d. The recall list, as provided by the manufacturer, must be verified

e. A clinical decision on patient management must be made (replacement or surveillance)

f. Patient must be notified and receive a full explanation of risk

g. Appropriate communication must take place with government, media, malpractice insurance agencies and with the hospital boards

h. Adequate follow-up facilities must be established (TTM, additional clinics, reimplant facility)

i. The explanted pacemaker must be returned to the manufacturer for analysis and report to confirm the failure mode

j. Warranty or financial adjustment must be made between the manufacturer and the implantation center

References

Bhatia S, Goldschlager N. Office evaluation of the pacemaker patient. JAMA. 254:10:1346–1352. 1985.

Garson A, Coyner T, Shannon CE, et al. A systematic approach to fully automatic (DDD) pacemaker electrocardiogram. In Practical Cardiac Pacing. PC Gillertte, JC Griffen, (Eds.). Baltimore: William & Wilkins, 181–270. 1986.

Levine P. Proceedings of the policy conference of the North America society of pacing and electrophysiology on programmability and pacemaker follow-up programs. Clin Prog Pacing Electrophysiol. 2:2:1984.

Levine PA, Lindenberg BS. Diagnostic data: an aid to the follow-up and assessment of the pacing system. J Electrophysiol. 1:396–403. 1987.

Luceri RM, Hayes DL. Follow-up of DDD pacemakers. PACE. 7:1187–1194. 1984.

Parsonnet V, Furman S, Smythe NPD, et al. Optimal resources for implantable cardiac pacemakers. Circulation. 68:224A-244A. 1983.

Schoenfeld MH. Follow-up of the pacemaker patient. In Principles of Cardiac Pacing. K. Ellenbogen, (Ed.), 1991.

Tyers GFO. FDA recalls: How to pacemaker manufacturers compare? Ann Thorac Surg. 48:390. 1989.

Fraser JA, Cameron D, Dependency Risk Score: A safe and consistent stratification for pacemaker follow-up. 1984. (Abstract)

U.S. Government Printing Office. Medicare Carriers Manual, Transmittal No. 1051, October, 1984.

Suggested Readings

Furman S. Pacemaker Follow-up. In A Practice of Cardiac Pacing. 1st edition. S Furman (Ed.). Mount Kisco: Futura Publishing Co, Inc., 379–412. 1986.

Griffin JC, Schuenemeyer TD. Pacemaker follow-up: an introduction and overview. Clin Prog Pacing and Electrophysiol. 1:1.30–39. 1983.

Harthorne J. Current Problems in Cardiology; Cardiac Pacemakers. St. Louis: Year Book Medical Publishers, Inc., 12:11. November, 1987.

Hayes D, Higano S. DDDR Pacing: Follow-up and Complications. In New Perspectives in Cardiac Pacing. 2nd edition. Barold D, Mugica J, (Eds.). Mount Kisco: Futura Publishing Co, Inc. 1991.

Parsonnet V, Myers G, Manhardt M. A pacemaker follow-up clinic: an analysis of detection of signs of impending pacemaker failure. In Cardiac Pacing. 2nd ed. Samet El-Sharif N, (Eds.). Philadelphia: WB Saunders Co, 255–270. 1980.

Sutton R, Bourgeois I.: The Foundations of Cardiac Pacing Pt. 1. The Bakken Research Center Series, Mount Kisco: Futura Publishing Co, Inc., 245–301. 1991.

CHAPTER 19

Pediatric Considerations

Vicki Zeigler

The use of pacemakers in the pediatric population is increasing. This is largely due to newer and better surgical techniques to correct congenital heart disease as well as better identification of pacing indications among pediatricians and family practitioners. The advances in surgical techniques for congenital cardiac lesions frequently causes damage to the conduction system requiring some form of pacemaker intervention.

Because these bradyarrhythmias and/or atrioventricular blocks occasionally resolve in the postoperative period, these patients may be temporarily paced.

Many of these patients will, however, require permanent cardiac pacemakers. A small portion of the pediatric population will require pacing for congenital conduction defects in the presence of an anatomically normal heart.

The following chapter will review the indications for pacemakers in children, temporary pacing in this population as well as the implantation requirements, nursing care, patient/family education, and follow-up of permanent pacemakers in the pediatric population.

From: Schurig L. *Educational Guidelines: Pacing and Electrophysiology.* Armonk, NY: Futura Publishing Co, Inc, © 1994.

Objectives

1. Identify the indications for a permanent pacemaker in the pediatric population.
2. Assess the interaction between the patient, the patient's family, and the treatment implemented.
3. Apply scientific knowledge to the implantation of pediatric pacing in clinical practice.
4. Define standards of care.
5. Recognize complications of pacemaker therapy.
6. Develop a plan of care for the patient/patient's family undergoing permanent cardiac pacemaker implantation.
7. Select safety/activity precautions for pacemaker recipients.
8. Set up for assisting with initiation of pacemaker therapy in pediatrics.
9. Apply the principles of cardiac pacing to the child who is temporarily paced.

   * Glossary and Abbreviations – refer to general pacing definitions.

Education Content

A. Indications

   1. Class I – definitely indicated

      a. Second or third degree AV block with symptomatic bradycardia

      b. Advanced second or third degree AV block with moderate to marked exercise intolerance

      c. External ophthalmoplegia with bifascicular block

      d. Sinus node dysfunction with symptomatic bradycardia

      e. Congenital AV block with wide QRS escape rhythm or with block below the His bundle

      f. Advanced second or third degree AV block persisting 10 to 14 days after cardiac surgery

   2. Class II – probably or possibly indicated

      a. Bradycardia-tachycardia syndrome with need for an antiarrhythmic drug other than digitalis or phenytoin

      b. Second or third degree AV block within the bundle of His in an asymptomatic patient

      c. Prolonged subsidiary pacemaker recovery time

      d. Transient surgical second or third degree AV block that reverts to bifascicular block

      e. Asymptomatic second or third degree AV block and a ventricular rate < 45 beats per min when awake

      f. Complete AV block when awake, with an average ventricular rate < 50 beats per min

      g. Complete AV block with double or triple resting cycle length pauses or minimal heart rate variability

      h. Asymptomatic neonate with congenital complete heart block and bradycardia in relation to age

      i. Complex ventricular arrhythmias associated with second or third degree AV block or sinus bradycardia

      j. Long QT syndrome

   3. Class III – not indicated

      a. Asymptomatic, postoperative bifascicular block.

      b. Asymptomatic postoperative bifascicular block with first degree AV block

      c. Transient surgical AV block that returns to normal conduction in < 1 week

      d. Asymptomatic type I second degree AV block

      e. Asymptomatic congenital heart block without profound bradycardia in relation to age

B. Contraindications

    1. There are no known contraindications for permanent pacemakers in children; however, those children with a right to left shunt (due to congenital anomalies) should NOT be candidates for transvenous leads but rather an epicardial approach should be taken.

C. Clinical and/or Electrophysiologic Identification of Arrhythmia

    1. Patient experiences atrial tachycardia after repair of congenital heart disease (CHD) as documented by:

        a. Transtelephonic monitoring

        b. 12 lead electrocardiogram

        c. 24 hour ambulatory monitor

        d. Continuous telemetric monitoring (while hospitalized)

    2. Atrial tachycardia is unresponsive to Digoxin and further action (i.e., antitachycardia pacing and/or antiarrhythmic medications) is required.

D. Congenital Complete Atrioventricular Block

    1. Upon birth, the ECG exhibits a regular P-P interval and a regular R-R interval with no relationship or synchrony between the atria and ventricles.

    2. Occurs in 1/15,000 live births and approximately one-half of these patients will become symptomatic and require permanent pacemakers prior to age 18. (Michaelson & Engle, 1972).

    3. The diagnosis can be made prior to birth in utero using fetal echocardiography. Additionally, it can be confirmed at birth by 12 lead ECG.

    4. In utero, fetus may exhibit hydrops fetalis. The child after birth to adolescence may experience syncope, congestive heart failure, and/or exercise intolerance.

    5. The treatment in the compromised fetus is permanent cardiac pacing immediately following birth. In the older child, treat with a permanent pacemaker if the rate criteria is met or associated symptoms occur.

E. Acquired Atrioventricular Block

    1. Second or third degree AVB that occurs after corrective surgery for CHD or symptomatic second or third degree AVB acquired via a viral or other infectious process

    2. 30/5000 children undergoing reparative surgery for CHD will develop AVB requiring permanent cardiac pacing (Driscoll, et al, 1979)

    3. Diagnosis

        a. Telemetric or bedside monitor

        b. 12 lead ECG

      c. 24 hour ambulatory monitor

      d. Transtelephonic monitor

  4. Symptoms

      a. Congestive heart failure (CHF)

      b. Syncope

  5. If postoperative block, treat with steroids to possibly decrease inflammation around AV node or His bundle.

      a. Temporary pacing – Part Two, Chapter 16

      b. If block persists for 10–14 days post surgery, permanent cardiac pacing is indicated

F. Sinus Node Dysfunction

  1. Sinus bradycardia with associated symptoms

      a. Acquired-sinus bradycardia, sinus exit block, rate < 40 when awake, rate < 30 when asleep, or > 3.0 second pause; most common after repair of congenital heart defect (CHD)

      b. Congenital-extremely rare

  2. Diagnosis

      a. Telemetric or bedside monitor

      b. 12 lead ECG

      c. 24 hour ambulatory monitor

      d. Electrophysiology study

  3. Symptoms

      a. Congestive heart failure

      b. Syncope

      c. Exercise intolerance

  4. Treatment

      a. Permanent cardiac pacing (atrial only if AV node function is normal)

G. Acquired Atrial Tachyarrhythmias

  1. Atrial reentry tachycardia that occurs after repair of CHD

  2. Occurs in CHD repairs that involves an atrial repair, particularly in Fontans, Mustards/Sennings and ASDs

  3. Diagnosis

      a. Telemetric or bedside monitor

      b. 12 lead ECG

      c. 24 hour ambulatory monitor

      d. Electrophysiology study (definitive)

  4. Symptoms

      a. Palpitations

    b. Dizziness

    c. Syncope

    d. Congestive heart failure

  5. Treatment

    a. Atrial antitachycardia pacing

H. Evaluation of the Pediatric Pacemaker Candidate

  1. History and physical examination

  2. Cardiovascular function

    a. Echocardiography

    b. Radiography

    c. Exercise tolerance testing

  3. Arrhythmia evaluation

    a. 12 lead ECG

    b. 24 hour ambulatory monitoring/heart rate variability

    c. Transtelephonic monitoring

    d. Exercise testing

  4. Hospital course

    a. Preadmission

      1. Financial review

      2. Parental/patient conference (optional)

    b. Admission

      1. Laboratory examination and preparation

      2. Chest radiograph

      3. Informed consent

      4. Stress test (if applicable)

      5. Cardiac catheterization with electrophysiology study (if applicable)

      6. 24 hour ambulatory monitor analysis

      7. Antiarrhythmic drug evaluation (if applicable)

      8. Consult with pediatric pacemaker associated professional

      9. Type and cross for 1 unit PRBC

    c. Pediatric pacemaker technology – utilizes basic principles covered under pacemaker hardware section

      1. Hardware (includes hardware covered in aforementioned section)

      2. Magnet operation

      3. Pacemaker complications (see complications, Part Two, Chapter 18)

      4. Troubleshooting a pediatric pacemaker:

      a) Inadequate tachycardia termination
      b) Far-field R-wave oversensing
      c) Inappropriate atrial overdrives
      d) Inappropriate sensing and/or pacing in bradycardia devices
      e) Upper rate limits and refractory periods
      f) Rate response behavior (if rate responsive device)
   5. Interaction with other devices
      a) Electrocautery
      b) External defibrillators
      c) Diathermy
      d) MRI
      e) Household devices

I. Operative Management (Implantation)

  1. Electrophysiology study (if applicable)
    a. Wenckebach rate if atrial pacemaker and retrograde conduction times
    b. Tachyarrhythmia evaluation (if applicable)
      1. Tachycardia induction
      2. Tachycardia morphology and typical behavior
      3. Tachycardia termination utilizing an external version of the soon to be implanted device
    c. Vein feasibility
      1. Contrast injection into intended venous access and subclavian puncture by aiming at catheter in subclavian vein
      2. Puncture subclavian as lateral as possible i.e., at radiographic chest wall
  2. Procedure room supplies
    a. Pacing system
      1. Appropriate pulse generator with one back-up device readily available
      2. Appropriate pacing lead or leads with at least one back-up available
      3. Use as physiologic a system as possible, including maintenance of AV synchrony
    b. Sterile equipment
      1. Bipolar/unipolar test cable/electrogram cable
      2. Sterile lead caps (if removal also)
      3. Magnet
      4. Appropriate programming wand
      5. Extra parts kits, adapters, etc.

      6. Additional, appropriate stylets

      7. Appropriate screwdrivers (if removal)

   c. Miscellaneous equipment

      1. Programmer back-up must be in hospital

      2. PSA back-up must be in hospital

      3. Back-up leads and pacemaker

      4. Accessory kit

   d. Case preparation

      1. Pre-programming of pulse generator with telemetry check

      2. Battery check for PSA

      3. Sterilize equipment

   e. Pulse oximeter, emergency equipment in procedure room

   f. Retain patient manual, registration forms, and device warranty

   g. Case documentation (Part Two, Chapter 17)

J. Patient Management

  1. Patient/family education

   a. Patient manual for the pacemaker – provided by company

   b. Preoperative instructions regarding procedure, devices, and post-operative care by staff nurse *and* pacemaker associated professional

   c. Temporary ID card

   d. Generator warranty

   e. Medic alert request form (if requested by patient and/or family)

   f. Pacemaker instruction sheets

      1. General guidelines

      2. Follow-up

      3. Subacute bacterial endocarditis (SBE) prophylaxis (when appropriate)

      4. Activity

      5. Site care

      6. Emergency plan

      7. Transtelephonic follow-up

   g. Medication (if applicable)

  2. Postoperative patient care standards

   a. The nurse will monitor/assess the patient for postoperative complications in addition to those related to the pacemaker

   b. The nurse will incorporate into his/her plan of care consideration for events which will effect the patient/family's response to the pacemaker

   c. The nurse will incorporate into his/her plan of care consideration for events which will affect the patient/family's response to the pacemaker

    d. The nurse will initiate appropriate intervention for actual or potential problems determined from the assessment

    e. The nurse will design a plan of care to identify and manage actual and/or potential problems for the pediatric pacemaker patient using nursing diagnoses

    f. The nurse will provide complete documentation for the care given to the pediatric pacemaker patient and his/her family

3. Long-term patient follow-up
   a. Outpatient appointment schedule
   b. Transtelephonic follow-up schedule
   c. ERI/replacement indicators

4. Safety program
   a. Electrical safety
   b. MRI
   c. Activity

5. Discharge plan
   a. Prescriptions and medication teaching (if applicable)
   b. Outpatient appointments
   c. Telephone transmitter instruction (verbal and written)
   d. SBE prophylaxis instructions (although not recommended by AHA, some physicians still observe)
   e. Emergency plan for unsuccessful device termination of tachyarrhythmia (if applicable).
   f. Referrals
      1. Home care
      2. Social services
      3. Other

K. Documentation

1. Patient care policies
2. Standards of care
3. Patient management
   a. Monitoring
   b. Assessment
   c. Plan of care
   d. Interventions
   e. Outcomes
   f. Evaluation
4. Patient education

5. Procedure room
    a. Pacing/sensing thresholds
    b. Magnet tests
    c. Generator/lead data
    d. Medications
    e. Real-time telemetry via programmer
6. Implant testing record
7. Equipment inventory
8. Follow-up
    a. Clinic worksheet
    b. Early replacement indicator (ERI) determination or end-of-service (EOS)
    c. ECG
    d. Programmers
9. Computer data-base

L. Computer Data-base

1. Data entry
2. Report generation
3. Trends
4. Tracking
5. Recalls
6. Manufacturer alerts

M. Temporary Pacing

1. Epicardial wires (postoperative)
    a. Most frequently used technique in children
    b. Should be bipolar
    c. Be aware that thresholds tend to rise rapidly postoperatively
2. Transvenous
    a. Must be done in ICU or catheterization lab
    b. In children, the femoral approach may be used more frequently than the subclavian or jugular
    c. Child should be sedated
    d. May be done under echocardiographic guidance
3. Transcutaneous/transthoracic
    a. Used only in emergency situations in most children
    b. For optimal results, keep child sedated, intubated and pharmacologically paralyzed
4. Esophageal

    a. Rarely used for temporary pacing in children for bradycardia, but may be used for overdriving atrial tachycardia

5. Modes

    a. Dual chamber

        1. If possible, use DDD (rather than DVI) to allow AV synchrony in the presence of high/fluctuating atrial rates and CHD

    b. Single chamber

        1. Atrial application can be used to overdrive atrial reentry tachycardia

        2. May also be used for intermittent AV block or sinus bradycardia, or when venous access allows only one lead

N. Pacemaker Follow-up in Pediatrics

  1. Transtelephonic

    a. Weekly phone ECGs during acute phase (first 6 weeks), then monthly for first year. Every 3 months after that until approaching ERI/EOL then increase to monthly again

    b. If phone ECG is abnormal 2 times, patient must come in for hands on follow-up

  2. Outpatient evaluation

    a. ECG

    b. Chest radiograph

        1. To evaluate lead placement, length and growth

    c. Echocardiogram

        1. In patients with CHD, function generally gets better after pacemaker placement.

    d. Exercise testing

        1. To evaluate heart rate response, exercise tolerance and rate response settings if rate responsive device

    e. Pacemaker check

        1. Pacing thresholds

        2. Sensing thresholds

        3. Underlying rhythms

        4. Battery status

        5. Lead impedances

        6. Re-programming for adequate safety margins and battery longevity

References

Daberkow, E. Permanent pacemakers in children. J Cardiovasc Nurs. 6(3): 56–64. 1992.

Dreifus LS, Fisch C, Griffin JC, Gillette PC, Mason JW, Parsonnet V. ACC/ AHA fast force report on guidelines for implantation of cardiac pacemakers and antiarrhythmia devices. J Am Coll Cardiol. 18:1–13. 1991.

Gillette PC. Transvenous implantation technique. In Practical Cardiac Pacing. Gillette, PC, Griffin, JC, (Eds.). Baltimore: Williams & Wilkins, 45–62. 1986.

Gillette PC, Wampler DG, Shannon C, Ott D. Use of atrial pacing in a young population. PACE. 8:94–100. 1985.

Gillette PC, Zeigler VL, Case CL, Harold M, Buchles DS. Atrial antitachycardia pacing in children and young adults. Am Heart J. 122(3):844–849. 1991.

Hayes DL, Holmes DR Jr, Maloney JD, et al. Permanent endocardial pacing in pediatric patients. J Thorac Cardiovasc Surg. 85:618–624. 1983.

Michaelson M, Engle MA. Congenital Complete heart block: an international study of the natural history. Cardiovasc Clin. 4:86–101. 1972.

Ott DA. The epicardial approach to cardiac pacing. In Practical Cardiac Pacing. Gillette PC, Griffin JC. (Eds.). Baltimore: Williams & Wilkins, 63. 1986.

Shannon CE. Pacing system follow-up. In Practical Cardiac Pacing. Gillette PC, Griffin JC. (Eds.). Baltimore: Williams & Wilkins, 137–160. 1986.

Smith RT. Pacemakers for children. In Pediatric Arrhythmias Electrophysiology and Pacing. Gillette PC, Garson, A, (Eds.). Philadelphia: WB Saunders, Co., 532–558. 1990.

CHAPTER 20

Research Requirements with Implanted Devices

Margaret Millis Faust

Subsections:
A. Reporting Mechanisms for Clinical Research
B. Adverse Effects Secondary to Medical Devices
C. Phases of Clinical Research
D. Medical Device Safety Act
E. Investigational Device Exemption (IDE)
F. Components of IDE
G. Reporting Responsibilities
H. Pre-Market Notification 510(K)
I. Pre-Market Application

Non-physician health care providers who practice cardiac pacing and electrophysiology monitor implanted devices for efficacy, adverse effects, and side effects as a part of routine practice. Frequently these skills are utilized in clinical trials with implanted devices. New medical devices must undergo clinical testing for safety and efficacy before they can be marketed.

The United States Congress passed a law in 1976 to amend the Federal Food, Drug and Cosmetic Act; its goal was to ensure that only safe and effective medical devices are used in patient treatment. The United States Food and Drug Administration (FDA) is responsible for regulating device testing and use. The FDA monitors testing and use of cardiovascular devices through the Center for Devices and Radiological Health (CDRH) in the Division of Cardiovascular Devices.

The process of medical device testing is carefully controlled by the CDRH.

From: Schurig L. *Educational Guidelines: Pacing and Electrophysiology.* Armonk, NY: Futura Publishing Co, Inc, © 1994.

Trials are performed in a phased manner with numbers of devices and staff limited in the first phase, then gradually increased in the second phase. When the testing is complete, all of the data is submitted to CDRH for evaluation.

Careful monitoring of medical devices continues even after approval of its use. The Medical Device Reporting regulation enacted in 1984 requires regular reporting regarding product performance and medical device problems for implanted cardiac pacemakers and defibrillators even after they have been approved. Recently more concern regarding under-reporting of injuries related to medical devices has prompted Congress to establish stricter regulations whenever complications or malfunctions related to medical device use cause serious injury or death to a patient. The "Safe Medical Device Act" was enacted to give the FDA more ability to monitor and to intervene when problems are detected. The Act now gives the FDA power to notify patients or problems and recall devices. Failure to comply with the Act will bring sanctions against facilities; additionally, the FDA will be allowed to inspect user facilities. The FDA plans to monitor facilities to ensure compliance with the Act.

Any serious injury or death which is suspected to be caused by a medical device or the improper use of a medical device must be reported to the FDA by the institution where the injury occurred. The written report must be received by the FDA within ten (10) working days. Serious injuries or deaths which are related to pacemaker, leads or implantable defibrillators should be reported immediately to the manufacturer as well. The definition of who should report problems includes hospitals, nursing homes, and ambulatory surgical facilities.

A serious injury or illness is defined as "life-threatening or that which results in permanent impairment of a body function or permanent damage to a body structure or necessitated immediate medical or surgical intervention to preclude permanent impairment of body function or permanent damage to a body structure." A medical device obviously includes pacemakers and defibrillators, but can even be a bandaid. It is any object which is used in the treatment of patients. Each institution should establish its reporting mechanism and the non-physician health provider should become familiar with it.

Research with implanted devices requires the non-physician health provider to be familiar with the regulations regarding investigational devices as well as regulations regarding responsibilities in reporting complications and problems with approved medical devices.

Objectives

1. Recognize the reporting mechanism for data collected in clinical research utilizing implanted medical devices.
2. List the phases of clinical research when testing medical devices.

3. Identify characteristics of each phase of clinical research utilizing medical devices.
4. Identify the circumstances for which an associated professional (AP) is required to report to the FDA under the recently enacted "Safe Medical Device Act."
5. Describe the Investigational Device Exemption (IDE) application.
6. Name the items which must be included in the IDE application.
7. Discuss responsibilities when an unanticipated adverse effect related to the medical device occurs.
8. Describe a pre-market 510 K notification.
9. Describe a premarket approval (PMA) application.

Note: Please refer to "Research Requirements" in Part Three for general information about clinical research.

Education Content

A. Reporting Mechanism for Clinical Research Utilizing Medical Devices

    1. United States Food and Drug Administration (FDA) is ultimately responsible

        a. Jurisdiction of Center for Devices and Radiological Health (CDRH) – one of six centers within the FDA

        b. Implanted pacemakers and defibrillators are under scientific review and surveillance by the Office of Device Evaluation in CDRH

    2. Sponsor reports data to FDA (via CDRH)

    3. Investigator reports to the sponsor

    4. Investigator is also responsible to FDA and may be audited by the FDA

B. Adverse Effects Secondary to Medical Devices

    1. Investigator must issue a report describing the event within 10 days to the sponsor

    2. The sponsor has an additional 10 days to investigate and issue a report to the CDRH

C. Phases of Clinical Research Utilizing Investigational Devices

    1. Phase 1

        a. Centers limited; up to 15 centers.

        b. Up to 30 devices total

        c. 1 month follow-up

        d. Data reported to CDRH

    2. Phase 2

        a. Phase 1 data reviewed and accepted

        b. Up to about 25 centers

        c. Up to 250 patients

        d. Quarterly progress reports or after each series of 30 patients have been treated with the investigational device

    3. Device changes

        a. Sponsor must submit supplement to IDE application

        b. Additional data may be required

        c. Each change reviewed case by case

D. Medical Device Safety Act

    1. Passed by United States Congress in 1990

2. Reporting mechanism is the responsibility of the institution, but non-medical providers should learn and utilize reporting mechanism.

3. Regulations written regarding reporting requirements when serious injury or death occurs secondary to malfunction or misuse of a medical device.

4. Reports must include
   a. Name of device
   b. Serial number
   c. Model number
   d. Name and address of manufacturer
   e. Description of the event

5. Reports are not admissible in court unless the parties involved knew the information given was false.

6. Suspension of PMAs. FDA, after an informal hearing, would be permitted to suspend the approval of a premarket approval application (PMA).

7. Use of PMA data to support other sponsor's PMA. One year after the fourth approval of a device having the same principles of operation and the same used as the device initially approved, FDA could use the safety and efficacy data in the approved PMAs to support other premarket approval applications.

8. Codification of FDA present criteria for evaluating 510(k)s and requirements for manufacturers to search for adverse safety and effectiveness information for some "predicate" devices listed in Section 510(k) notifications.

E. Investigational Device Exemption (IDE) Application

1. Must be used if the device is considered a "significant risk" device

2. "Significant risk" means that the patient would be at risk for serious injury or death if the device malfunctions. (From Code of Federal Regulations)
   a. Implants
   b. Life-supporting
   c. Life-sustaining
   d. Used to diagnose, cure, mitigate, or treat disease

F. Components of IDE Application (From Code of Federal Regulations, Title 21, part 812)

1. Name and address of product sponsor

2. Complete report of prior testing
   a. Laboratory
   b. Animal

      c. Prior clinical

      d. Bibliography of all publications relevant to device investigation and a summary of all unpublished material.

3. Complete investigational plan
   a. Name of device
   b. Intended use
   c. Study duration
   d. Study objective
4. Written protocol
   a. Methods
   b. Analysis of protocol demonstrating that scientific reasoning is sound
5. Description and analysis of all risks incurred by exposure to investigation.
   a. Describe how risks will be minimized
6. Justification for investigation
7. Description of patient population
8. Name and address of the principal investigator
9. Description of each component, property and principle of operation of device and of each anticipated change during investigation
10. Written procedure for monitoring the investigation
11. Description of methods, facilities and controls used for manufacture, processing, packing, storing and installation (if applicable) of device
12. Copies of all labeling and instructions for device use
13. Copies of all information distributed to patients; including consent forms

G. Responsibilities for Reporting Adverse Effects and Serious Complications Related to Device Use and Testing

    1. Manufacturers must report to the Center for Devices and Radiological Health
   a. All adverse device experiences (including malfunctions) that result in serious injury or death
   b. Annual report for PMA devices (includes adverse experiences)
    2. Investigators must immediately report device related injury or death to manufacturer and their institutional review board

H. Pre-Market 510(K) Notification

    1. Application to commercially market device
    2. Must be submitted to FDA (CDRH) if a similar device has already been approved

   3. Submitted only after clinical trial is complete
   4. Supporting data
      a. Pre-trial data and literature
      b. Clinical trial data and literature
   5. Reviewed by CDRH staff
      a. Must be reviewed within 90 days

I. Pre-Market Approval Application (PMA)

   1. Application to commercially market device
   2. Must be submitted to FDA (CDRH) if a similar device is not already approved
   3. Submitted after clinical trial is complete
   4. Supporting data
      a. Clinical trial data and literature
      b. Pertinent related literature (published and unpublished)
   5. Review process
      a. Reviewed by CDRH staff within 180 days
      b. Also reviewed by an advisory panel
         1. Composed of individuals with diverse backgrounds
            a) Physicians with different specialties, engineers, industry representative and a consumer representative
         2. Review hearing is open to the public
         3. Panel sends recommendation to CDRH for final decision
   6. Device approval is contingent upon submission and review of annual reports
      a. Annual report must contain
         1. Changes made to device that affect efficacy and safety
         2. Bibliography of all published and unpublished reports about device since it was approved
         3. Adverse reactions and device malfunctions
      b. After approval for use
         1. Adverse effects that do not cause serious injury or death
            a) User can report to CDRH through the Medical Device and Laboratory Product Reporting system
            b) Helps to assess how the device is functioning in the marketplace
         2. Reporting by manufacturers is in addition to the requirements of the "Safe Medical Devices Act"

References

Palmer PN. Nursing organizations discuss health care reform, Safe Medical Device Act, AIDS. AORN. 55:(594). 1991.

Scott WL. Medical-device complication reporting: a quality assurance mechanism. J Intraven Nurs. 13:178–182. 1990.

Code of Federal Regulations, (1991) Food & Drugs, Book 21, Parts 800 to 1299, Subsection 809.20, Part 812 – Investigational Device Exemptions, pp 75–88.

Code of Federal Regulations, (1991) Food & Drugs, Book 21, Parts 800 to 1299, Subsection 813.170, Part 814 – Premarket Approval of Medical Devices, pp 110–124.

Code of Federal Regulations, (1991), Food & Drugs, Book 21, Parts 800 to 1299, Subsection 803.3, Part 803 – Medical Device Reporting, pp 41–46.

Code of Federal Regulations, (1991) Food & Drugs, Book 21, Parts 800 to 1299, Subsection 803.33, Part 805 – Cardiac Pacemaker Registry, pp 46–48.

Code of Federal Regulations, (1991) Food & Drugs, Book 21, Parts 800 to 1299, Subsection 860.1 Part 860 – Medical Device Classification Procedures, pp 134–145.

Code of Federal Regulations, (1991) Food & Drugs, Book 21, Parts 800 to 1299, Subsection 868.6225, Part 870 – Cardiovascular Devices, pp 252–271.

Code of Federal Regulations, (1991) Food & Drugs, Book 21, Parts 800 to 1299, Subsection 809.20, Part 812 – Investigational Device Exemptions, pp 75–88.

Code of Federal Regulations, (1991) Food & Drugs, Book 21, Parts 800 to 1299, Subsection 813.170, Part 814 – Premarket Approval of Medical Devices, pp 110–124.

For more information on the Safe Medical Device Act, call US Pharmacopeia Practitioners Reporting Network 1–800–638–6725. The address is: 12601 Twinbrook Parkway, Rockville, MD 20852.

CHAPTER 21

Other Topics

Chea Haran

Subsection:
A. Pacemaker Patient Education

In order to identify and/or see impending problems involving the permanent pacemaker and the patient, one must be able to effectively communicate and manage the health care of that individual. It is important to design and implement a patient education program which is tailored to each individual patient's needs.

The educational program should begin as soon as the determination is made that a pacemaker is indicated. It should encompass aspects such as the historical events, present day technology, terminology, the cardiac system, quality of life and long-term care post-implantation of the device. The patients' perception of pacemaker surgery is also a vital component. The final outcome on how they will cope or adjust in the future with their pacemaker will depend on their understanding and acceptance of the pacemaker.

Ideally, the whole health care team, patient, family, physician, nurse or pacemaker follow-up person, social worker and any significant other, should be an active participant within the pacemaker educational system.

Objectives

1. Identify the educational needs of the pacemaker patient.
2. Discuss therapeutic ways to decrease patient anxiety and facilitate improved coping mechanisms post-implant.

From: Schurig L. *Educational Guidelines: Pacing and Electrophysiology.* Armonk, NY: Futura Publishing Co, Inc, © 1994.

3. Outline a patient care plan tailored to their individual needs.
4. Illustrate components of the conduction system.
5. Identify the content of an educational program specific to the pacemaker patient recognizing their needs and limitations.
6. List current educational information sources available for pacemaker patients.

Glossary and Abbreviations

Angina: (pectoris): An episode of severe paroxysmal chest pain radiating from the heart to the shoulder and down the left arm due to ischemia of the heart muscle.

Anticoagulants: Preventing coagulation. An agent that prevents coagulation.

Asynchronous pacemaker: Pacemaker with fixed rate; rate is independent of the heart's electrical or mechanical activity, as it contains no mechanism capable of sensing cardiac activity.

Asystole: Period in which the heart does not contract, standstill.

Bipolar: Having two electrodes or contacts within the heart.

Capture: Consistent control of heart rate with an artificial pacemaker, each artificial pacing impulse results in one effective contraction of the heart.

Demand pacemaker: Pacemaker that senses spontaneous cardiac activity and responds by inhibiting the pacemaker output impulse.

Diaphragmatic stimulation: Stimulation of the phrenic nerve or diaphragm by the pacing stimulus, causing a hiccough-like reaction.

Diuretics: Promoting the excretion of urine. An agent that increases the output of urine.

Electrode: Electrically conductive element (usually the end of a lead) which contacts body tissue.

Endocardial lead: Lead inserted so the electrode contacts the endocardium.

Epicardial: The outer layer of the heart muscle. In pacing, describes the attachment of the pacing lead to the outer layer of heart muscle.

Erosion: Externalization of the pacemaker generator through the skin related to poor tissue healing, pressure against the skin from inside the pocket or lack of adequate muscle mass to cover the device.

Fine tuning: Decreasing voltage and pulse width in order to increase pacemaker longevity. Programming the pacemaker for optimal operation over a long period of time.

Fluoroscopy: Examination of an internal structure by a continuous viewing of shadows formed by differential transmission of x-rays through the objects. The type of x-ray utilized for pacemaker insertions.

Hematoma: A localized mass of extravasated blood that is relatively or completely confined within an organ or tissue. The blood is usually clotted and, depending on how long it has been there, may manifest various degrees of organization and discolorization.

Increased longevity (pacer): Extending pacemaker battery life through fine tuning.

Infection: Endoparasitism; multiplication of microorganisms in the body proper, especially in the pocket made for the generator.

Myopotential inhibition: Those electric potentials generated by the contraction of skeletal muscles.

Non-invasive: Description of diagnostic procedures which do not involve the insertion of needles, cannulas or other devices that require penetration of the skin.

Pectoral stimulation: Muscle twitching which can occur after implantation; usually occurs with unipolar system and can be corrected with programming.

Phrenic nerve: The nerve which innervates the muscles in the diaphragm.

Pneumohemothorax: The presence of air or gas and blood in the thoracic cavity.

Repolarization: Electrical recovery of the heart.

Sensing: The ability of the pacemaker to acknowledge an intrinsic heart beat.

Telemetry: The circuitry required to monitor, measure and transmit various parameters within the pulse generator. Types of data retrieved include: real-time measurements, stored data, programmed data, diagnostic data, event markers, histograms and intracardiac electrograms.

Education Content

A. Pacemaker Patient Education

1. Benefits
   a. Increase understanding of the pacemaker
   b. Decrease patient anxiety
   c. Increase knowledge of patient and family about living with a pacemaker, of pending problems, and prevention of unnecessary hospitalization
   d. Decrease cost to the consumer and the health care delivery system
   e. Increase awareness and continuity of education
      1. To promote a sense of well-being
      2. To enhance the quality of care
      3. To enhance the quality of life
   f. Increase longevity of patient and pacemaker

2. Goals
   a. Establish proper guidelines to use in pacemaker education
   b. Assure that the patient is aware of the proper channels to follow when a suspected problem arises
   c. Allow time for verbalization
   d. Discuss common concerns pertaining to the pacemaker (i.e., lifestyle, sex, safety, how the heart functions, pacemaker failure, etc.)
   d. Provide the patient with a list of resources on how to retrieve pacemaker information
   e. Improved patient compliance
   f. Increase pacemaker longevity through timely fine tuning

3. Concerns to address specific to the pacemaker patient
   a. Denial. Do I really need this pacemaker?
   b. Concern over cost of the pacemaker and their ability to pay for it
   c. Fear of dying and/or electrocution – "How long can I expect to live with this pacemaker?"
   d. Change in self image, physical changes, disfigurement, scars – what will people think?
   e. Misconceptions that the pacemaker will correct and cure diseased hearts
   f. Employment, type of work, frequent travel, sports and exposure to electromagnetic fields (EMI) that would interfere with the pacemaker
   g. Over-the-counter medications and prescriptions
   h. Exposure to the health care system for other treatments

4. Access individual needs specific to that patient – Refer to Part One, Chapter 7 (Patient education, general).
5. Teaching plan and methods
   a. Develop a teaching plan.
      1. Goals
      2. Objectives
      3. Methods
         a) Discussion
         b) Flip charts
         c) Audio-visual aides
         d) Booklets/pamphlets
         e) Tapes
         f) Charts
         g) Methods specific to the patient's level of understanding
      4. Resources
   b. Conduct patient interviews to define content
   c. Design education program
   d. Conduct teaching sessions
   e. Evaluate teaching process
   f. Make necessary changes to the program or for each patient as they proceed through the program
   g. Document teaching process
      1. Medical record
      2. Teaching check list

B. Preoperative
   1. Patient interview
      a. Lifestyle
      b. Support system
      c. Medications
      d. Indication for pacemaker
      e. Symptoms
      f. Past medical history
      g. Previous surgery
      h. Allergies
      i. Travel and leisure activities
      j. Occupation
      k. Financial status
      l. Medical insurance

   m. Other resources

   n. Diagnostic work-up (labs, etc.)

2. Education content (will vary with time available prior to implantation)

   a. Review lifestyle and potential interaction with the pacemaker

   b. List names and telephone numbers of individuals in their support system who will be actively involved in their long-term care

   c. Trace the normal pathway of blood through the heart and name the anatomy

   d. Draw a single channel and dual channel pacemaker and lead system on a heart diagram

   e. State briefly what a pacemaker does once implanted

   f. List present medications and be aware of the ones held prior to surgery and why held

   g. Understand the importance of returning for follow-up (review often)

      1. Clinic

      2. Transtelephonic monitoring

   i. Review basic terminology and ask questions to understand level of patient's comprehension

   l. Demonstrate how to take radial pulse correctly (will need to repeat this)

   m. Distinguish between the types of rates possible in current pacemaker technology

   n. Understand how longevity varies in devices and between individuals

   o. Discuss indication for pacemaker

C. Surgical Procedure

  1. Informed consent

  2. Pacemaker implantation

   a. Physical needs

      1. Position on operative table, include potential duration

      2. Urinate prior to the procedure

      3. Pain medications

      4. Local anesthetic agent

      5. Breathing under the drapes

      6. Room temperature

      7. Skin preparation

      8. Inability to move

      9. Sterile area

   b. Psychological needs

   1. Reassurance
   2. Participate in procedure by following instructions
   3. Terminology patient can understand
   4. Communication
   5. Repeat instructions if needed
   6. Avoid terms such as "end of life, pacemaker jargon"
   7. Holding patient's hand
 c. Procedure
   1. Routine, minor procedure
   2. Transvenous
   3. Small pocket made for generator and location
   4. Monitoring
   5. Room set up
   6. Fluoroscopy (Patient safety)

D. Postoperative and Pre-Hospital Discharge Instructions

   1. Care of wound
      a. Review size, depth and pocket with patient and local anesthetic and suture removal if indicated
      b. Review hematomas, if patient notices any swelling or discharge, heat or increased tenderness on pacer site, they are to notify their care giver as soon as possible
      c. Review site discomfort, can persist for up to 2 months
      d. Review signs of infection
      e. Report any visible or subjective sign of muscle stimulation in pocket at pacer site, or hiccoughs should be brought to the attention of the care giver to rule out perforation or to decrease high outputs
      f. Auscutate the lungs to rule out pneumothorax secondary to traumatic needle stick
      g. Report presence of pre-implant symptoms, can signify lead displacement or loss of capture
      h. Review that essentially there is no care for the wound only if there is slight oozing, cleanse area well without rubbing or causing irritation to the incision
      i. Removal of external sutures (if used) in 7–10 days postoperatively
   2. Lifestyle
      a. Take and record pulse
      b. Carry pacemaker identification card
      c. Report recurrence of previous symptoms
      d. Continue diet

    e. Continue medications unless changed or discontinued by the physician

    f. Notify physician of travel plans

    g. Discuss home electrical safety

    h. Resume sexual activity

    i. Resume work per physician's instructions

    j. Adhere to treatment programs in effect for other health care problems

3. Follow-up

    a. Transtelephonic follow-up (TTM)

        1. Telephone communication

        2. Locations

            a) Hospital

            b) Physician office

            c) Commercial service

    b. Clinic

        1. On site visit vs. the telephone

        2. Locations

            a) Hospital

            b) Physician office

        3. Refer to Part Two, Chapter 18, for specifics of pacemaker follow-up to provide for the patient

4. Do's and don'ts

    a. Do's

        1. Review electromagnetic fields, i.e., electrical generators in factories, magnetic resonance imaging, microwave ovens and other electromagnetic interference

        2. Reassure the patient that today's pacemakers are highly reliable and if a systematic routine follow-up schedule is maintained, problems will remain at a minimum and if schedule is maintained, pacer will last longer

        3. Instruct the patient to write down questions they think of and bring the list to the next follow-up visit

        4. Review the benefits of programmability

    b. Don'ts

        1. Compare yourself with other pacemaker patients. Each one is unique and requires a follow-up schedule tailored to individual needs. Review pacemaker dependent at this time.

        2. Do not put a magnet over the telemetry box, it depletes battery life of transmitter battery

        3. Do not hold a magnet over the pacemaker longer than 30 seconds. Only place magnet on pacer when testing.

5. Postoperative complications
    1. Hematoma, bleeding in the pulse generator pocket with skin discoloration in breast area and under arm, can extend to waist
    2. Infection
    3. Diaphragmatic and pectoralis major stimultation
    4. Hiccoughs with inadvertent stimulation of phrenic nerve
    5. Lead fracture, dislodgement or insullation fracture
    6. Myocardial perforation
    7. Pneumothorax, R/O by chest x-ray
    8. Venous thrombosis/embolism
    9. Tricuspid valve insufficiency
    10. Electromagnetic interference (EMI)
    11. Poor wound healing
    12. Arrhythmias
    13. Battery migration
    14. Congestive heart failure
    15. Externalization of the power pack (generator)

E. Psychological Needs

   1. Anxiety
      a. Allow for verbalization of concerns and discuss ways to help decrease anxiety
      b. Stress the positive aspects of having a pacemaker.
   2. Sense of security
      a. Review reliability of pacer back-up with current literature
   3. Dependency
      a. Only take pulse if you feel dizzy, weak or if pre-pacer symptoms reappear
   4. Sexuality
      a. All sexual activities can be as before, don't change lifestyle
   5. Reliability of pacemaker and battery failure with FDA guideline
      a. With FDA guidelines over the years, today's pacemakers are highly reliable. Leads are smaller, flexible and more durable, tine and screw-ins provide reliable fixation.
      b. Batteries are smaller and last longer, less erosion noted. With proper programming, reliability and battery performance are assured.
      c. Built-in safety features and filters protect against EMI. Therefore, today's pacemakers are very reliable and failure, if the patient is properly monitored, should not be an issue.
   6. Warranties

    a. Every company has its own policy on warranties.

    b. Encourage patients to request a copy of the warranty upon discharge

F. Patient Education for Generator Replacement

  1. Content to explain the need for replacement

    a. The pacemaker battery registers end-of-service (EOS) indications, usually following 8–10 years of service.

    b. EOS means end-of-service for the battery.

    c. At this time the initial implant procedure will be repeated.

    d. The existing lead or leads will be tested and the majority will remain. On some occasions the lead system needs to be removed with the old pacemaker generator.

    e. Reimplantation is the removal of the old pacemaker battery and attachment of a new generator to the existing lead system. The replacement implantation procedure is much quicker than the initial implant.

  2. Length of stay

    a. The procedure can be done as an out-patient (23 hour admission). Side effects are minimal if any. In some cases, when an atrial lead is to be added, the patient will stay 1 or 2 days.

    b. Safety

      1. Recommend 24 hour Holter to evaluate operation of the system especially if it has been upgraded.

      2. Review components of the patient education program done following initial implantation.

G. Patient Educational Services

  1. International Association of Pacemaker Patients, Inc., P.O. Box 54305, Atlanta, GA 30308. This is a non-profit association which supports the emotional and psychological needs of pacemaker recipients.

  2. Hospital Pacemaker Clubs or support groups – check your local hospitals

  3. Individual pacemaker companies provide educational materials

  4. Individual patient education manuals given to patients at discharge

  5. Video tapes

  6. American Heart Association

  7. Finally, a good resource person would be anyone in the health care team.

References

Furman S, Hayes D, Holmes D. A Practice of Cardiac Pacing. New York: Futura Publishing Co, Inc., 379. 1986.

Moses S, Miller T. A Practical Guide to Cardiac Pacing. 3rd edition. Boston: Little, Brown. 1991.

Riegel P, Brest D. Dreifus' Pacemaker Therapy: an Interprofessional Approach. Philadelphia: FA Davis. 1986.

Silverman H. Elements of informed consent. Clin Rev. 2:8:115. 1992.

Vallario L, Lemon R, Gillette P, Kratz J. Charleston SC. Pacemaker follow-up and adequacy of Medicare guidelines. Am Heart J. 116:11. 1988.

Part 3

ELECTROPHYSIOLOGY CURRICULUM

CHAPTER 22

Basic Electrophysiology

Elizabeth Darling
Lois Schurig

Subsection:
A. Membrane Potentials
B. Action Potentials
C. Ion Channels
D. Automaticity
E. Conduction Velocity
F. Refractoriness
G. Reentry
H. Triggered Activity
I. Other Concepts
J. Basic Electrophysiology of Antiarrhythmic Medications

Historically, electrophysiology has been a field of rapidly expanding knowledge as to the diagnosis and management of patients with arrhythmias. The field can be divided into two basic areas; diagnostic and therapeutic electrophysiology. From a diagnostic stand point, the discovery by Einthoven that the heart's electrical potentials can be recorded, establishes the true basis of electrophysiology. If you expand the theory that you can record electrical signals from the heart, intracardiac recordings are a natural extension of Einthoven's discovery. A doctor by the name of His discovered that you could record an electrical potential from the area distal to the AV node. The area was then identified as the bundle of His. The discovery by His opened countless doors to the analysis of normal and abnormal conduction within the heart leading to explanations as to where arrhythmias originate and then to also serve as a marker for therapeutic intervention.

From: Schurig L. *Educational Guidelines: Pacing and Electrophysiology.* Armonk, NY: Futura Publishing Co, Inc, © 1994.

From the stand point of therapeutic electrophysiology, there have been great strides taken recently with ablation of cardiac tissue for the treatment of arrhythmias. However, therapeutic electrophysiology began several years ago with the termination of reentrant tachycardias using overdrive pacing or entrainment of the arrhythmia. Ablation of cardiac tissue has been accomplished by several methods such as surgical, direct current, chemical and radiofrequency, all with varying degrees of success and risk benefit ratio for the patient. Therapeutic electrophysiology can be considered as a first line therapy for many cardiac arrhythmias in the 1990s.

Chapter 22 of Part Three, the Electrophysiology Curriculum is designed to further define the basic concepts of cardiac electrophysiology presented in Part One, the Core Curriculum. The chapter begins with an explanation of the cardiac cell, action potentials, cell refractoriness and ends with the mechanisms as they relate to the action potential.

Due to the nature of the rapidly expanding field of cardiac electrophysiology and the potential for new knowledge, it is hoped that the basics of electrophysiology will help us understand the developments as they arise.

Objectives

1. Differentiate between early and late afterdepolarizations.
2. Describe the components of reentry.
3. Identify the characteristics of various mechanisms of arrhythmias.
4. Differentiate between active and passive impulse formation.
5. Describe the ECG criteria for recognition of various mechanisms of arrhythmias.
6. Identify normal characteristics of cardiac cells.

Glossary and Abbreviations

Abnormal automaticity: The result of an abnormal acceleration of Phase 4 activity of the action potential; the property of a fiber to initiate an impulse. Accounts for less than 10% of tachyarrhythmias.

Action potential: With an appropriate stimulus, the membrane potential of a cardiac cell will decrease resulting in a sudden rapid depolarization followed by repolarization back to the resting potential. The action potential is a result of the transport of ions across the cell membrane causing voltage changes. When the voltage changes are plotted with time, they are reflected as an action potential.

Anion: Negatively charged ions.

Antegrade conduction: Transmission of the impulse down the conduction system starting with the SA node generating the impulse down to the Purkinje network (orthograde).

Arrhythmia: An irregular rhythm due to a disturbance in impulse formation, impulse conduction or a combination of both.

Ashman's phenomenon: Long-short cycle during atrial fibrillation results in aberrant conduction.

Automaticity: The ability of a cardiac cell to spontaneously initiate an action potential resulting in the depolarization of the cell.

Calcium channels: Ion channels that mediate the plateau phase of the action potential by allowing positively charged ions to slowly enter the intracellular space. The action potential of the SA and AV node are dependent on the slow calcium channels.

Cation: Positively charged ions.

Cell membrane: The wall surrounding a single cell.

Combined disorders: The interaction between disorders of impulse conduction and disorders of impulse formation that results in initiation of a tachyarrhythmia. One type of disorder causes the other to occur.

Compensatory pause: Time following a premature beat. Recovery time of the SA node in preparation for the next impulse. The SA node is depolarized by previous beat, therefore, must start over.

Delayed afterdepolarizations: A delayed afterdepolarization (late potential) occurs during Phase 4 of the action potential.

Depolarization: The first phase of a cardiac action potential. The result of a cell being excited beyond -80 to -90 mV causes the cell membrane to allow the passage of positive ion current across the cell membrane.

Disorders of impulse conduction: Inappropriate conduction of an impulse as a result of a conduction delay or clock that controls the atrial or ventricular rate for one or more complexes, it can occur in all cardiac tissue.

Disorders of impulse formation: Inappropriate discharge rate of the sinus node or discharge from an ectopic focus that controls rhythm for one or more impulses. Can occur in most cardiac tissue, but it does not normally reach threshold due to overdrive suppression of the sinus node. Ectopic activity can occur when the sinus discharge rate is abnormally slow or the normal impulse is blocked allowing the escape of the abnormal rhythm. Ectopic activity can occur when the rate of ectopic activity exceeds the normal sinus rate.

Early afterdepolarizations: An early afterdepolarization occurs before full repolarization of the cardiac cell, Phase 2 or 3 of the action potential.

Ectopic origin: Cardiac rhythms which originate outside the SA node are referred to as ectopic rhythms. Mechanisms involved in abnormal impulse formation are passive (escape) and active (ectopic) impulse formation.

Ectopic rhythm: A rhythm that originates outside the SA node.

Excitability: The ability of a cardiac muscle to generate an action potential.

Extracellular: Outside the cell membrane.

Heart block: Failure of an impulse initiated in the SA node to conduct normally to the ventricles usually as a result of an abnormality in conduction velocity or refractoriness within the AV node, distal to the AV node or infra-Hisian.

Hyperpolarization: Accumulation of intracellular sodium causing a more negative diastolic membrane potential.

Intracellular: Within the cell membrane.

Ions: Charged molecules.

Ion transport: The movement of ions across the cell membrane which is controlled by specialized protein channels.

Ion channels: Channels found within the cell membrane that regulate the passage of ions across the cell membrane during the process of depolarization and repolarization.

Membrane potential: Voltage difference across the cell membrane as a result of negatively charged ions within the cell, -80 to -90 millivolts in cardiac muscle.

Normal origin: The property of impulse formation (automaticity) is not confined to a single cardiac center. This capability is shared by the SA node, AV node and the Purkinje network. Every focal collection of P cells has the potential of functioning as pacemaker of the heart, but one dominates. The SA node is the primary pacemaker due to its faster rate of automaticity.

Overdrive suppression: Inhibition by a faster pacemaker of a slower pacemaker as a result of hyperpolarization.

Parasystole: A fixed rate asynchronously discharging pacemaker which is not altered by the dominant rhythm. The ectopic focus is insulated by entrance block and depolarization only occurs when the myocardium is excitable.

Reentry: The most common mechanism responsible for tachyarrhythmia initiation. A result of three properties (1) two or more paths, (2) one of the paths must conduct more quickly than the other, and (3) one path must have unidirectional block.

Refractoriness: The inability of a cell or a group of cells to depolarize due to incomplete repolarization.

Repolarization: The gradual return of a cell to its original state by a reversal of the ion flux that occurs during depolarization, phase 1 through 3 of the action potential.

Retrograde conduction: Transmission of the impulse from a site in the heart other than the SA node. Conduction goes from Purkinje network area back up to the atrium (VA conduction).

Sodium channels: Ion channels that mediate phase 0 of the action potential by allowing positively charged sodium ions to rapidly enter the intracellular space resulting in a change in the transmembrane potential.

Sodium-potassium pump: The pump maintains an osmotic balance between intracellular and extracellular fluid by transporting three ions of sodium out of the cell in exchange for two potassium ions. The result is a low intracellular sodium concentration and a high intracellular potassium concentration.

Stimulus: Delivery of a small electrical current.

Triggered activity: A leakage of voltage during Phase 3 or 4 of the action potential resulting in an afterdepolarization which is caused by a preceding impulse.

Education Content

A. Membrane Potentials

    1. Determines cellular excitability

    2. Restricts movement of ions between the intracellular to the extracellular space

    3. Selective ion transport maintains ion distribution.

    4. Intracellular, negatively charged ions (anions) cannot cross the cell membrane

    5. Positively charged ions (cations) balance the anions to maintain electrical neutrality

    6. Activation of the sodium-potassium pump (principle cations in the extracellular space) maintains electrical neutrality by allowing $Na+$ + and $K+$ to cross the cell membrane

    7. Resting cell membrane potential is -90 millivolts primarily based on $K+$ gradient across the cell wall

B. Action Potential

    1. Result of a stimulus decreasing membrane potential

    2. 5 phases

        a. Phase O – *rapid depolarization*, sodium channels open allowing a rapid influx of sodium

        b. Phase 1 – *early rapid repolarization*, calcium channels open allowing calcium to enter the cell at the same time the sodium influx decreases

        c. Phase 2 – *plateau*, decrease in the conductance of ions resulting in a state of equilibrium

        d. Phase 3 – *repolarization*, increasing outward flow of potassium

        e. Phase 4 – *resting*, ions have returned to their original balance awaiting the next stimulus to decrease the membrane potential

C. Ion Channels

    1. Sodium-potassium pump

    2. Calcium channels

    3. Sodium channels

    4. Potassium channels

D. Automaticity

    1. The mechanisms by which the normal heart rhythm is generated.

    2. Cardiac cells capable of impulse formation are found throughout the conduction system.

3. A leakage of ions back and forth across the cell membrane results in spontaneous phase 4 diastolic depolarization.

E. Conduction Velocity
  1. The speed of conduction of an electrical impulse across cardiac tissue.
  2. Related to the rate of rise during depolarization in phase 0 of the action potential.

F. Refractoriness
  1. The period of time after a depolarization during which the cell cannot depolarize again
  2. Refractory periods
     a. Effective refractory period (ERP) – The period of time when an action potential cannot be initiated by a normal electrical stimulus.
     b. Relative refractory period (RRP) – The period of time when only a stimulus greater than that normally used will initiate an action potential.
     c. Absolute refractory period (ARP) – The period of time when the initiation of an action potential is impossible no matter how strong the stimulus.
     d. Functional refractory period (FRP) – The shortest period of time that allows for the initiation of an action potential.

G. Reentry
  1. An impulse once conducted through the heart returns to reactivate the atria or ventricles. Activation of the same cardiac tissue occurs.
  2. Reentry schematic → ectopic foci with localized refractoriness → NSR beat travels non-refractory path → localized refractory area recovers → NSR beat triggers another response.

H. Triggered Activity
  1. Early potentials (afterdepolarizations)
     a. Occur during final stage of repolarization
     b. Likely to trigger arrhythmias with bradycardias
     c. Termination occurs with hyperpolarization
     d. Torsades de pointes (Tdp)
     e. Rate stability after a few beats
  2. Delayed potentials (afterdepolarizations)
     a. Second depolarizations occurring after full repolarization, after phase 3 of the action potential (T wave)
     b. Produces ectopic atrial, junctional, or ventricular tachycardias
     c. ↑ intracellular calcium

d. ↓ cycle lengths and catecholamines have a tendency to aggravate environments susceptible to the effects of late potentials

e. Result from digitalis, reperfusion, catecholamines

I. Other Concepts

1. Mechanisms

   a. Active impulse formation

   Active (ectopic) – results when cells in the heart capable of pacing experience a change in automaticity. They become irritable due to the changes in excitability, experience an increase in cell membrane permeability with an increased rate and override the SA node to assume the role of pacemaker. The alterations can be due to anoxia, tissue damage, drugs or other situations which disrupt the normal cardiac environment.

   An ectopic beat on the rhythm strip is identified by its relationship to the sinus beats. It occurs early in the cardiac cycle.

   1. Enhanced normal automaticity
      a) Acceleration of phase 4
      b) Cause of arrhythmia from Purkinje fibers with high membrane potential
      c) Suppressed by overdrive pacing, when potential becomes less negative, overdrive pacing is diminished
      d) Ectopic beats or rhythms
      e) Emerge at slower rate
      f) Warm up period
      g) Treat with class I antiarrhythmics

   2. Abnormal automaticity
      a) Existence of a low membrane potential, < 60 mV, action potential more CA dependent
      b) Not responsive to overdrive pacing or lidocaine
      c) Generates VT as seen in first 24 hours post-MI
      d) Emerge even with satisfactory sinus rhythm
      e) Treat with CA channel blockers.

   b. Passive impulse formation

   Passive (escape) – results when the SA node fails to produce an impulse, slowing the rate of impulse formation, or the impulse formed cannot be conducted to the AV node. Therefore, the alternate centers assume the role of pacemaker for one or more beats due to their superior rate. The alterations can be due to ischemia, increased K or depletion of catecholamines.

   An escape beat on the rhythm strip is identified by its relationship to the sinus beats. It comes late in the cardiac cycle or replaces the expected sinus beat. If the escape mechanism is able to remain dominate, it continues at its own rate and rhythm. This is an automatic, physiologic response not to be treated without evaluation of the cause.

c. Dissociation – condition where the atria and ventricles beat independently. It is not a diagnosis in itself, but a syndrome. Follows an alteration in rhythm or conduction. Produced under the following conditions:

1. Default – slowing or impairment of SA node impulse or conduction at SA junction

2. Usurption – acceleration in AV node or ventricles of impulse formation.

3. AV conduction disturbance

   On the ECG, there is a loss of the normal P to QRS relationship for a variable period of time. The number of QRS complexes usually exceeds the number of P waves. Occurs with sinus bradycardia, sinus arrhythmia, pacing, VT, digitalis.

d. Aberrant conduction – refers to the distortion of the QRS complex of a supraventricular impulse. An alternate pathway of ventricular conduction. Related to the impulse invading the ventricles during the relative refractory period.

e. Reciprocal or echo beat – a beat that results when the same impulse activates the heart for a second time. It is helpful to remember conduction is possible both antegrade and retrograde.

f. Concealed conduction – alteration in impulse formation or conduction caused by electrophysiologic events not recorded on the ECG. The AV junction is partially penetrated by an atrial impulse and not completely conducted. The refractoriness created prevents the conduction of the following beat. ECG findings include:

1. A prolonged P-R interval or a blocked P wave occurs at a time conduction should be possible.

2. As the AV node is the usual site affected, the AV node will not produce the expected escape beat after a long pause. Seen with interpolated beats, pacing, ventricular standstill.

J. Basic Electrophysiology of Antiarrhythmic Medications – Also refer to Chapter 28.A.

1. Effect change in cardiac tissue by altering the shape of the action potential.

2. Antiarrhythmics fall into 5 different classes

   a. Class I – bind to the sodium channel and decrease the rate of depolarization.

   1. Ia – slow conduction velocity and increase refractory period.

   2. Ib – decrease action potential duration and shorten refractory periods

   3. Ic – depress conduction velocity

b. Class II – decrease sympathetic tone
c. Class III – increase action potential duration and as a result refractory periods
d. Class IV – block calcium channels
e. Class V – increases parasympathetic activity

References

Fogoros N. Electrophysiology Testing: Practical Cardiac Diagnosis. Boston: Blackwell Scientific Publications. 1991.

Horowitz LN. Current Management of Arrhythmias. Philadelphia: BC Decker, Inc. 1991.

Josephson ME, Seides SF. Clinical Cardiac Electrophysiology: Techniques and Interpretations. Philadelphia: Lea & Febiger. 1979.

Josephson M. Clinical Cardiac Electrophysiology: Techniques and Interpretations. Philadelphia: Lea & Febiger. 1993.

Naccarelli GV. Cardiac Arrhythmias: A Practical Approach. New York: Futura Publishing Co, Inc. 1991.

Ward DE, Camm A. Clinical Electrophysiology of the Heart. London: Edward Arnold. 1987.

Zipes DP, Jalife J. Cardiac Electrophysiology: From Cell to Bedside. Philadelphia: WB Saunders Co. 1990.

CHAPTER 23

Clinical Electrophysiology

Joni Baxter
Elizabeth Darling

Subsection:
A. Clinical Electrophysiology
  1. Initial Clinical Assessment
  2. Clinical Evaluation
  3. Indications for Diagnostic Electrophysiologic Study
B. Contraindications and Precautions

Cardiac electrophysiology is developing an expanding role in the medical community. Diagnostic electrophysiologic (EP) studies assist physicians with risk stratification and choice of appropriate interventions. This method of patient management enables a significant reduction in symptom recurrence, arrhythmia recurrence and mortality rate.

Prior to the presentation to the EP laboratory, a thorough history and physical must be completed. The information most helpful when referring a patient for an EP study includes a history of symptoms, surrounding events, documented arrhythmias, underlying heart disease, and left ventricular function. Evaluation of these patients frequently includes an extensive general cardiac workup. The arrhythmia evaluation often includes non-invasive testing such as event monitors, signal averaged ECG, telemetry and Holter monitoring prior to the risk and expense of an EP study.

The indications for EP studies used in this chapter are based on the recommendations of the ACC/AHA Task Force Report on Guidelines for Clinical Intracardiac Electrophysiology Studies: Assessment of Diagnostic and Therapeutic Cardiovascular Procedures (Subcommittee to Assess Clinical In-

---

From: Schurig L. *Educational Guidelines: Pacing and Electrophysiology*. Armonk, NY: Futura Publishing Co, Inc, © 1994.

tracardiac Electrophysiology Studies), published in the *Journal American College of Cardiology*, 1989.

The population undergoing EP studies is changing. This is in part due to the advent and success rate of therapeutic EP guided procedures such as ablation, surgery, and implantable devices compared to the ineffectiveness, intolerance, and adverse complications associated with antiarrhythmic drug therapy.

Objectives

1. Describe the portion of a history and physical assessment needed prior to referring a patient for an electrophysiology study.
2. List methods of evaluating intermittent symptoms.
3. Describe patients that are definitely indicated, probably or possibly indicated and not indicated for an EP study to evaluate a patient for documented or suspected atrioventricular heart block.
4. Describe patients that are definitely indicated, probably or possibly indicated and not indicated for an EP study to evaluate a patient with sinus node dysfunction.
5. Describe patients that are definitely indicated, probably or possibly indicated and not indicated for an EP study to evaluate a patient for syncope.
6. Describe patients that are definitely indicated, probably or possibly indicated and not indicated for an EP study to evaluate a patient after a cardiac arrest.
7. Describe patients that are definitely indicated, probably or possibly indicated and not indicated for an EP study to evaluate a patient for documented or suspected narrow or wide complex tachycardia.
8. Describe patients that are definitely indicated, probably or possibly indicated and not indicated for an EP study to evaluate a patient for unexplained palpitations.
9. Describe patients that are definitely indicated, probably or possibly indicated and not indicated for an EP study to evaluate a patient for documented or suspected Wolff-Parkinson-White syndrome (WPW).
10. Describe patients that are definitely indicated, probably or possibly indicated and not indicated for an EP study to evaluate patients with premature ventricular beats (PVCs) and couplets.

Education Content

A. Clinical Electrophysiology

  1. Initial clinical assessment

    a. Heart disease

      1. CAD

      2. Cardiomyopathy

      3. Valvular disease

      4. Primary electrical disease

      5. Previous surgery

    b. New York Heart Association

      1. Class I – cardiac disease without resulting limitations

      2. Class II – cardiac disease with slight limitations

      3. Class III – cardiac disease with marked limitations

      4. Class IV – cardiac disease with inability to carry out physical activity without discomfort (may have symptoms at rest)

    c. Clinical history

      1. Presenting symptoms

        a) Palpitations

        b) Diaphoresis

        c) Dyspnea

        d) Lightheaded/dizziness

        e) Pre-syncope

        f) Syncope

        g) Angina

      2. Arrhythmia event history

        a) Frequency

        b) Duration

        c) Patient tolerance

        d) Previous therapy tried

        e) Date of diagnosis

        f) Due to reversible factors

        g) Patient activity pre-event

        h) Patient activity post-event

        i) Mode of termination

    d. Documentation of arrhythmia

      1. EMT rhythm strip

      2. ER documentation

       3. Cardiac telemetry

       4. Holter or event recorder

2. Clinical evaluation

   a. Electrocardiographic

       1. 12 lead ECG

       2. Telemetry

       3. Event recorder

       4. Esophageal

       5. SAECG

       6. Holter

   b. Cardiac function

       1. Echo

       2. MUGA

       3. Cardiac catheterization

       4. Thallium stress

       5. MIBG

       6. Treadmill exercise test

3. Indications for Diagnostic Electrophysiologic Study

   a. Atrioventricular (AV) heart block

       1. Class I – definitely indicated

          a) When His-Purkinje block is suspected and cannot be diagnosed by scalar ECG

          b) Pacemaker patients with syncope or near syncope in whom VT is suspected

       2. Class II – probably or possibly indicated

          a) Concealed junctional extrasystoles suspected as the cause of AV block

          b) AV block when there is a need to assess treatment options

       3. Class III – not indicated

          a) When symptoms and presence of AV block are correlated by the ECG

          b) Asymptomatic patients with AV nodal Wenckebach

          c) Asymptomatic patients with periodic AV block or short duration often associated with sinus slowing

   b. Wide complex tachycardias (QRS > 0.12 sec)

       1. Class I – definitely indicated

          a) Patients with wide complex tachycardias that are sustained and/or symptomatic when the diagnosis is unclear

       2. Class II – probably or possibly indicated

          a) Patients with pre-excitation syndromes with suspected antidromic tachycardia to evaluate mulitple bypass tracts

    3. Class III – not indicated

      a) Patients with VT or SVT with aberration or pre-excitation seen on the ECG

c. Sinus node function

    1. Class I – definitely indicated

      a) When a casual relationship between the presence of sinus bradycardia, sinus pauses, and patients symptoms has not been established

    2. Class II – probably or possibly indicated

      a) In patients with known sinus node dysfunction and the need for pacemaker insertion, to assess appropriate site and modality of pacing

      b) In patients with known sinus node dysfunction to determine severity or mechanism and response to drugs

      c) Symptomatic patients to exclude other arrhythmic mechanisms

      d) Patients in the above categories when the information will facilitate treatment.

    3. Class III – not indicated

      a) Asymptomatic patients with sinus bradycardia during sleep

      b) When symptoms are clearly related to sinus dysfunction

d. Syncope, unexplained

    1. Class I – definitely indicated

      a) Patients with unexplainled syncope, especially those with structural heart disease

    2. Class II – probably or possibly indicated

      a) Patients with unexplained syncope without structural heart disease

    3. Class III – not indicated

      a) Syncope explained by another cause

e. Cardiac arrest, survivors

    1. Class I – definitely indicated

      a) All patients who have survived a cardiac arrest without an acute Q wave MI

      b) Patients surviving and episode of cardiac arrest occurring > 48 hrs after acute MI

    2. Class II – probably or possibly indicated

      a) Patients surviving a cardiac arrest due to bradycardia

    3. Class III – not indicated

      a) Patients with cardiac arrest occurring only within the first 48 hrs of acute MI

  b) Patients with cardiac arrest resulting from acute reversible ischemia or other identifiable cause

f. Narrow complex tachycardia (QRS < 0.12 sec)

 1. Class I – definitely indicated

  a) Patients who have recurrent drug resistant tachycardia

  b) To evaluate therapeutic efficacy for 1)

  c) Patients who prefer ablative therapy to drugs

 2. Class II – probably or possibly indicated

  a) Patients with recurrent tachycardia who are less symptomatic requiring therapy in whom there is concern of the effect of drugs on the conduction system

 3. Class III – not indicated

  a) Patients whose ECG gives sufficient information about the tachycardia to permit treatment

  b) Patients whose tachycardias can be controlled by vagal maneuvers or drugs without precise arrhythmia analysis

g. Wolff-Parkinson-White Syndrome (WPW)

 1. Class I – definitely indicated

  a) Patients who are considered for nonpharmacologic treatment for life-threatening or incapacitating arrhythmias

  b) Patients intolerent of drug interventions

 2. Class II – probably or possibly indicated

  a) Patients with arrhythmias requiring treatment in whom additional information is needed:

   1) Type of arrhythmia

   2) Localization

   3) Number and electrophysiologic properties of accessory pathways

   4) Effects of drugs

  b) Asymptomatic patients with ECG evidence of WPW during sinus rhythm in whom additional information is needed

   1) guidance to remain in a high-risk occupation or activities

  c) WPW syndrome and a family history of premature sudden death

  d) WPW patient undergoing cardiac surgery for another reason

 3. Class III – not indicated

  a) Asymptomatic patients without arrhythmias who are not in class II, 2) and 3)

h. Chronic intraventricular conduction delay (IVCD)

 1. Class I – definitely indicated

  a) Symptomatic patients with BBB whose ventricular arrhythmia is suspected to be the cause for the symptoms

2. Class II – probably or possibly indicated
   a) Symptomatic patients with BBB in whom additional information will help treatment or assess prognosis
      1) Site
      2) Severity of conduction delay
      3) Drug response
3. Class III – not indicated
   a) Asymptomatic patients with IVCD
   b) Symptomatic patients with IVCD whose symptoms can be related to the ECG

i. Prolonged QT syndrome
   1. Class I – definitely indicated
      a) None
   2. Class II – probably or possibly indicated
      a) Identify proarrhythmic effects of drugs in patients experiencing their first episode of sustained VT or cardiac arrest while receiving and antiarrhythmic drug
   3. Class III – not indicated
      a) Congenital QT prolongation
      b) Acquired QT syndrome with symptomes related to an identifiable cause or mechanism

j. Ventricular premature complexes and couplets
   1. Class I – definitely indicated
      a) None
   2. Class II – probably or possibly indicated
      a) Patients with PVCs and unexplained pre-syncope or syncope
   3. Class III – not indicated
      a) Asymptomatic patients with PVCs

k. Unexplained palpitations
   1. Class I – definitely indicated
      a) Patients with palpitations who have a heart rate documented by medical personnel to be > 150 bpm and the ECG fails to document the cause of the symptoms
   2. Class II – probably or possibly indicated
      a) Patients with clinically significant palpitations
         1) Cardiac origin suspected
         2) Symptoms sporadic
         3) Symptoms not documented on repeated ECG or event recordings
         4) Determine mechanism of arrhythmia

     5) Direct treatment

     6) Assess prognosis

   3. Class III – not indicated

    a) Patients with palpitations due to extracardiac causes

l. Guide drug therapy

  1. Class I – definitely indicated

   a) Patients with sustained VT or cardiac arrest related to VT or VF, not associated with:

    1) Long QT syndrome

    2) Appearing within 48 hrs of an acute MI

    3) Spontaneous PVCs are not able to be documented on ECG recordings

  2. Class II – probably or possibly not indicated

   a) Recurrent, symptomatic paroxysmal AFib unresponsive to empiric antiarrhythmic therapy

   b) Recurrent, symptomatic, inducible SA node reentry, intra-atrial reentry and ectopic atrial tachycardias unresponsive to empiric antiarrhythmic therapy

   c) Recurrent, nonsustained VT not associated with MI or long QT syndrome

   d) Identify proarrhythmic effects in patients experiencing the first episodes of sustained VT or cardiac arrest while on antiarrhythmic drugs

   e) Risk stratification and consideration of therapy post-MI with decreased LV function, frequent PVCs or episodes of nonsustained VT or both, and the SAECG shows late potentials

  3. Class III – not indicated

   a) Isolated ectopics, atrial or ventricular

   b) Multifocal atrial tachycardia

   c) VT or cardiac arrest occurring only < 48 hrs after an acute MI

   d) Asymptomatic, nonrecurrent, or drug-responsive supraventricular or nonsustained ventricular tachycardias

   e) Ventricular arrhythmias with congenital long QT syndrome

m. Candidates for implanted electrical devices

  1. Class I – definitely indicated

   a) Candidates who require a device to treat arrhythmias

   b) Patients with a device in whom treatment changes may influence the safety or efficacy of the device

  2. Class II – probably or possibly indicated

   a) Patients with antitachycardia devices to validate device operation during follow-up

      b) Patients with antibradycardia devices to test for appropriate pacing site(s) and the capability of the conduction system

   3. Class III – not indicated

      a) Patients who are not candidates for implanted electrical devices

n. Candidates for ablative therapy

   1. Class I – definitely indicated

      a) Patient evaluation prior to arrhythmia surgery or other ablative procedures

      b) Assessment of procedure efficacy

      c) Evaluation of the need for additional intervention

   2. Class II – probably or possibly indicated

      a) Patients with symptoms from arrhythmias and an identified cause appropriate for surgery or other ablative procedures

   3. Class III – not indicated

      a) Patients with arrhythmias not candidates for surgical or ablative procedures

o. Electrophysiology procedures in children

   1. Class I – definitely indicated

      a) Similar to those described in previous sections for adults

      b) Undiagnosed "narrow QRS" tachycardia and sinus tachycardia cannot be determined

   2. Class II – probably or possibly indicated

      a) Similar to those described in previous sections for adults

      b) Patients without symptoms at high risk for sudden death

      c) Congenital complete heart block and escape rhythms with wide QRS complexes

   3. Class III – not indicated

      a) Similar to those described in previous sections for adults

      b) Congential complete heart block with escape rhythms with narrow QRS complexes

      c) Acquired complete heart block

      d) Patients without symptoms and surgically induced bifascicular block

p. New Indications

   1. New indications are evolving

   2. Future recommendations may be forthcoming

q. Safety

   1. Morbidity and mortality from EPS will vary, depending on the degree of cardiac compensation of the patients studied

   2. Adverse complications occur in $< 2\%$ of the EPS study population

3. The risk of death is difficult to assess because there are few reports of death, but it is estimated at < 0.01%.

4. Since rhythm disturbances are often a desired end point of the study, such rhythm disturbances may result.

B. Contraindications and Precautions

    1. Contraindications

        a. Unstable angina

        b. Uncontrolled CHF

        c. Bleeding disorder

        d. Uncooperative patient

        e. Severe PVD

        f. Severely debilitated patient

        g. Valvular or subvalvular aortic stenosis (LV entry)

        h. Thrombophlebitis (femoral)

        i. Groin infections (femoral)

        j. Bilateral amputee (femoral)

    2. Precautions

        a. Draw coagulation studies prior to procedure

        b. Draw electrolytes and magnesium level prior to procedure, if indicated

        c. Request monitored bed for patients with acute life-threatening arrhythmias

        d. Evaluate status of antiarrhythmic drugs (off 5 half lives of the drug if baseline study)

        e. Evaluate emotional status prior to procedure

References

Akhtar M, Fisher JD, Gillette PC. NASPE Ad Hoc Committee on guidelines for cardiac electrophysiology. PACE. 8:611–618. 1985.

Zipes DP, Akhtar M, Denes P. Guidelines for clinical intracardiac electrophysiology studies. Circulation. 80:1925–1939. 1989.

Zipes DP, Akhtar M, Denes P. Guidelines for clinical intracardiac electrophysiologic studies: a report of the ACC/AHA task force on assessment of diagnostic and therapeutic cardiovascular procedures (subcommittee to assess clinical intracardiac electrophysiology studies). JACC. 14: 1827–1842. 1989.

CHAPTER 24

Laboratory Procedures

Brenda L. Rosenberg

Subsection:
A. Patient Preparation
B. Catheterization Techniques
C. Recording Techniques
D. Risks and Complications
E. Patient and Family Support

The electrophysiology study (EPS) is an invasive study which is done using intracardiac electrode catheters placed in the right side of the heart to try to recreate arrhythmias a patient has been symptomatic with in the past. It is an objective treatment, as the actual arrhythmia is recreated and drugs are used to control the arrhythmia in a laboratory setting as opposed to the empirical (trial and error) treatment previously used.

This chapter describes the preparation and support of the patient and the laboratory environment for an electrophysiology study.

The EPS, being an invasive study, has its own inherent risks, but with careful patient preparation and meticulous attention to detail that risk can be minimized. The important information obtained can be used to tailor the treatment program to the patient's specific needs.

Objectives

1. Identify components of a care plan for pre-operative and post-operative management of the electrophysiology (EP) patient.

From: Schurig L. *Educational Guidelines: Pacing and Electrophysiology*. Armonk, NY: Futura Publishing Co, Inc, © 1994.

2. Identify risk factors of an electrophysiology study (EPS).
3. Define the differences between an initial EP study and a follow-up EP study.
4. List sites used for catheter placement and rationale.
5. Identify principles of sterile technique in the laboratory setting.
6. Explain the difference in EP catheters and their applications.
7. Evaluate patient comprehension of an EP test and the results.
8. Identify needs of the patient and family members related to the treatment protocols implemented following and EP study.
9. Explain the role of medications for the electrophysiology study.
10. Identify ways to reduce electrical interference in the electrophysiology lab.

Glossary and Abbreviations

Cardioversion: Delivery of energy (measured in joules) through the chest wall, synchronizing with the R-wave to stop ventricular tachycardia and restore a normal rhythm in the heart.

Cor sinus: Appendage of the right atrium that lies over the left atrium.

Cournand: Curve that is shaped into the catheter used in the EPS. Commonly used for RV and HIS placements.

Damato: Deep "C" curve to the catheter. It sometimes helps with placement in the cor sinus.

Defibrillation: Delivery of energy (measured in joules) through the chest wall to stop ventricular fibrillation and restore a normal rhythm in the heart.

Electrophysiology study (EPS): The study of the electrical conduction of the heart.

Half life: Refers to the time it takes a drug to decrease its effectiveness in the body.

Intracardiac: Contained within the heart.

IVPB: Intravenous piggy back, a method of drug administration.

Josephson: Another catheter curve. This is straighter than the Cournand. Often used for right ventricular placement.

NPO: Nothing by mouth.

Quadripolar: A catheter which has four (4) pacing electrodes at its tip.

RA: Right atrium.

RV: Right ventricle.

RVA: Right ventricular apex.

RVOT: Right ventricular outflow tract.

Steady state: The body when free of drugs and electrolytes are in normal quantities.

Tripolar: Catheter with 3 pacing electrodes at its tip.

VF: Ventricular fibrillation.

VT: Ventricular tachycardia.

Education Content

A. Patient Preparation

1. Sterile technique and preparation of the patient.

   a. NPO a minimum of 6 hours prior to the procedure, (clear liquid breakfast if procedure is late in the afternoon)

   b. Have a patent IV in place

   c. Shave right (and left) groin depending on the procedure and number of catheters to be used

   d. Receive cardiac medications prior to the study with sips of water as the doctor orders them

      1. For an initial study

         a) The patient should be in as close to a normal or drug-free state as possible

         b) All antiarrhythmics should be weaned from the body for at least 5 half lives of the drug

            1) Using a table that lists drug half lives, it can be figured when to stop the drug prior to the EPS

      2. For a repeat study

         a) If testing the oral equivalent of an IV drug tested in the previous EPS, the drug should be given on the prearranged schedule even though patient is held NPO

         b) If a previous oral form failed, then the patient should be treated as an initial study patient and drug-free of the failed drug

2. ECG monitoring technique

   a. It is essential to have sharp waveforms in your surface ECG leads. Things that may help:

      1. Carefull skin preparation using a skin defoliant-sandpaper, gritty lotion or gauze to provide good electrode contact with the skin

      2. Isolate electrode wires from other electrical wires

      3. Fresh electrodes

      4. Have chest area dry and free of any oils or creams

   b. A 12 lead ECG needs to be available at a moment's notice

      1. This can be achieved through some monitoring systems

      2. Have the patient hooked up to a 12 lead ECG monitor if not available through the monitoring system

   c. The monitor's skin leads must be clean as these are the reference points for the intracardiac electrogram. The leads used will depend on the doctor's preference.

   d. When placed over the chest, radiolucent wires and electrodes are helpful to eliminate excessive wires visible under the fluoroscopy and to avoid confusion for placement of pacing leads.

3. Defibrillation techniques

   a. Quick defibrillation is the secret in the EP lab!

   b. Have the defibrillator checked routinely by the biomedical department to be sure it is delivering the correct amount of energy.

   c. Check the defibrillator prior to its use during a case to be sure it is working properly.

   d. The use of adhesive defibrillator pads is a plus. One does not have to disturb the sterile field to defibrillate.

   e. Defibrillate/cardiovert only on the doctor's instructions

      1. It is necessary to see if the ventricular tachycardia is sustained or non-sustained and whether or not the patient can be paced out of the rhythm.

      2. It is usually acceptable to wait until the patient loses consciousness before giving the shock, but this will depend on the circumstances.

   f. Be ready for quick defibrillation in the event ventricular fibrillation is stimulated.

   g. Cardioversion may be used for ventricular tachycardia or atrial fibrillation.

B. Catheterization Techniques

   1. Site preparation

      a. The patient's groin should be shaved.

      b. Care must be taken to avoid nicks or scratches from the razor, these could be sites of infection.

      c. Check the patient's pedal and post-tibial pulses on the leg the catheters will be inserted in.

      d. An antiseptic solution is used to clean the site.

      e. The solution is applied to the skin, working in circular motion.

      f. Always move outward without going back over a previously cleaned site.

      g. Dry the area with a sterile towel.

      h. Surround the site with sterile towels.

         1. This serves to define the sterile area and to catch any excess blood during the catheter insertion.

      i. Drape the patient with the sterile drape. This should reach from the patient's neck down to the feet.

         1. Some drapes have an adhesive that keeps the hole directly over the site and this should be placed directly on the patient's skin not on the sterile towels.

    j. Check with the doctor about sites to prep

        1. Possible sites are the right femoral, left femoral and left jugular

2. Entry sites

    a. The right femoral vein is the main site used in EPS.

        1. Generally up to three 6F introducers can be inserted into that site

    b. The right femoral artery can be used to obtain a constant arterial blood pressure throughout the study.

        1. This is very helpful in the event VT is stimulated to indicate how well the patient tolerates the rhythm based on BP.

    c. The left femoral vein is generally used as a second site in the event more than three catheters will be used or if the patient's vasculature on the right makes it difficult to pass the catheters.

    d. The internal jugular vein is usually used in the event the cor sinus needs to be accessed.

3. Catheter selection (physician preference)

    a. For an adult EPS, a 5–7F catheter is generally used.

    b. Introducers should be 1F size larger to accommodate catheter manipulation.

    c. Woven Dacron has been the material of choice with proven torque. Maneuverability is its primary function.

    d. Quadripolar catheters are the workhorse of the EPS.

        1. They allow 2 electrodes for monitoring and 2 electrodes for stimulation at the same site.

    e. Bipolar catheters and tripolar catheters can also be used.

    f. The catheters may have a "bend" at the end that helps placement in different areas in the heart.

        1. The basic shapes are:

            a) Straight – for use in the RA or RV

            b) Cournand – a gentle "J" for use in the His bundle site, RV and cor sinus

            c) Josephson – "J" – for use in the His bundle site, RV or cor sinus

            d) Damato or cor sinus – a deep "J" – for use in the cor sinus

    g. Electrodes are normally placed 5 mm or 10 mm from each other. They may be more widely spaced or more closely spaced.

    h. Catheters can be special ordered if you have a specific need.

    i. Most EP catheters have a solid core without a lumen.

    j. These catheters are commonly reused-either a set amount of times or until the pacing electrodes no longer function.

    k. They should be soaked in a cleaning solution, gas sterilized, aired for 24 hours prior to being reused.

l. They should be checked with an ohmmeter after the soaking procedure to assure that the pacing electrode is intact.

C. Recording Technique
    1. Techniques for electrical interference reduction:
        a. Biomedical engineering should test equipment on a routine basis to assure no current leakage exists (must be less than 10 microamps). Greater than 10 microamps can be an electrical hazard to the patients or to the staff.
        b. Staff must also be aware of electrical hazards and have them taken care of before they become problems – Refer to Part One, Chapter 8, Safety.
        c. Turning off fluoroscopy equipment when catheters are in place will help with excessive "noise" on waveforms.
        d. Isolating catheter wires and wire connections from each other will also help reduce interference on waveforms and monitoring.
        e. Good skin preparation prior to electrode placement and careful anatomical placement will cut down most interference seen on the waveforms.

D. Risks and Complications
    1. The overall mortality rate for EPS is 0.6%. This is slightly less than that for coronary angiography studies.
    2. The complications for EPS depend on the site used. They are:
        a. Hypotension
        b. Hemorrhage
        c. Arterial injury
        d. Thrombophlebitis
        e. Emboli – systemic or pulmonic
        f. Cardiac perforation
        g. Tamponade
        h. Infection – systemic or at entry site
        i. Pneumothorax
        j. Transient or intermittent arrhythmias
        k. Proarrhythmic effects of drugs
        l. Death

E. Patient and Family Support
    1. Pre-procedure education
        a. Pamphlets and handouts that describe in "English" what EPS is about and what to expect. Obtain copies appropriate to other languages in the area.

b. A tour of the EPS laboratory or pictures taken to show the equipment and the standard attire of personnel.

c. Allow time for both patient and family to ask questions and receive the answers.

d. It is ideal if the EPS nurse can do the education. The patient and family will then have a bond with someone from the lab before the procedure occurs.

2. Emotional support

    a. The patient has the lab staff to help them relax and understand the procedure as it occurs.

    b. Medications may also be given to achieve sedation.

    c. The family should be encouraged to wait in the designated waiting area or the patient's room.

        1. This facilitates communication during and after the procedure.

        2. Everyone is aware of where they can be reached.

        3. These locations are more comfortable.

    d. The waiting area should be a pleasant with refreshments available if possible.

    e. Inform the family of the location of the vending machines or cafeteria.

    e. The family should be updated as often as possible during the study and especially if there are any delays – difficult catheter placement, drug infusion, doctor delays, etc.

3. Medications

    a. Sedation helps the patient to lay on the table for extended periods of time, to relax and not remember the unpleasant treatment modalities, ex: defibrillation.

    b. Valium, Versed and Fentanyl may be used without effects on the outcome of the study.

    c. Oxygen saturation should be monitored and patients should be on nasal oxygen during sedation.

    d. The sedation should be deep enough to provide amnesia but the patient needs to be arousable to answer questions.

    e. Antiarrhythmic drugs will be used in the event an arrhythmia is stimulated to identify their effects on the arrhythmia.

        1. Ventricular tachycardia: Pronestyl, Quinidine and Lidocaine are used in the IV form. Amiodarone is usually only tested in the oral form, however studies on the IV administration are being done.

        2. Supraventricular tachycardia: Inderal, Verapamil, Adenosine and Pronestyl may be used in the IV form.

    f. The drug chosen is given in a loading dose and then maintained with a drip (if appropriate).

1. The previous stimulation is repeated to see if the arrhythmia can be restimulated while the drug is on-board.

2. If the arrhythmias can be restimulated, then the patient has failed that drug.

3. If it is harder to restimulate the arrhythmia or it is at a slower rate, they have still failed the drug, but it provides some help to determine the method of treatment.

4. If the arrhythmia is not restimulated, the drug is determined to be effective. The patient will be placed on an oral equivalent of the drug and retested when a therapeutic level has been achieved.

g. Stimulants may be used if the arrhythmia is difficult to recreate with normal stimulation techniques or is normally occurring during physical activity.

1. Usually Isuprel is added in either a drip or bolus administration

4. Post-procedure education and emotional support

a. The patient needs to comply with bedrest and not moving the affected leg for 6–8 hours after the procedure. The family can assist by encouraging the patient during the recovery phase.

1. A sandbag may be used for 1–4 hours if the artery was cannulated.

2. A leg immobilizer can be used if the patient has difficulty complying with the movement restrictions.

3. Medications should be ordered to help the patient with back pain or general aches induced by prolonged procedure times or bedrest.

b. The patient and family should be informed of the test results and treatments available. The patient should have the information repeated on the next day when sedatives have worn off and they are more alert.

c. It is helpful to meet with the patient and family (if available) each day of the stay to answer questions and explain things one more time. It is best to correct any misconceptions at this time!

d. Detailed (but in English – or other language) handouts should be given for post-operative care and treatments.

e. Medications should be explained. Give the patient medication cards listing common uses of the drug, desired effects, side effects and any follow-up treatment needed.

f. Teaching for any implantable device, surgical treatment or ablations should begin now.

g. Provide the patient and family with phone numbers to use once they are home for questions that arise following discharge. It is helpful for them to be able to reach the EP staff if at all possible

h. A follow-up phone call 3–5 days after discharge is helpful to find out how the patient is, if there are any post-procedure complications, and to answer any questions.

i. Schedule appointments for follow-up and treatments as necessary.

References

Bashore TM. Invasive Cardiology: Principles and Techniques. BC Decker: Philadelphia. 1990.

Connelly A. An Examination of stressors in the patient undergoing electrophysiologic studies. Heart Lung. 335–342. 1992.

Josephson ME. Clinical Cardiac Electrophysiology: Techniques and Interpretations. 2nd edition. Lea and Febiger: Philadelphia. 1990.

Lubell DL. The Cath Lab: An Introduction. Lea and Febiger: Philadelphia. 1993.

Monroe D. Patient teaching for x-ray and other diagnostics. RN. February: 44–46. 1991.

Schurig L. Management of the patient requiring a cardiac electrophysiology study – Adult. Oakwood Hospital Policy and Procedure Manual. September, 1992.

Underhill SL. Cardiac Nursing. 2nd edition. JB Lippincott: Philadelphia. 1989.

Yee BH. Cardiac Critical Care Nursing. Boston: Little, Brown and Co. 1986.

Zipes DP, Jalife J. Cardiac Electrophysiology: from Cell to Bedside. Philadelphia. WB Saunders Co., 1990.

CHAPTER 25

Instrumentation

Jeanne Shewchik
Michelle G. Tobin

Subsection:
A. Laboratory Supplies
B. Laboratory Equipment
C. Maintenance

The electrophysiologic study is used to assess the conduction system of the heart, including the SA node, AV junction and Purkinje system function. It is also a tool to assess and determine the characteristics of arrhythmias. Efficacy of anti-arrhythmic drugs and devices can be tested as well as mapping procedures to locate arrhythmogenic foci.

Since many EP studies have the potential to induce hemodynamically unstable arrhythmias, they require personnel trained to deal with any cardiac emergencies. In addition to having a strong cardiology-knowledge base, the associated professional should be able to operate all equipment used in the laboratory. Their responsibilities may include, but are not limited to: physical and psychological assessment of patient condition, preparation of the patient for procedure, administration of medication, operation of the stimulator, intubation and other duties as per laboratory and hospital policy.

The EP study may appear complicated, requiring sophisticated equipment, however, the practitioner assessing cardiac electrical system function can accomplish this with basic equipment and supplies.

From: Schurig L. *Educational Guidelines: Pacing and Electrophysiology.* Armonk, NY: Futura Publishing Co, Inc, © 1994.

Objectives

1. List four pieces of equipment needed for the basic electrophysiology laboratory.
2. Identify the equipment and supplies needed for a basic electrophysiologic study.
3. Recognize the safety precautions for patients undergoing an electrophysiologic study.
4. Recognize equipment failure and report it to the appropriate resources.
5. Describe components of a preventive maintenance program for an electrophysiology department.
6. List emergency equipment required for an EP study.

Glossary and Abbreviations

Burst pacing: Delivery of multiple fast stimuli.

Decremental stimulation: Delivery of programmed electrical extrastimuli at progressively longer cycle lengths.

Electrode catheters: Consist of insulated wires attached to an electrode, which is exposed to the intracardiac surface. It is capable of being unipolar to multipolar and designed to record and pace intracardiac tissue.

Electrograms: Unipolar or bipolar recording of electrical wave forms from electrodes in contact with the myocardium.

Fluoroscopy: A technique used for examining deep structures by means of roentgen rays.

Incremental pacing: Delivery of programmed electrical extrastimuli at progressively shorter cycle lengths.

Multi-Channel switch box (junction box controls): The device that controls the connections from the electrode catheters to various recording and pacing devices.

Oscilloscope: An instrument that displays a visual representation of electrical variations on a fluorescent screen.

Physiologic recorder: A recorder that records three to four surface ECG leads and has the capability of recording multiple intracardiac leads.

Premature stimulus: A programmed electrical stimulus specifically timed from a preceding stimulus or from an intrinsic spontaneous event.

Programmed stimulator: A specialized pacing unit. It can be programmed to introduce complex sequences of paced beats to within 1 ms. It can also synchronize pacing to intrinsic heart rhythms. It can deliver one or several electrical stimuli at specifically timed intervals. i.e., premature stimuli, burst stimuli, incremental/decremental, trained stimulation.

Education Content

A. Laboratory Equipment

1. Fluoroscopy – should have the ability to record fluoroscopic data permanently for future reference
   a. Cine
   b. Video
   c. Mobility – it is desirable to be able to manipulate fluoroscopy in different positions for improved position and documentation.
2. Radiographic table
   a. Mobility – should be easily manipulated into multiple positions, ideally by the person changing the catheter position
3. Physiologic recorder
   a. Ability to record different speeds from 25 to 500 mm/sec.
   b. Capability to record three to four surface ECGs with multiple intracardiac electrograms
   c. Equipped with a variable signal limiter
   d. Hard copy recorder
   e. Long-term storage device, ex: optical discs
4. 12 Lead ECG – ability to document 12 surface leads simultaneously
   a. Free standing
   b. Capability of the recording system
5. Oscilloscope
6. Emergency equipment
   a. Oxygen
   b. Suction
   c. Cardioverter/defibrillator – portable with battery pack.
   d. Back-up cardioverter/defibrillator – available in case the other fails
   e. External pacemaker either as a separate unit or as part of the defibrillator
   f. Intubation equipment
   g. Standard emergency cart
   h. Emergency drug box
   i. Capability of emergency cardiac surgery
   j. Monitoring device
7. Programmable stimulator – has the ability to deliver sensed and paced extrastimuli
8. Multichannel lead switching box or junction box
   a. Multiple catheter capabilities
   b. Record and pace switch

      1. Extrastimuli with a minimum of S_4, ideally expanded S_4
      2. Incremental pacing
      3. Decremental pacing
      4. High-rate pacing
  9. Hemodynamic monitoring capability
    a. Arterial line
    b. Swan Ganz
    c. Cardiac output measurements (optional)
    d. Pulse oximetry

B. Laboratory Supplies
  1. Sterile trays
    a. Sterile drapes
    b. Sterile needles and syringes
    c. Sterile containers for anti-microbial scrub, saline and local anesthesia
    d. Hemostats
    e. Sponges
    f. Disposable container for contaminated materials
    g. Sterile tubing for IV
  2. Instrumentation for gaining vascular access
    a. Introducers
    b. Sheaths
    c. Cook or Potts needle
  3. Electrode catneters
    a. Bipolar
    b. Tripolar
    c. Quadrapolar (most common)
    d. Multipolar (used for mappings)
  4. Medications (per individual lab policy)
    a. Emergency
    b. Anti-arrhythmics
    c. Local anesthesia
    d. Anti-anxiety agents
    e. Anesthetic agents
    f. Antagonist drugs for standard drugs administered
  5. Documentation record
    a. Equipment charge record
    b. Vital-sign record
    c. Physician record

    d. Procedure record

    e. Physician order sheet

    f. Associated professional documentation sheet

C. Maintenance

  1. Emergency check list done at routine intervals with documentation

  2. Resterilization of instruments and catheters under local guidelines

  3. If reusing catheter, verify catheters

    a. Electrical integrity (ohmmeter)

    b. Catheter integrity (visual inspection)

    c. Sterility

    d. Chemical absorption from multiple sterilizations

  4. Safety equipment inspection per Joint Commission, OSHA or other established standards per state or country

  5. Equipment maintenance by manufacturer's warranty

  6. Complete electrical isolation and defibrillation protection

  7. Radiation exposure per radiation safety guidelines

  8. Limitation of patient exposure to radiation

  9. Establish a preventive maintenance program for all equipment in the laboratory

    a. Inspection by bio-med upon receipt of any new equipment

    b. Track any maintenance done on each piece of equipment

    c. Set up PM schedule for all equipment

References

Fogoros RN. Practical Cardiac Diagnosis: Electrophysiology Testing. Boston: Blackwell Scientific. 1991.

Josephson ME. Clinical Cardiac Electrophysiology: Techniques and Interpretations. Philadelphia: Lea and Febiger. 1993.

CHAPTER 26

Invasive Electrophysiology Testing

Carol J. Gilbert

Subsection:
A. Baseline Assumptions
B. Baseline Assessments
C. Evaluation of Tachycardias

Invasive electrophysiology studies (EPS) are usually performed in a specially equipped procedure room such as a cardiac catheterization or electrophysiology laboratory. Intracardiac electrodes are introduced through veins, and less frequently arteries, to be positioned under fluoroscopic guidance to various sites for recording and/or pacing depending upon the reason for study. Electrodes are used to record intracardiac electrograms (IEG) and to perform programmed electrical stimulation (PES).

The purposes of the electrophysiology study (EPS) are multiple:

1. To characterize physiologic and pathological properties of the atria and ventricles, study the conduction characteristics of the atrioventricular conduction system (AVCS), identify additional accessory pathways, and determine the sites and mechanisms of arrhythmias.
2. To correlate patient symptoms with arrhythmias and evaluate risks for life-threatening events and/or differentiate arrhythmias.
3. To define arrhythmia induction and termination methods for EPS guided interventions, i.e., drugs, antitachycardia pacing, antiarrhythmia surgery, implantable cardioverter defibrillation, ablation, etc., and for reference during subsequent EPS evaluating efficacy of therapies.

From: Schurig L. *Educational Guidelines: Pacing and Electrophysiology.* Armonk, NY: Futura Publishing Co, Inc, © 1994.

The following chapter is designed to identify the basic components of the EPS including methods of determining normal and abnormal responses through, but not limited to, PES.

Objectives

1. Identify the purpose of an electrophysiology study (EPS) and types of EPS guided therapies.
2. Identify sequences of activation to differentiate normal and abnormal mechanisms and conduction.
3. Measure conduction times, anterograde and retrograde refractory periods, and tachycardia rates.
4. Explain procedural intent, techniques and potential risks.
5. Track the EPS to be ready to respond with appropriate cardiac life support as needed.
6. Anticipate supplies and actions necessary to perform EP studies based on knowledge of anticipated outcomes.

Glossary and Abbreviations

A: Atrial deflection of the intracardiac electrogram (IEG), representative of atrial muscle depolarization.

H: His bundle deflection of the IEG representative of His depolarization.

V: Ventricular deflection of IEG representative of ventricular muscle depolarization.

HBE: His bundle electrogram, The IEG recorded from the anatomical location of the His bundle.

A-H: Measurement approximating anterograde intranodal conduction time. Made from the beginning of the A to the onset of the H on the HBE.

H-V: Measurement approximating anterograde conduction time along the His bundle/Purkinje system to the ventricular muscle. Made from the beginning of the H on the HBE to the onset of the earliest ventricular depolarization as seen on any recording whether surface or intracardiac.

V-H: Measurement approximating retrograde conduction time from the ventricles to the His bundle along the Purkinje/Bundle branch system. In most instances this measurement is short such that the H is concealed within the V electrogram, i.e., the V-H < QRS duration.

H-A: Retrograde measurement approximating intranodal conduction made from the beginning of the H to the A. Note that the H-A differs from the A-H by the inclusion of the His duration and exclusion of the atrial electrogram duration.

S: Stimulus artifact.

S_1: The first stimulus artifact in a protocol, usually repeated in a constant cycle length for a number of beats as a drive or train. May be set to increment (increase cycle length, slowing) or decrement (decrease cycle length, accelerating). Often referred to as continuous or drive pacing.

A_1, H_1, V_1: Stimulus artifact; atrial, His bundle and ventricular depolarizations, respectively, resulting from stimulation by S_1 or basic drive.

S_2: Stimulus artifact of the second paced beat of a protocol, (the first premature stimulus) following S_1, having a coupling interval or cycle length different than the S_1-S_1 interval. Usually this is a single premature where S_1-S_2 < S_1-S_1.

A_2, H_2, V_2: Atrial, His bundle and ventricular depolarizations, respectively, secondary to S_2.

S_3, S_4: The third and forth extrastimuli with differing coupling intervals following S_1 and S_2.

A_3, H_3, V_3: Atrial, His bundle and ventricular depolarizations, respectively, secondary to S_3.

A_4, H_4, V_4: Atrial, His bundle and ventricular depolarizations, repectively, secondary to S_4.

Anterograde conduction times: A-H, H-V.

CI: Coupling interval.

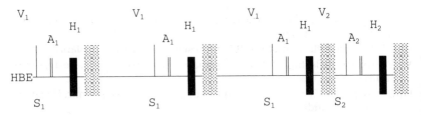

Figure 1. Recordings from intracardiac electrode pair positioned in the area of the His Bundle are schematically represented to illustrate atrial pacing. Three S_1 stimulus artifacts at constant basic cycle length (BCL) and the single premature extrastimulus, S_2, are illustrated with subsequent atrial capture (A_1 and A_2, respectively), conduction through the AV node to the His (H_1 and H_2) and the ventricles (V_1 and V_2). Similar schemma are used to illustrate other points throughout this section.

CL: Cycle length: Measured in milliseconds (ms), these CL are reciprocal to heart rate in beats per minute, i.e., increasing CL yield slower heart rates.

Extrastimuli: Premature stimuli, S_n, i.e., stimuli outside the basic drive or intrinsic rhythm.

Entrainment: Transient increase in rate of a tachycardia to the rate of pacing. All tissue responsible for sustaining the tachyarrhythmia must be included.

Retrograde conduction times: V-H, H-A.

Sinoatrial conduction time (SACT): Time for impulse to exit from the sinus node to the atria.

Sinus node recovery time (SNRT): Time for the sinus node to recover, generate an impulse and depolarize the atria, following penetration by stimuli.

Effective refractory period (ERP): Longest premature coupling interval that fails to propagate through the tissue. It is measured proximal to the refractory tissue.

Relative refractory period (RRP): Longest coupling interval of a premature impulse that results in prolonged conduction relative to that of the basic drive. The RRP marks the end of the full recovery period, the zone during which the conduction of the premature impulse and the basic drive impulses are identical.

Functional refractory period (FRP): The minimal interval between two consecutive conducted impulses. Since the FRP is a measure of conduction, it is described as points distal to the tissue.

Anterograde Refractory Periods:

Effective refractory period (ERP) of the atrium: longest S_1-S_2 interval that fails to result in atrial depolarization (A_2).

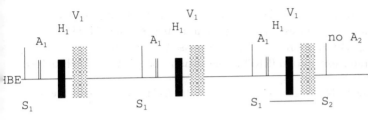

Figure 2. ERP of the atrium. S_2 is not followed by A_2.

ERP of the atrioventricular node (AVN): longest A_1-A_2 interval measured at the His bundle electrogram that fails to propagate to the His bundle.

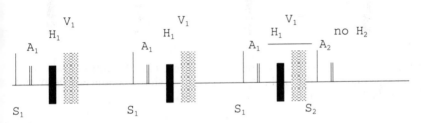

Figure 3. ERP of the AVN is shown. A_1-A_2 fails to propagate through the AVN to the His bundle. No H_2 follows A_2.

ERP of the His Purkinje System (HPS): longest H_1-H_2 that fails to propagate to the ventricles.

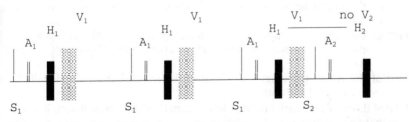

Figure 4. ERP of the HPS is shown. H_1-H_2 fails to propagate through the His bundle to the ventricles. No V_2 follows H_2.

ERP of the atrioventricular conduction system (AVCS): longest A_1-A_2 that fails to result in ventricular depolarization.

Functional refractory period (FRP) of the atrium: shortest A_1-A_2 in response to any S_1-S_2.

FRP of the AVN: shortest H_1-H_2 interval in response to any A_1-A_2.

FRP of the HPS: shortest V_1-V_2 interval in response to any H_1-H_2.

FRP of the AVCS: shortest V_1-V_2 in response to any S_1-S_2.

Relative refractory period (RRP) of the atrium: longest S_1-S_2 at which S_2-A_2 exceeds S_1-A_1 (latency).

RRP of the AVN: longest A_1-A_2 at which the A_2-H_2 ( ) exceeds the A_1-H_1 ( ).

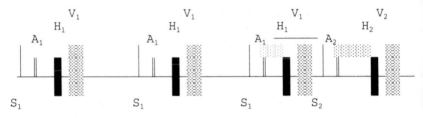

Figure 5. RRP of the AVN is shown. An S_2 results in A_2 sufficiently close to impinge upon the RRP of the AVN. A_2-H_2 ( ) shows conduction delay and exceeds A_1-H_1 ( ).

RRP of the HPS: longest H_1-H_2 interval at which the H_2-V_2 interval exceeds the H_1-V_1 interval or results in an aberrant QRS complex.

Retrograde Refractory Periods:

ERP of the ventricle: longest S_1-S_2 interval that fails to evoke a ventricle response.

ERP of the HPS: the longest V_1-V_2 interval at which V_2 blocks below the bundle of His. (Identifiable only if H_2 is recorded prior to the occurrence of block.)

ERP of the AVN: the longest S_1-H_2 or H_1-H_2 interval at which H_2 fails to propagate to the atrium.

ERP of the ventriculoatrial conduction system (VACS): longest S_1-S_2 interval that fails to propagate to the atrium.

FRP of the ventricle: shortest V_1-V_2 interval measured on surface ECG or ventricular electrogram in response to any S_1-S_2.

FRP of the HPS: shortest S_1-H_2 or H_1-H_2 interval in response to any V_1-V_2 interval.

FRP of the AVN: shortest A_1-A_2 interval in response to any H_1-H_2 interval.

FRP of the VACS: shortest A_1-A_2 interval in response to any S_1-S_2 interval.

RRP of the ventricle: longest S_1-S_2 interval at which the S_2-V_2 interval exceeds the S_1-V_1 interval (latency). The onset of V is measured on surface ECG or local electrogram at the site of stimulation.

RRP of the VACS: longest S_1-S_2 interval at which the S_2-A_2 interval exceeds the S_1-A_2 interval.

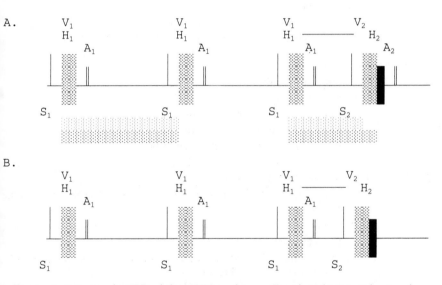

Figure 6. Retrograde ERP of the AVN is shown. Panel A depicts 3 beats of basic cycle length ventricular pacing (S_1-S_1) followed by a single extrastimulus (S_2). All basic cycle beats are followed by atrial depolarizations (A_1) in the retrograde direction. The H_1 is not visualized as it is obscured by the ventricular depolarization (V_1). S_2 results in V_2 with V_1-V_2 interval sufficiently short to impinge on the RRP of the HPS retrogradely and H_2 emerges from the V_2, i.e., V_2-$H_2 > V_1H_1$. Note on basic drive H_1-H_1 (▒) = V_1-V_1 (■) whereas H_1-$H_2 > V_1$-V_2.

Education Content

A. Baseline Assumptions

   1. Reentry is the basis for most arrhythmias therefore PES is a useful tool utilized in initiation and termination of arrhythmias as pacing schemes can effect changes in refractoriness which are the underlying mechanisms.

      a. Physicians should be board certified in Cardiac Electrophysiology (or board eligible).

      b. See previous chapters on basic electrophysiology and mechanisms of arrhythmias.

   2. The EPS has a low complication rate.

      a. Lab supplies and equipment should be sufficient to carry out all emergency procedures.

      b. Institution should have back-up cardiovascular, open heart surgery, anesthesiology, echocardiography and other ancillary supports.

B. Baseline Assessment

   1. Physiologic monitoring.

      a. Surface ECGs

         1. Minimum of three continuously recorded leads

            a) Lead I and II or avF: document axis

            b) V_1: differentiate bundle branch blocks

         2. Intermittently, 12 leads standard ECG

      b. Intracardiac electrograms

         1. Atrial (A): high right atrial (HRA) near sinus node unless specified

         2. His bundle (HB)

         3. Ventricular (V), right ventricular apex unless specified.

         4. Coronary sinus (CS)

            a) CSd and CSp = distal and proximal recordings are deep and shallow in the CS respectively

            b) Most CS recordings show both left atrial and left ventricular electrograms.

         5. Left ventricular (LV)

      c. Hemodynamic monitoring

         1. Noninvasive blood pressure

         2. Oximeter

         3. Arterial line pressure monitoring

   2. Measurement of conduction intervals.

      a. All intervals are measured in milliseconds (msec)

         1. 1 second = 1000 msec.

    2. Paper speeds = 100–150 millimeters per second to provide accuracy of within 4–5 msec.

b. Intra-atrial conduction sequence of sinus rhythm

    1. High right atrium (HRA)/mid-lateral RA

    2. Low lateral RA

    3. Low septal RA at AV junction on HBE

    4. Left atrium (LA), laterally

    5. LA, posterolaterally on CSd

c. Atrioventricular nodal (AVN) conduction: AH interval

    1. Approximation of conduction time through the atrioventricular node

    2. Measured from the beginning of the low right atrial (LRA) to the beginning of the H on the HBE.

    3. Normal value = 45–140 msec.

    4. Validation of the His includes exploration to assure most proximal recording excluding right bundle potentials, identifying split potentials, etc.

    5. Variations in AH: wire movement, basal state changes (up to 20 msec), responses to pacing, defibrillation, drugs, etc.

d. His Purkinje system (HPS) conduction: HV interval

    1. Approximation of conduction time through the His and along the right and left bundle branches to exit and activate the ventricular muscle.

    2. Measured from the beginning of the His on the proximal HBE to the earliest identified ventricular activity whether on the HB, ventricular or surface electrograms (HV).

    3. Normal value = 35–55 msec.

    4. His validation as above.

    5. Stability of HV: not effected by changes autonomic tone, basal state, pacing; possibly effected by defibrillation. Effected by medications and abruptly changed pacing cycles.

3. Methods of cardiac stimulation

a. Thresholds

    1. Measured in milliamperes (mA)

    2. 2 × threshold utilized for programmed electrical stimulation studies.

b. Sites

    1. Atria: HRA, La from CS.

    2. Ventricles:

        a) Right (RV), apex and outflow

        b) LV from distal CS, (CSd) or from an endocardial left ventricular wire.

c. Deliver techniques
   1. Transvenous, endocardial is most common
   2. Epicardial or heart wires either during or post-open heart surgery
   3. Esophageal: swallowed "pills" or nasopharangeal introduced transvenous or esophageal wires
   4. Transcutaneous, transthoracic: uncommon for EPS.
4. Programmed electrical stimulation (PES) protocols
   a. Extrastimulus testing
      1. Sinoatrial conduction time
         a) Method: Introduction of atrial premature beats (A_2) following 8–10 beats of sinus rhythm (A_1) to evaluate the effect of these extrastimuli on subsequent sinus rhythm, the first escape beat of which is A_3.

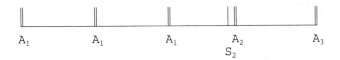

Figure 7. SACT pacing is illustrated. Single extrastimuli (S_2) are introduced and the effect on atrial escapes evaluated.

b) Evaluation: As premature coupling interval (A_1-A_2) is shortened, four zones of interaction noted.
   1) Zone 1, collision: A_1-A_2 plus A_2-A_3 = $2(A_1$-$A_1)$, fully compensatory, usually when A_1-A_2 is 70–80% of A_1-A_1, i.e., 70–80% of the sinus cycle length (see above).
   2) Zone 2, reset: A_1-A_2 resets the sinus pacemaker so that resulting A_2-A_3 exceeds sinus cycle length. Typically occurs at A_1-A_2 is 40–50% premature.

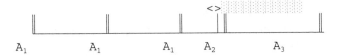

Figure 8. Reset: Conduction time into and out of the sinus node is estimated by the difference (<>) between A_2-A_3 (▒) and A_1-A_1 (▒).

• A_2-A_3 usually remains constant throughout the zone and its duration depends on conduction into (<) and out of (>) the sinus node plus sinus automaticity (▒).

- The difference between A_2-A_3 and A_1-A_1 is an estimate of total sinoatrial conduction time

$$(SACT) = \frac{(A_2\text{-}A_3 \text{ minus } A_1\text{-}A_1)}{2}$$

3) Zone 3, interpolated: A_1-A_2 plus A_2-A_3 = A_1-A_1, sinus entrance block.

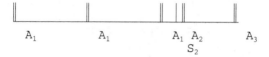

Figure 9. Interpolation: A_2 does not change the sinus rhythm. A_1-A_1 equals A_1-A_3.

4) Zone 4: A_1-A_2 plus A_2-A_3 < A_1-A_1, sinus node reentry.

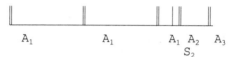

Figure 10. Sinus node reentry. A_1-A_3 is less than the A_1-A_1 or BCL.

2. Determination of antegrade refractory periods
   a) Method: Atrial pacing at a site close to the sinus node usually at the high right atrium (HRA) for 6–10 beats at a constant basic cycle length (BCL) followed by introduction of single, premature atrial extrastimuli.
      1) The S_1-S_1 or BCL is usually at or near the patient's intrinsic sinus cycle length, or is one of several standard CL used, e.g., 400, 450, 500 or 600 msec for reproducibility.
      2) BCL usually requires 8–10 beats to stabilize conduction.
      3) The S_1-S_2 = S_1-S_1 minus 50 msec. and decrement by 10–20 msec per repetition until ERP of the tissue
   b) Response: see definitions above
3. Determination of ventricular refractory periods
   a) Method: As above except pacing is performed at the right ventricular apex. Should absent retrograde conduction (no ventriculoatrial [VA] conduction) prevents stabilized BCL, simultaneous atrial and ventricular pacing might be helpful.
   b) Response: see definitions above

b. Rapid pacing protocols

    1. Incremental atrial pacing: analyze functional properties of the atria, sinus node and AVCS

        a) Method: Pacing of the atrium at a CL just less than the patient's sinus CL with progressive shortening cycles (20–50 msec) to increment the rate.

        b) Normal response:

            1) AH prolongation until AV Wenckebach type AV block appears, usually at CL 500–350 msec.

            2) HV interval remains stable although sudden increases in CL (burst pacing at CL < 350 msec) may show infra-His blocks which are not abnormal.

    2. Sinus node recovery time (SNRT)

        a) Method

            1) Continuous atrial pacing at various cycle lengths beginning at a cycle length just faster (shorter) than that of sinus down to about 400 msec. Presence of AV block is inconsequential. Pacing is for 30–60 seconds at a site as close as possible to the sinus node, i.e., HRA.

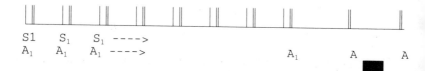

Figure 11. Continuous atrial pacing is shown. It stops abruptly and spontaneous atrial escape beats occur. The A_1-A (■) interval is evaluated as listed below.

        b) Evaluation: Measure escaping sinus beats and evaluate rhythms following cessation of pacing. (see below)

            1) Maximum sinus node recovery time (SNRT): longest pause from last paced atrial depolarization (A_1) to the first return sinus beat (A). (see above ■)

            2) Corrected sinus recovery time (CSNRT) = SNRT-sinus cycle length (SCL). Normal CSNRT < 550 msec.

            3) %SNRT/SCL for normals is = < 150%.

            4) Total recovery time (TRT): duration after last paced A_1-A_1 before return to basic sinus cycle length. Normal < 5 sec, usually 4–6 seconds.

    3. Incremental ventricular pacing: identify presence or absence of retrograde conduction and pattern of retrograde activation.

        a) Method: Pacing of the ventricle at a CL just less than the patient's sinus rate with progressive shortening in 50–100 msec increments.

b) Evaluation: Normal responses

    1) 40–90% of patients have retrograde conduction.

    2) A gradual increase in VA interval with retrograde (VA) Wenckebach type blocks at short CL.

    3) Retrograde His is identified in only 10% of patients.

C. Evaluation of Tachyarrhythmias

  1. Supraventricular tachyarrhythmias

    a. Sinus node function studies

      1. Assessment of autonomic tone

        a) Methods

          1) Exercise testing

          2) Carotid sinus massage (in absence of carotid bruits)

          3) Atropine (1–3 mg) = acceleration to 90 bpm.

          4) Isoproterenol (1–3 μg/min) = sinus acceleration to 25% of baseline in normals.

          5) Propranolol (0.1 mg/kg up to 10 mg) = 16–22.5% increase in BCL.

          6) Pharmacologic denervation (atropine 0.04 mg/kg and propranolol 0.2 mg/kg) to determine intrinsic heart rate (IHR) defined by the following equation IHR = 117.2 (0.53 $\times$ age) bpm.

      2. Extrastimulus, incremental and continuous pacing as described above.

    b. Attempted induction of atrial, atrioventricular, and/or junctional arrhythmias.

      1. Programmed electrical stimulation (PES) techniques to permit disparity of refractoriness within cardiac tissues to establish delays and blocks requisite permit

        a) Methods:

          1) Straight, continuous atrial and ventricular pacing at several BCL (Atrial pacing may induce Wenkebach cycle lengths at slower rates [longer cycles] than the SVT rate of a given patient).

          2) Extrastimulus pacing with single (A_2 or V_2), double ($A_2 + A_3$ or $V_2 + V_3$), triple (A_2, $A_3 + A_4$ or V_2, $V_3 + V_4$) extrastimuli. (Ventricular extrastimuli useful in inducing uncommon AVN reentry and tachycardias utilizing accessory pathways.)

          3) Burst pacing at short cycle lengths.

      4) Repetition of the above at multiple cardiac sites including but not limited to:
- Right atrium
- Left atrium
- Coronary sinus (left atrium or left ventricle)
- Right ventricle

      5) Induction of functional bundle branch blocks (BBB)
- Evaluation of configuration and axis to compare to spontaneous tachycardias.
- To test the effect or absence of effect of these BBBs on retrograde conduction times during SVT when retrograde conduction over an accessory pathway suspected: BBB ipsilateral to accessory pathways increases retrograde conduction times and slows cycle lengths while BBB contralateral do not.

      6) Identify QRS alterans: seen in approximately 1/3 orthodromic SVT compared to less tham 1/10th AVN reentrant SVT.

c. Mapping of tachyarrhythmia: catheter map, review for sequences

d. Medication challenges:
1. Isoproterenol may be given to improve conduction facilitating induction.
2. Procainamide may be given to increase refractoriness to increase dispersion of refractoriness, to induce block below the His or to slow and organize polymorphic tachycardias.

e. Evaluation
1. Differentiation of triggered activity, reentry and abnormal automaticity
   - **a)** Initiation by basic drive/rapid pacing
     - **1)** Triggered activity:
       - Frequency of decreases as BCL decreases
       - First coupling interval (CI) decreases as BCL decreases
     - **2)** Automatic rhythms:
       - Spontaneous, not initiated by pacing
       - More manifest at slow rates
     - **3)** Reentry:
       - Highly reproducible
       - First CI tends to be unchanged or to increase as BCL decreases
   - **b)** Initiation by BCL and S_2
     - **1)** Triggered activity: none
     - **2)** Automatic rhythms: none

    3) Reentry:
- Highly reproducible
- Narrow range of critical S_1-S_2
- First CI tends to be unchanged or increase as S_1-S_2 decreases

  c) Response of tachycardia to overdrive (OD) pacing
    1) Triggered activity
- No termination
- First escape CI resets or shows overdrive suppression

    2) Automatic rhythms
- No termination
- First escape CI shows overdrive suppression

    3) Reentry
- High frequency of termination
- Narrow range of OD CL
- First escape CI resets or increases as OD CL decreases
- Entrainment

  d) Response of tachycardia to extrastimuli (S_2)
    1) Triggered activity: 10–75% termination
    2) Automatic rhythms
- No termination
- Return CI resets or increases as S_2 CI decreases (may decrease with abnormal automaticity)

    3) Reentry
- High frequency of termination
- Narrow range of critical S_2 CI

2. Differentiation of SVTs
  a) SVT originating in the atria
    1) Sinus tachycardia
- Mechanism: enhanced automaticity produced by sympathetic stimulation or vagal withdrawal
- Characteristics:
  — Rates rarely above 150 bpm
  — AV conduction unchanged from normal
  — Gradual onset
  — Neither induced nor terminated by PES

    2) Sinus node reentry
- Mechanism: Reentry from the sinus node or adjacent atrial muscle
- Characteristics:

— Initiated and terminated by critically timed atrial premature beats

— Cycle length usually greater than 350 msec.

— Initial delays or blocks in AVN prior to stimulation of sympathetic system (anxiety, decreased blood flow, etc.) and facilitation of AVN conduction

— P waves identical to normal sinus

3) Atrial tachycardia

• Mechanism: differentiated by responses to PES as above, ie., if induced by PES then termed reentrant, etc (see e,1., above)

• Characteristics

— P waves not similar to sinus P waves in morphology

— Unifocal: beat-to-beat P waves are the same, unchanging morphology.

— Multifocal: different P waves identified

— Persistence of SVT despite AV block

• Types:

— Atrial flutter: Reentrant atrial tachycardia with atrial rate 250–350 bpm

— Atrial fibrillation: Reentrant atrial tachycardia with disorganized or chaotic atrial depolarizations.

— Intraatrial reentry.

b) Junctional tachycardias

1) AVN Reentry

• Mechanism:

— Common AVN reentry: Anterograde block of an atrial impulse in an AV nodal fast pathway is accompanied by simultaeous anterograde conduction along a slow pathway to the ventricles. During the course of slow anterograde conduction, the fast pathway recovers excitability and conducts retrogradely to reexcite the atria.

— Uncommon AVN reentry: Anterograde conduction is over the fast pathway and retrograde over the slow pathway.

• Characteristics:

— Dissociation of refractoriness within the AVN, slow conducting pathway and fast conducting pathway with longer refractoriness, as identified during extrastimulus pacing. (Demonstration of 2 or more AV nodal pathways with differing conduction and refractoriness.)

342

— Common AVN reentry:

Long PR (AH) – short RP (HA)
Initiated by atrial extrastimuli more frequently than ventricular pacing
CL: $357.5 +/- 56.8$
Atrial activation sequence: low interatrial septum anteriorly is first

Most common form of all SVTs

— Uncommon AVN reentry:

Short PR (AH) – long RP (HA)
Frequently requires ventricular extrastimuli to induce
Atrial activation sequence: low interatrial septum posteriorly is first
CL $510 +/- 10$

2) AV reentry utilizing accessory pathway (AP)

- Mechanism: Incorporation of an acessory AV pathway within a reentrant circuit.

  — Orthodromic: Initial block anterogradely over an accessory pathway, conduction anterogradely over the AVN and subsequent conduction retrogradely to the atrium via the AP.

  — Antidromic: Anterograde conduction over the AP, retrograde conduction via the AVN

- Characteristics:

  — Atrial activations, dependent on AP atrial insert site, usually eccentric except for septal AP

  — CL: $321.25 +/- 60$

  — QRS alterans in about 1/3 of cases.

  — BBB ipsilateral to AP insertion site increases VA conduction time and increasing CL demonstrating which ventricle is part of circuit

  — Anterograde conduction over the AP (manifest Wolff-Parkinson-White syndrome) need not be present

  — May require ventricular extrastimuli for induction

2. Ventricular tachyarrhythmias

   a. Attempted induction

   1. Programmed electrical stimulation (PES) techniques to permit disparity of refractoriness within cardiac tissues to establish delays and blocks requisite permit

      a) Methods

      1) Straight, continuous atrial and ventricular pacing at several BCL

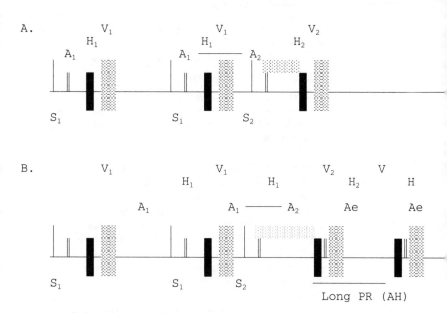

Figure 12. Elicitation of Dual AVN pathways and induction of common AVN reentrant SVT. An S_2 results in A_2 sufficiently close to impinge upon the RRP of the AVN. A_2-H_2 ( ) shows conduction delay and exceeds A_1-H_1 (Panel A). A closer premature (Panel b) conducts with longer A_2-H_2 ( ) demonstrating that the A_2 has blocked in the fast pathway (ERP-AVN fast pathway) but continues to conduct over the slow pathway. Recovery of excitability of the fast pathway in the retrograde direction is apparent as there is an atrial echo (Ae) of the common AVN reentrant type.

2) Extrastimulus pacing with single (V_2), double (V_2 + V_3), triple (V_2, V_3 + V_4) extrastimuli.

3) Burst pacing at short cycle lengths.

4) Repetition of the above at multiple cardiac sites including but not limited to:
   • Right atrium
   • Left atrium
   • Coronary sinus (left atrium or left ventricle)
   • Right ventricle

b) Evaluation
  1) Sensitivity increases with
   • Number of extrastimuli
   • Number of ventricular pacing sites
   • Rapid drive cycle length
   • Higher current stimuli
   • Sustained VT compared to cardiac arrest patients
  2) Specificity
   • Decreases with the above 1. a–d
   • Induction is rare in patients without structural heart disease and no history of VT
   • Decreases with nonsustained polymorphic VT inductions
c) Differential diagnosis: macroreentry (intraventricular) versus microreentry
  1) Macrorentry: 5–7% of sustained VT
   • Mechanism: Utilizes one bundle branch retrogradely and the alternate bundle anterogradely to the ventricle
   • Characteristics:
    — Frequently associated with dilated cardiomyopathy and prolonged HV
    — Terminates with block below the His
    — Block above the His (no AV conduction) is inconsequential
    — HH cycles correlate to succeeding QRS cycles
    — Constant HV despite varying cycle lengths
    — H-RB sequence indicates impulse propagation through the HPS prior to each QRS.
    — Localized ablation of one of the bundle branches (usually right) eliminates tachycardia
  2) Microreentry: Most common form
   • Mechanism: Alteration of transmembrane action potentials of myocardial cells caused by ischemia, electrolyte imbalance, drug effects, etc.
   • Characteristics:
    — Frequently associated with previous myocardial infarct
    — Block above or below the His is inconsequental to the maintenance of tachycardia
  3) Long QT syndrome: torsades de pointes
   • Mechanism
    — Early afterpotential
    — Triggered

- — Strongly dependent upon adrenergic stimulation
- — Pause dependent
- Characteristics:
  - — Adrenergic dependent

    Jevell and Lange-Nielsen syndome
    Congenital deafness
    Autosomal recessive inheritance
    Romano-Ward syndrome
    Autosomal dominant inheritance
    Sporadic type, nonfamilial
    Atypical:
    Intracranial disease
    Mitral valve prolapse
    Sudden infant death syndrome

  - — Pause dependent

    Drug induced: antiarrhythmics, phenothiazines, antidepressants, IV erythromycin, insecticides
    Electrolyte abnormalities
    Altered nutritional states, e.g, liquid protein diet, starvation, anorexia nervosa
    Severe bradyarrhythmias
    Idiopathic

2. Induction of functional bundle branch blocks (BBB)
   a) Evaluation of configuration
   b) Evaluation of axis
   c) Compare a and b above to spontaneous tachycardia

References

Akhtar M, Mahmud M, Tchou P, Denker S, Gilbert C. Normal electrophysiologic responses of the human heart. In Cardiology Clinics: Electrophysiologic evaluation of arrhythmias. Horowitz LN (Ed.). Philadelphia: WB Saunders Co., 365–386. 1986.

Akhtar M. Clinical spectrum of ventricular tachycardia. Circulation. 82:5: 1561–1573. 1990.

Bauernfiend RA, Welch WJ, Brownstein SL. Distal atrioventricular conduction system function. In Cardiology Clinics: Electrophysiologic evaluation of arrhythmias. Horowitz LN (Ed.). Philadelphia: WB Saunders Co., 417–428. 1986.

Caceres J, Jazayeri M, McKinnie J, et al. Sustained bundle branch reentry as a mechanism of clinical tachycardia. Circulation. 79:2:256–270. 1989.

Greenspan AM. Indications for electrophysiologic studies. In Cardiology Clinics: Electrophysiologic evaluation of arrhythmias. Horowitz LN (Ed.). Philadelphia: WB Saunders Co. 1986.

Josephson ME, Seides SF. Clinical cardiac electrophysiology: techniques and interpretations. Philadelphia: Lea & Febiger. 1979.

Mason JW, Winkle RA. Electrode-catheter arrhythmia induction in the selection and assessment of antiarrhythmic drug therapy for recurrent ventricular tachycardia. Circulation. 58:6:971–985. 1978.

Morady F. The spectrum of tachyarrhythmias in preexcitation syndromes. In Cardiac Preexcitation Syndromes. Benditt DG, Benson DW, (Eds.). Martinus Nijhoff. 119–199. 1986.

Reiffel JA. Electrophysiologic evaluation of sinus node function. In Cardiology Clinics: Electrophysiologic evaluation of arrhythmias. Horowitz LN (Ed.). Philadelphia: WB Saunders Co., 387–400. 1986.

Wellens HJ, Ross DL, Farré J, Brugada P. Functional bundle branch block during supraventricular tachycardia in man: observations on mechanisms and their incidence. In Cardiac Electrophysiology and Arrhythmias. Zipes DP and Jalife, J. (Eds.). Orlando: Grune & Stratton. 1985.

Woosley RL. (Ed.). The role of programmed electrical stimulation in evaluation of investigational antiarrhythmic drugs. Circulation. (Suppl II) 73:2: 1986.

Zipes DP, Akhtar M, et al. Guidelines for clinical intracardiac electrophysiologic studies. ACC/AHA. March. 1989.

CHAPTER 27

Mapping Techniques

Margaret Millis Faust

Subsection:
A. Indications
B. Procedure Considerations
C. Transesophageal Electrocardiography

Mapping techniques are used to localize the site of origin of a reentrant tachycardia. Historically, this technique has been clinically important if drug and/or pacemaker therapy fails. Initial cases involved those patients for whom all existing therapies had failed. Mapping techniques were developed to help locate the reentrant circuit for surgical ablation. Mapping techniques have been refined and options for ablation now include endocardial catheter ablation as well as surgical ablation. These advancements are improving the success in treating dysrhythmias. The best results have been seen in patients who have accessory pathways and AV node reentrant pathways. Mapping and ablation of reentrant ventricular tachycardia has been less successful, although it is hoped that catheter ablation using radiofrequency energy will achieve greater results. Defining an accurate "map" of the reentrant tachycardia circuit can be very tedious and time consuming, but determining the accurate location of the reentrant tachycardia is the most vital ingredient for the success of any ablative therapy.

Many patients will proceed to mapping and ablative therapy after drug and/or pacemaker therapy fails; however, the development of radiofrequency energy to ablate certain reentrant tachycardias has made mapping and ablation a "first choice" therapy in many cases. Patients need to receive information about the mapping and ablation techniques. Mapping a reentrant tachycardia is a lengthy procedure and the patient should be made aware of the need to be very still for prolonged periods of time. Acceptable comfort mea-

From: Schurig L. *Educational Guidelines: Pacing and Electrophysiology*. Armonk, NY: Futura Publishing Co, Inc, © 1994.

sures should be explored with the patient and close attention to the patient's comfort should be given during the procedure. Women of childbearing age should be informed of the necessity of fluoroscopy in the procedure.

Associated professionals should be aware of the importance of determining the exact location of the reentrant tachycardia and be prepared for long procedure times. Mapping techniques require the use of more radiation than any other technique currently used in diagnosing arrhythmias. The invasive lab should be equipped to perform biplane fluoroscopy; sometimes even cine fluoroscopy is necessary to define anatomical locations. Personnel should assure proper use of radiation badges and lead protective coverings. Lead protective coverings may include aprons, throat protectors, goggles, and hand protectors.

Associated professionals who are involved with management of arrhythmia services need to understand that mapping and ablation are time and personnel intensive procedures requiring special fluoroscopy equipment, multiple specialized endocardial catheters and/or specialized surgical equipment. All of these factors need to be considered in calculating the cost of the procedure, managing staff schedules and forecasting annual operating and capital equipment expenses.

This chapter will deal with invasive mapping techniques.

Objectives

1. Identify three different invasive mapping techniques.
2. Plan for management of patient undergoing a mapping procedure.
3. Select safety precautions necessary for the staff assisting in mapping procedures.
4. Identify special equipment necessary for mapping procedures.
5. Name arrhythmias commonly mapped.
6. Discuss the general procedure for endocardial catheter mapping.
7. Discuss advantages and disadvantages of unipolar electrograms.
8. Discuss advantages and disadvantages of bipolar electrograms.
9. Become familiar with mapping schemas for different reentrant pathways.
10. Discuss the general procedure for epicardial mapping.
11. Discuss the patient considerations for transesophageal electrocardiography.
12. Name four uses for transesophageal electrocardiography.
13. Identify the advantages and disadvantages of transesophageal electrocardiography.
14. Identify special equipment for transesophageal electrocardiography.

Glossary and Abbreviations

Accessory pathway: Muscular tissue composed of working myocardial tissue connecting the atrium and the ventricle outside of the normal conduction system.

Cardiac probe: Insulated wire attached to an electrode which is directly exposed to cardiac tissue. It may record unipolar or multipolar electrograms from the epicardial surface or intracavitary surfaces of the heart. It is not designed to pace the myocardium. The probe may be in ring form to fit around the surgeon's finger, stick form or rectangular plaque to be placed on the area desired. Signals are generally directed to a paper recorder for measurement.

Electrode catheter: Insulated wire attached to an electrode, which is exposed to the intracardiac surface. It may record unipolar or multipolar intracardiac electrograms and is designed to record and pace intracardiac tissue.

Mapping sock: Surgical mesh material with electrodes snapped onto the material. Designed to be placed around the surface of the heart to record multiple electrograms simultaneously. Signals may be directed to a computer which color code and draw electrical signals based on their conduction times. Selected signals may also be sent to a paper recorder for measurement.

Pace mapping: Catheter manipulation with pacing to assist in localization of arrhythmogenic focus. Pacing near the focus will produce an ECG morphology similar to that of the arrhythmia. Should be used as an adjunct to mapping during the arrhythmia.

Reentrant tachycardia: A rhythm whose substrate is electrophysiologic inhomogeneous cardiac tissue. Initiation and maintenance of a reentrant tachycardia require: "(1) at least two functionally distinct pathways that join proximally and distally to form a closed circuit of conduction, (2) a unidirectional block in one of the pathways, and (3) slow conduction down the unblocked pathway (the conduction time down the alternate pathway must exceed the refractory period of the initially blocked pathway)" (Josephson, 1979).

Transesophageal lead: An insulated wire attached to an electrode designed to record cardiac electrical signals from the esophagus. It may be encapsulated in a gelatinous "pill" to assist in placement of the catheter in the esophagus. The electrode may also pace the heart.

Education Content

A. Indications for Mapping Procedures
  1. Symptomatic reentrant tachycardias
    a. Accessory pathways
      1. Wolf-Parkinson-White may not be symptomatic
    b. AV node
    c. Concealed bypass tracts
    d. Ventricular (less successful)
    e. Atrial flutter (recurrences have been observed)
  2. Tachycardia should be able to be induced by programmed stimulation
  3. Tachycardia should be hemodynamically stable
    a. Antiarrhythmic agents may be used to slow rate

B. Procedural Considerations
  1. Endocardial mapping (non-surgical)
    a. Time intensive procedure
    b. Increased exposure to radiation through fluoroscopy
    c. Patient comfort
    d. Specialized catheters may be used
      1. Usually requires 3 or more catheters
      2. Electrode spacing < 5 mm may be helpful
      3. Coronary sinus catheter may be placed
      4. Small French size may be helpful
      5. Steerable catheters may be used
    e. Reference electrodes placed
      1. Usually two reference electrodes (not moved during procedure)
    f. Arterial line
      1. Needed for ventricular tachycardia
        a) To determine hemodynamic stability
        b) To determine systole and diastole
      2. May be used for other tachycardias
    g. Electrograms
      1. During tachycardia
        a) Unipolar
          1) Filter .05 −greater or = 400 Hz
          2) More precise measure of local activation
          3) Poor signal/noise ratio
          4) Can record distant signal (especially a problem with infarct areas)

    b) Bipolar

       1) Filter 30–40 and 400–500 HZ

       2) Better signal/noise ratio

       3) High-frequency components better seen

       4) Standard electrograms between distal and third electrode (1 cm intra-electrode distance with 5 mm spacing and a quadrapolar catheter)

       5) May use second and fourth electrode

       6) Electrodes must be in contact with myocardium for reliable results

  h. Mapping schemas

    1. Accessory pathways

      a) Anatomical correlation

       1) Cross-section at midatrial level

        • Numbers used to define anatomical location

      b) Coronary sinus catheter

       1) Electrode pairings used to designate site

    2. AV node

      a) Catheter placement used to locate site

    3. Ventricular

      a) 15–20 sites mapped

      b) Positions should be verified using multiple planes of fluoroscopy

      c) At least six consecutive stable electrograms from each site are recorded

      d) Beat to beat variation should be < or = 5 msec

      e) Multiple tachycardias significantly prolong the procedure

      f) Anatomical correlation

       1) Longitudinal sections

        • Left ventricle

         — Numbered 1–12

        • Right ventricle

         — Numbered 13–17

 i. Pace mapping

   1. Should be used with mapping during the tachycardia to confirm location

   2. QRS complex will resemble morphology during the tachycardia when paced from the site of the pathway

   3. Can be performed during catheter mapping or intraoperative mapping

2. Epicardial mapping

a. Performed during cardiac surgery
b. May be done in conjunction with other cardiac procedures
   1. Coronary artery bypass
   2. Ventricular aneurysmectomy
   3. ICD implant
c. Anesthesia and cardioplegia may affect ability to induce arrhythmia
   1. Accurate endocardial mapping should be done prior to procedure to pinpoint location of reentrant pathway
   2. May need to rely on pace mapping
   3. Antiarrhythmic agents should be avoided unless needed for hemodynamic stability
d. Equipment
   1. Electrodes
      a) Ring probe
      b) Ring plaque
      c) Stick probe
      d) Rectangular plaque electrode
      e) Sock electrodes
      f) Endocavitary balloon electrode (used to endocardial signals during surgical ablation)
      g) "Plunge electrodes" (Kramer, et al.)
   2. Junction box
   3. Filtering capabilities – signal may be filtered or unfiltered
   4. Paper recorder
   5. Possible computerized recording and analysis
   6. Pacing capability needed
e. Patient selection
   1. Other therapies have failed
   2. Anatomical location inaccessible by endocardial ablation techniques
   3. Patients with infarcts
      a) Aneurysms are frequently site of reentrant circuit
f. Mapping schema
   1. Ventricular
      a) Epicardial 54 sites
         1) Anterior view
         2) Left lateral view
         3) Inferoposterior view
      b) Endocardial (during surgical ablation)
         1) Anatomic areas

- Inferior view
- Septal view
- Anterior view
    2) Clockwise fashion at 12 sites
      - 1 cm spacing
      - Site designations differ with anatomical location
  2. Accessory pathways
    a) Epicardial-anatomical landmarks used
      1) Left sided pathways almost always epicardial along mitral annulus
      2) Right sided pathways may be epicardial or endocardial across AV ring
      3) Posteroseptal
        - RA to LV
        - LA to LV
        - RA to RV
    b) Mapping performed while pre-excited
  3. AV node modification – used only when catheter ablation fails
  4. Right atrial tachycardia
    a) Mapping schema uses anatomical landmarks

C. Transesophageal Electrocardiography
  1. Electrode placement
    a. Atrial pacing
      1. 7–11 cm above gastroesophageal junction
    b. Ventricular pacing
      1. 2–4 cm above gastroesophageal junction
    c. Quadrapolar electrodes may be used
    d. Current levels
      1. 25 mA effective
      2. Greater than 60 mA causes injury in animals
      3. Need *esophageal* pacemaker
  2. Indications
    a. Initiate and terminate various supraventricular tachycardias
    b. Distinguish between different types of supraventricular tachycardias, atrial flutter and sinus tachycardia
    c. Test sinoatrial conduction
    d. Test AV node function
    e. Unmask accessory bypass tracts
    f. Serially test antiarrhythmic agents

g. Stress the myocardium to detect pacing induced wall motion abnormalities

3. Patient preparation
   a. Lead may need to be inserted through a nasogastric tube
   b. Lead may be swallowed in special gelatin "pill" which dissolves leaving the electrode in the esophagus
   c. Pacing with currents less than 20mA is tolerated
   d. Patient may feel substernal or epigastric pain similar to indigestion when paced

4. Advantages
   a. Less invasive
   b. Complications are rare

5. Disadvantages
   a. Ventricular pacing not reliable
   b. Electrode relatively easy to dislodge

References

Josephson ME, Seides SF. Clinical Cardiac Electrophysiology: Techniques and Interpretations. Philadelphia: Lea and Febiger, 147–148. 1979.

Josephson ME. Clinical Cardiac Electrophysiology: Techniques and Interpretations. Philadelphia: Lea and Febiger. 1993.

Saksena S, Goldschlager N. Electrical Therapy for Cardiac Arrhythmias: Pacing, Antitachycardia Devices, Catheter Ablation. Philadelphia: WB Saunders Co., 109–111. 1990.

CHAPTER 28.A

Therapeutic Modalities
Pharmacotherapy

Katharine Irene Faitel

Subsection:
1. Cardioactive Effects
2. Drug Dosage and Blood Levels
3. Adverse Effects
4. Interactions with Other Drugs
5. Contraindications
6. Patient Education
7. General Patient Drug Information

During the 1970s and early 1980s, although alternative therapies were being explored, pharmacologic treatment was the most frequently used treatment of lethal and potentially lethal ventricular arrhythmias.

Epidemiologic studies conducted during this time supported the increased incidence of sudden death in patients with repetative and complex ventricular arrhythmias. Patients with ejection fractions of 30% or less, and a previous history of myocardial infarction, were found at high risk for sudden death.

It was presumed that pharmacologic treatment of ventricular arrhythmias would prolong life.

The results of a large, multicenter study, the Cardiac Arrhythmia Suppression Trial (CAST), demonstrated that this presumption was not valid. Specifically, data from CAST showed treatment of ventricular arrhythmias with encainide (no longer commercially available), flecainide, and ethmozine, in asymptomatic or mildly symptomatic patients following a myocardial in-

---

From: Schurig L. *Educational Guidelines: Pacing and Electrophysiology.* Armonk, NY: Futura Publishing Co, Inc, © 1994.

farction was associated with an increase in sudden death and overall mortality. This information when compared to the extremely low incidence of sudden death in the placebo group of that same study has brought about a hesitancy to treat all but the most complex and symptomatic ventricular arrhythmias.

Once the decision is made to treat patients with antiarrhythmic agents careful consideration must be given to possible interactions with other cardiac and non-cardiac drugs. Non-potassium sparing diuretics may cause hypokalemia and acquired long QT syndrome.

Combinations of antiarrhythmics each known to cause QT prolongation will have an additive effect on the QT interval. Generally, class IB agents combine well with class IA and class III agents that are known to cause QT prolongation.

Patients with advanced coronary disease or ventricular dysfunction with refractory arrhythmias have a lower success rate for suppression of the arrhythmia and higher potential for side effects with the use of pharmacologic agents.

Patients requiring higher antiarrhythmic drug dosages tend to experience more pronounced side effects. Some side effects can be diminished by reduced doses. Combination therapy may be effective with two antiarrhythmics at reduced dosages, minimizing side effects.

Another important fact to consider is that negative inotropic effects that may be negligible in patients with normal myocardial function, may have a significant effect in patients with an already depressed myocardium.

Before initiating any pharmacologic agent any electrolyte abnormality must be corrected. A hypersensitivity to any drug is a contraindication to its usage.

At present, class 1a agents (quinidine, procainamide, and disopyramide) continue to be used as standard treatment for lethal and potentially lethal symptomatic arrhythmias. Class 1b agents (mexiletine) are used as alternatives or in combination with class 1a agents. Class 1c agents (flecainide, propafenone, and ethmozine) are reserved for patients with life-threatening sustained ventricular tachycardia/fibrillation. Because of the increased mortality rate associated with use of these drugs, they should not be used in patients with recent myocardial infarction, and should only be initiated in the hospital while on continuous telemetry observation. It is important to note, however, that all antiarrhythmics are capable of worsening arrhythmia (proarrhythmia) with little predictability. Patients with sustained ventricular tachycardia and reduced ejection fractions are most likely to have this potentially lethal adverse effect.

The class III agents (amiodarone, bretylium and sotalol) are used only for life-threatening sustained ventricular tachycardia and/or fibrillation when other anti-arrhythmics are unsuccessful.

The treatment of symptomatic, benign arrhythmia is difficult to resolve. Treatment of severe symptoms is acceptable, and use of β-blocking agents followed by class 1a or 1b drugs would be appropriate.

The CAST trial has caused the medical community to reassess the usage of pharmacologic intervention for ventricular arrhythmias. In the wake of the

CAST results, other treatment modalities are coming into more common usage, often in combination with pharmacologic therapy.

Objectives

1. Name ECG changes that one may expect to see with quinidine like drugs. Flecainide type drugs.
2. State the dosage of IV lidocaine used to treat sustained ventricular tachycardia.
3. State which of the following antiarrhythmics have a strong proarrhythmia profile: quinidine, pronestyl, norpace, flecainide.
4. State two factors known to enhance the incidence of proarrhythmia in patients with reduced left ventricular function and sustained ventricular arrhythmia.
5. State the rationale for using combination antiarrhythmics. What caution must be considered?
6. State why propranolol, being a β-blocker, is not an ideal drug for patients with bronchospasm or peripheral vascular disease.
7. State the dosage of IV verapamil used to treat acute supraventricular tachycardia.
8. Review ECG conduction disorders that contraindicate the use of antiarrhythmics unless an artificial pacemaker is present.
9. Patients are often the first source of information to the health care provider. Tell what they can do to be an active participants in their own health care.

Glossary and Abbreviations

Anticholinergic effect: Drug effect that impedes the impulses of the parasympathetic nerves.

Benign, potentially lethal, and lethal ventricular arrhythmias: Benign ventricular arrhythmias occur in the absence of structural heart disease and pose negligible risk of sudden cardiac death. They do not require treatment unless accompanied by debilitating symptoms.

Potentially lethal ventricular arrhythmias include multifocal PVDs, couplets, and non-sustained ventricular tachycardia occurring in the presence of organic heart disease and pose a moderate risk for cardiac sudden death.

Lethal ventricular arrhythmias include life-threatening ventricular tachycardia or fibrillation posing a high risk of sudden cardiac death.

CAST: The Cardiac Arrhythmia Suppression Trial (CAST) was designed to examine the hypothesis that suppressing asymptomatic or mildly symptomatic ventricular ectopic activity after myocardial infarction would reduce the risk of sudden death. Patients in whom ventricular ectopy could be suppressed with encainide, flecainide, or moricizine were randomly assigned to receive either active drug or placebo. The outcome showed an increase in deaths in patients treated with encainide, flecainide or moricizine compared with those who received placebo.

Cholinergic receptors: One of the two basic receptors of the peripheral nervous system which mediate responses to acetylcholine. The peripheral nervous system is further divided into the somatic motor system (controls voluntary muscles) and the autonomic nervous system (parasympathetic and sympathetic nervous systems). Stimulation of the parasympathetic nervous system slows the heart rate, increases gastric secretions, controls emptying of the bladder and bowel, focuses the eye for near vision, and constricts the pupil of the eye. Stimulation of sympathetic nervous system regulates cardiovascular system, body temperature, and implements "fight or flight" reaction.

Lown-Ganong-Levine syndrome: Characterized by a short PR interval and a normal QRS, associated with a tendency to supraventricular tachycardia.

Sudden cardiac death: Unexpected death that is witnessed to occur within 1 hour of the onset of new symptoms and is assumed to have been caused by a lethal ventricular arrhythmia.

Sympathetic receptors: Sympathetic nerves have two kinds of receptors, alpha (α) and beta (β). α-receptors are located in the peripheral arteries. Their stimulation causes arterial vasoconstriction. β-receptors are subdivided into β_1 and β_2-receptors. β_1-receptors are located in the heart. β_1-receptor stimulation is responsible for increase in heart rate, enhanced AV conduction, and increased myocardial contractility. β_2-receptors are located in the lungs and arterial walls. Their stimulation causes bronchodilation and arterial vasodilation.

Sympathomimetics: Drugs that produce their effects by stimulation of the adrenergic receptors. Since the sympathetic nervous system acts through these same receptors, the effects are very similar (also referred to as adrenergic agonists).

Torsades de pointes (twisting of the points): Ventricular tachycardia so named because of the way the QRS complexes appear to twist around the baseline of the ECG. This arrhythmia is associated with a prolonged QT interval.

Wolff-Parkinson-White Syndrome: Accessory pathway characterized by a short PR interval, a broad QRS, widened by a slurring of the initial part of the ventricular complex, called a delta wave.

Education Content

A. Pharmacotherapy
Antiarrhythmics have effects common to the class to which they belong, as well as some that are characteristic of the individual agent.

1. ECG effects

	PR	QRS	QT
Class IA	o/ +	+	+
Class IB	o	o	o/ −
Class IC	+ +	+ +	o/ +
Class II	o/ +	o	o
Class III	+ +	+	+ +
Class IV	o/ +	o	o

key:
+	mild	o/ +	no effect or mild
+ +	marked	o/ −	no effect or suppression
o	no effect		

2. Drug dosages and blood levels:

Drug	Dose/Administration	Therapeutic Drug Levels
quinidine* sulfate	maintenance 200–600 mg q 6 h	(in patients with impaired renal function, the rate of elimination is decreased with concurrent increase in the steady state plasma level of any dosage regimen)
quinidine* gluconate	treatment of acute tachyarrhythmias in: 0.4–0.6 g followed by 0.4 g q 2–4 h, not to exceed 2.6 g (rarely used, produces painful necrosis)	
	maintenance: SR (sustained release): 324 mg 1–2 tabs q 8–12 h although q 6 h dosing may be required	antacids and food may delay the absorption of quinidine products
quinidex	maintenance: 300 mg 1–2 tabs 8–12 h	3.0–6.0 μg/mL
	caution in patients with renal, hepatic, cardiac impairment to avoid potential accumulation/ toxicity	

* Note: Quinidine is not recommended for the IV route related to accompanying hypotension.

Drug	Dose/Administration	Therapeutic Drug Levels
procainamide (Pronestyl)	treatment of acute arrhythmias IV: 1–2 g/200 mL d₅w 100 mg q 2–4 min (1 g in ½–1 h total: 2 g) PO: loading 1 g followed by maintenance 250–1000 mg q 4–6 h available: 250, 375, 50, 750 mg capsules	3–10 μg/mL metabolite NAPA 5–20 μg/mL
Procan SR	available: 250, 500, 750, 1000 mg tablets maintenance: 500–1000 mg q 6 h caution in patients with renal, hepatic, cardiac impairment to avoid potential accumulation/ toxicity	
disopyramide (Norpace)	300 mg PO loading dose followed by maintenance of 100–300 mg q 6–12 h SR (sustained release) 400–800 mg qd caution in patients with renal, hepatic, cardiac impairment to avoid potential accumulation/ toxicity	2–5 μg/mL
ethmozine (Moricizine)	PO available: 200, 250, 300 mg tabs 200–300 mg q 8 h	due to its many metabolites (at least 30), plasma monitoring is not of much value

Drug	Dose/Administration	Therapeutic Drug Levels
lidocaine	parenteral treatment acute life-threatening ventricular arrhythmias administered prophylactically to new onset MI patients available in IV form only 1–2 mg/kg at 50 mg/min rebolus 2–10 min if needed to a total dose of 3 mg/kg maintenance: 1–4 mg/min; give only half the standard dosage in patients with liver disease, heart failure, shock, to avoid accumulation/toxicity	2–5 μg/mL
mexiletine	PO available: 150, 200, 250 mg capsules for rapid control: 400 mg initially followed by 200 mg q 8 h PO maintenance: 100–400 mg q 8 h observe closely for signs of toxicity especially in patients with hepatic impairment To decrease side effects: give lower doses more frequently; administering with food may reduce GI side effects	.5–2 μg/mL
tocainide (Tonocard)	PO available: 50, 100, 150 mg tab starting dose: 200–400 mg q 8 h maintenance: 200–600 mg q 8 h (increase dose cautiously in patients with renal impairment or significant hepatic impairment)	3–5 μg/mL

Drug	Dose/Administration	Therapeutic Drug Levels
flecainide (Tambocor)	To decrease side effects: administer with food; will decrease peak plasma concentration but does not alter absorption PO available: 50, 100, 150 mg tabs initial dose: 100 mg q 12 h; titration upward in increments of 50 mg q 4 h until optimal response caution in patients with hepatic/renal/cardiac impairment to avoid potential accumulation/toxicity; loading dose is not recommended	0.2–1.0 µg/mL
propafanone (Rythmol)	PO available: 150, 300 mg tabs loading dose not recommended initial dose: 150 mg q 8 h; titration upward 3–4 d to 300 mg q 8 h (doses to 1200 mg/d have been used) Caution in patients with hepatic impairment	0.6–1.0 µg/mL after 3 d
propranolol (Inderal)	acute treatment: IV 1–3 mg slowly 1 mg/min observing ECG for AV block; may be repeated in 2 min; wait at least 4 h before giving additional dose PO available: 10, 20, 40, 60, 80, 90 mg tabs, usual PO dose 10–40 mg tid or qid (LA (long-acting) 60, 80, 120, 160 mg capsules for once daily dosing) Gradually reduce dose prior to discontinuing	50–100 µg/mL

Drug	Dose/Administration	Therapeutic Drug Levels
bretylium	treatment of immediately life threatening ventricular arrhythmias refractory to first line antiarrhythmic treatment such as lidocaine available IV, IM only: 5–10 mg/kg IV or IM slowly IV can be repeated in 15–30 min IM can be repeated q 6–8 h maintenance: 1–2 mg/min con't infusion	not available
amiodarone (Cordarone)	1) IV available investigationally only; for life-threatening ventricular arrhythmias refractory to first line treatment with lidocaine and bretylium IV bolus: 5 mg/kg over 10 min IV maintenance: up to 1 mg/min 2) *Delayed onset of action of oral formulation* • deposition of metabolites in fat stores responsible for long half-life • oral loading commonly given for 1 w to 10 d to saturate fat stores and speed onset of action • half-life is from 26–107 d, an average of 54 d (some antiarrhythmic effect may be apparent in 2–3 d; peak effect seen in 4–6 w)	1–2.5 μg/mL

Drug	Dose/Administration	Therapeutic Drug Levels
	• cumulative effects require close dosage adjustment for long-term therapy PO available: 200 mg tabs initial dose: 600–800 mg q d for up to 1 mo followed by 200–400 mg q d (can give single or two divided daily doses)	
sotalol	PO: 80, 160, 480 mg tablets starting dose: 80 mg q 12 h, incremental dosage increase q 3 h until optimal response	not available
verapamil (Isoptin, Calan)	IV: treatment of acute supraventricular tachyarrhythmias should not be used for chronic therapy in Wolff-Parkinson-White syndrome since it can accelerate conduction in the accessory bypass tract IV: 5–10 mg over 1–3 min (give cautiously in patients with reduced myocardial function) can be repeated in 10–20 min PO: 40, 80, 120 mg tablets usual dose: 240–480 mg q h in tid or qid doses caution in patients with hepatic impairment, not to be administered to patients with severe ventricular dysfunction	.1–.4 µg/mL

3. Sodium channel blockers (class I)
   a. Quinidine sulfate, quinidine gluconate, quinidex
      1. Inotropic effect
         a) Minor negative effect
      2. Acute/chronic side effects
         a) GI most common side effects: nausea, vomiting, diarrhea during initial and chronic therapy
            1) quinidex (1/3 absorption in the stomach and 2/3 in the intestinal tract over 8–12 hours)
            2) quinidine gluconate (release of the drug in intestinal tract over 8–12 hours) – minimizing GI effects
         b) Cinchonism, tinnitus, headache, and visual disturbances can occur after a single dose
            Acute hemolytic anemia, thrombocytopenia (purpura), agranulocytosis
            confusion, delirium, restlessness
            rash, dermatologic reactions, fever, arthritic syndromes
         c) When used for conversion from atrial fibrillation to sinus rhythm the indirect cholinergic effect of quinidine (blockage of vagal stimulation) may enhance AV conduction resulting in 1:1 AV conduction at rapid ventricular rates. (Can be avoided by digitalizing the patient prior to the administration of quinidine).
         d) Rare dramatic QT prolongation, polymorphic ventricular tachycardia during initial dosing period.
            1) Syncopal episodes frequently terminate spontaneously, but may be fatal
            2) QT prolongation 25% of corrected QT warrants discontinuation
      3. Proarrhythmia
         2% incidence in patients with minimal structural heart disease and stable arrhythmia and up to 16% in patients with potentially lethal and lethal arrhythmias.
         Incidences more commonly occur during the first week of therapy.
      4. Interactions
         a) Other anticholinergic agents increase vagolytic effects – many antisecretory, antispasmotic and anti-Parkinson drugs, antiemetic drugs (induce vomiting) and mydriatic drugs (cause pupils to dilate) have predominant anticholinergic properties
         b) Other cholinergic drugs may have reduced cholinergic effects – quinidine's anticholinergic effect may reduce effects of drugs used in the treatment of myasthenia gravis (Prostigmin, Tensilon)

c) Digoxin causes increased digoxin levels – displacement of digoxin from tissue binding sites, reduces its distribution volume

d) Carbonic anhydrose inhibitors, thiazide diuretics, sodium bicarbonate decrease the excretion of quinidine due to alkalinization of urine

e) Anticoagulants (Coumadin) may have a decreased clotting factor and should be carefully monitored for additive hypoprothrombinemia

f) Skeletal muscle relaxants may have increased neuromuscular blockade

g) Phenothiazides, reserpine, have an additive effect causing an increase in cardiac depression

h) Phenobarbital, phenytoin, and rifampin decrease serum half-life of quinidine

i) Antihypertensives may cause additive hypotensive effects

j) Amiodarone causes increased serum concentration of quinidine; theoretically may cause additive QT prolongation

k) Cimetidine causes prolonged quinidine half-life and increase in serum quinidine levels

l) Ranitidine has been known to cause premature ventricular contractions and/or bigeminy

m) Verapamil increases the half-life and serum plasma levels of quinidine – potentiates hypotensive reactions

n) Nifedipine decreases serum concentrations of quinidine

o) IV solution is incompatible with alkaline drug solutions, iodides and tannic acid – haze, cloudiness, precipitate, which may not be apparent immediately

5. Contraindications

a) Digitalis toxicity with AV conduction disorders

b) Complete AV block or other severe intraventricular conduction defects, especially those causing marked QRS widening (unless an artificial pacemaker is present)

c) Ectopic impulses and abnormal rhythms due to escape mechanisms

d) Myasthenia gravis

6. Patient education

a) Promptly report skin rash, fever, unusual bleeding, bruising, ringing in the ears, visual disturbances, nausea, vomiting, diarrhea, difficulty breathing; unusual, irregular fast or slow heart beat

b) Quinidine products may be taken with food or milk to lessen gastrointestinal irritation

b. Procainamide, pronestyl, Procan SR

  1. Inotropic effect

    a) Minor negative effect

  2. Acute/chronic side effects

    a) Hypotension, marked bradycardia, AV block, asystole, ventricular tachycardia – increased risk with rapid IV infusion
Nausea, vomiting, diarrhea
Agranulocytosis (rare, but the most serious side effect) – mostly seen within the first 3 months of therapy
Thrombocytopenia, neutropenia (especially with sustained release forms), hemolytic anemia, + ANA titer, myalgia, muscle and joint pain
Lupus erythematosus syndrome characterized by polyarthralgia, arthritis, and pleuritic pain
Fever, skin lesions, pleural effusion, and pericarditis – Symptoms resolve in about 2 weeks following discontinuance. – Monitor CBC, ANA titer during long-term therapy
Bitter taste
Mental depression, hallucinations
Hypersensitive reactions such as angioneurotic edema and maculopopular rash
Hepatomegaly with increased SGOT, SGPT.
Increase in ventricular rate with slowing of the atrial rate in patients with atrial fibrillation or flutter due to enhanced AV conduction – Pre-digitalization reduces this risk.

  3. Proarrhythmia

    a) Low incidence of proarrhythmia; induction of torsades de pointes

        1) QT prolongation 25% of corrected QT or widening of the QRS warrants discontinuation.

  4. Interactions

    a) Other antiarrhythmic drugs may cause additive toxicities necessitating a dosage decrease

    b) Antihypertensive drugs and thiazide diuretics may cause additive hypotensive effects – more likely with IV therapy

    c) Other anticholinergic agents increase anticholenergic effects (see quinidine – other anticholinergic agents)

    d) Other cholinergic drugs may have reduced cholinergic effect (see quinidine – other cholinergic drugs)

    e) Cimetidine increases the serum level of procainamide and its parent compound N-acetylprocainamide

    f) IV solution is incompatible with phenytoin sodium – if required they should be given separately

5. Contraindications
   a) Complete heart block (because of its effect on suppression of nodal and ventricular pacemakers and potential hazard for asystole)
   b) Systemic lupus erythematosus (with oral forms)
   c) Torsades de pointes, long QT syndrome

6. Patient education
   a) Promptly report fever, chills, joint pain or swelling, unusual tiredness or weakness, unusual bleeding or bruising, nausea, vomiting
   difficult breathing: unusual, irregular fast or slow heart beat
   b) Swallow extended release tablets whole without breaking, crushing or chewing – the special wax coating on the extended release tablets passes out of the body and may be seen in the stool, this is normal
   c) Pronestyl products may be taken with food or milk to lessen gastrointestinal irritation

c. Disopyramide (Norpace)

1. Inotropic effects
   a) Moderate to marked negative effects

2. Acute/chronic side effects
   Worsening of heart failure especially in patients with pre-existing condition or reduced myocardial function
   Hypotension, AV block, conduction disturbances, syncope, bradycardia
   Dizziness, agitation, depression
   Nausea, vomiting, anorexia, bloating, flatulence, weight gain
   Cholestatic jaundice, hypoglycemia, thrombocytopenia, dry mouth, nose, throat, eyes, blurred vision, urinary hesitancy, urinary retention – due to potent anticholinergic effects
   Other side effects include: fatigue, muscle weakness, headache, rash

3. Proarrhythmia
   a) Low incidence of proarrhythmia; induction of torsades de pointes
      1) QT prolongation 25% of corrected QT or widening of the QRS warrants discontinuation

4. Interactions
   a) Other antiarrhythmics increase conduction time, decrease contractility
   b) Phenytoin decreases disopyramide plasma levels; – plasma level of the parent compound, mono-N-dealkydisopyramide increase, although antiarrhythmic effectiveness may be reduced

371

    c) Rifampicin increases the metabolism of disopyramide; – disopyramide plasma levels decrease, although mono-N-dealkydisopyramide are increased, and effectiveness of standard doses may be reduced

5. Contraindications

    a) Cardiogenic shock

    b) Second or third degree AV block (unless an artificial pacemaker is present)

    c) Uncompensated or marginally compensated congestive heart failure

    d) Long QT syndrome or history of torsades de pointes

    e) Untreated urinary retention, glaucoma

    f) Myasthenia gravis

    g) Relative contraindications – concomitant use of β-blockers, verapamil and other medications which may precipitate congestive heart failure

6. Patient education

    a) Promptly report chest pain, shortness of breath, difficult urination, eye pain, sore throat, fever, muscle weakness, swelling of feet or ankles, unusual rapid weight gain, mental depression; unusual, irregular, fast or slow heart beat

    b) Some side effects may improve during treatment – constipation may be managed with increased bran in the diet or bulk laxatives; – dry mouth may be relieved by chewing gum or hard candy

d. Ethmozine (Moricizine)

1. Inotropic effect

    a) none or mildly negative effect

2. Acute/chronic side effects
Nausea, indigestion, diarrhea
Dizziness/vertigo, headache, fatigue, confusion, nervousness, euphoria, insomnia
Common CV side effects: ECG abnormalities, (sinus pause, AV block, junctional rhythm, intraventricular conduction disturbances), worsening of heart failure especially in patients with pre-existing condition or reduced myocardial function, palpitations, dyspnea
Urinary retention, skin reactions

3. Chronic (also see acute) side effects
Dry mouth, lessened sensitivity to touch, blurred vision

4. Proarrhythmia
3.7% incidence; torsades can occur, but is very uncommon

5. Interactions

    a) Digitalis causes additive effect – may cause prolongation of

PR interval but is not associated with an increased risk of second or third degree heart block

    b) Cimetidine decreases moricizine clearance and increases plasma levels – no significant change shown in efficacy or tolerance of moricizine – patients should be carefully monitored when cimetidine is initiated or discontinued or the moricizine dosage is changed

    c) Theophylline in combination with moricizine increases theophylline clearance and decreases theophylline half-life – plasma theophylline levels should be monitored at the initiation or discontinuance of moricizine

    d) Pacemakers

        1) The effect on pacing and sensing thresholds has not been sufficiently studied – warrants careful monitoring of pacing parameters prior to initiation of moricize and at regular intervals during therapy

6. Contraindications

    a) Cardiogenic shock

    b) Second or third degree AV block and RBBB associated with a left hemiblock (unless an artificial pacemaker is present)

7. Patient education

    a) Promptly report signs of congestive heart failure (shortness of breath, swelling of feet or lower legs), unusual, irregular, fast or slow heart beat

    b) Report the addition of new medications, especially cimetidine (Tagamet) or theophylline

    c) Side effects are usually transient – dizziness and gastrointestinal side effects are most common

e. Lidocaine

  1. Inotropic effects

    a) None or mildly negative effect

  2. Acute side effects
Bradycardia, hypotension, cardiac arrest
Central nervous system effects are most common and are dose related: lightheadedness, dizziness, lethargy, drowsiness, stupor, unconsciousness, respiratory depression and arrest, confusion, apprehension, euphoria, twitching, tremors, slurred speech, convulsions, double or blurred vision, and parasthesia
Vomiting
Allergic reaction – rare

  3. Proarrhythmia

    a) Rarely causes arrhythmia aggravation

    b) Does not induce torsades de pointes

4. Interactions
   a) β-blocking drugs reduce metabolic clearance of lidocaine, increasing the likelihood of toxicity
   b) Cimetidine also reduces metabolic clearance of lidocaine
   c) Succinylcholine (adjunct to anesthesia to induce skeletal muscle relaxation) increases neuromuscular blockade
   d) Incompatible in solution with ampicillin, amphotericin, methohexitone, sulphadiazine – precipitation may not be immediately apparent and may develop slowly

5. Contraindications
   a) Hypersensitivity to amide-type local anesthetics
   b) Significant AV node blocks, or intraventricular block
   c) Wolff-Parkinson White syndrome
   d) Stokes-Adams syndrome because of complete AV block or asystole

6. Patient education
   a) Instruct patient to report early signs of toxicity – central nervous system side effects

f. Mexiletine (Mexitil)
   1. Inotropic effect
      a) None to mildly negative effect
   2. Acute/chronic side effects
      Common GI side effects: nausea, vomiting, heartburn, diarrhea, abdominal pain
      Less common: peptic ulcer, GI bleed, esophageal ulceration, digestive disorders
      Common CNS side effects: dizziness, lightheadedness, tremor, ataxia, nervousness, speech difficulties, sleep disturbances, headaches, weakness, confusion, clouded sensorium, parasthesia
      Less common: hallucinations, psychosis, convulsions/seizures, nervousness, speech difficulties, memory impairment, blurred vision, visual disturbances
      Thrombocytopenia, leukopenia, myelofibrosis
      Hepatitis
      Positive ANA
      Rash
      Rare cardiac side effects: hypotension, bradycardia, AV block, conduction disturbances, atrial arrhythmia, widened QRS complex, increased arrhythmia, palpitations, chest pain
   3. Proarrhythmia
      Low incidence of proarrhythmia similar to lidocaine
   4. Interactions
      a) Phenytoin, rifampin, phenobarbital, and other hepatic-inducing drugs decrease serum mexiletine levels – monitor

plasma levels as well as patients' response to mexilitene to avoid ineffective therapy

b) Ammonium chloride and other agents that acidify the urine (e.g., potassium acid phosphate, sodium biphosphate, sodium acid phosphate) decrease renal reabsorption of Mexitil resulting in increased excretion of unchanged drug – monitor plasma levels as well as patients' response to mexitil

c) Atropine and narcotics decrease the rate of absorption due to decrease in gastric emptying rate – may be significant during initial mexiletine therapy due to variations in antiarrhythmic effect of initial doses

d) Theophylline may lead to increased theophylline levels – monitor theophylline levels during mexiletine therapy, particularly when mexiletine dose is changed

e) GI side effects are common with mexiletine and patients may take antacids and gastrointestinal drugs to treat these symptoms

   1) Aluminum hydroxide, and magnesium hydroxide, decrease the gastric emptying rate, prolonging the time to peak concentration of mexilitene – the bioavailability of mexilitene is unchanged – it is unlikely that the antiarrhythmic effect of mexiletine is altered

5. Contraindications

a) Cardiogenic shock

b) Second or third degree AV block (unless an artificial pacemaker is present)

6. Patient education

a) May be taken with meals/snack, or aluminum hydroxide gels to reduce gastrointestinal irritation

b) Early sign of mexitil toxicity is usually a fine tremor of the hands – may progress to dizziness, ataxia, nystagmus

g. Tocainide (Tonocard)

   1) Inotropic effect

      a) None to mildly negative effect

   2. Acute/chronic side effects

Common CNS side effects: dizziness, tremor, ataxia, nervousness, confusion, drowsiness, parasthesia, hallucinations, disorientation, headache, nystagmus

Less common: psychosis, convulsions, seizures, speech difficulties, agitation, depression, sleep abnormalities

Common GI side effects: nausea, vomiting, anorexia, diarrhea

Less common: abdominal pain, pancreatitis, difficulty swallowing, digestive disorders, constipation

Rare cardiac side effects: exacerbation of CHF, hypotension,

bradycardia, conduction disturbances, AV block, palpitations, chest pain, prolonged QT interval, claudication
Rare pulmonary side effects: respiratory arrest, pulmonary fibrosis, pneumonia
Other side effects:
Agranulocytosis
Increased ANA titer
Rash, lupus-like syndrome
Fever
Tinnitus, hearing loss
Dry mouth, thirst

3. Proarrhythmia
Low incidence of proarrhythmia similar to lidocaine

4. Interactions

   a) Lidocaine increases risk of central nervous system reactions – Although no known other major drug interactions, caution should be used in multiple drug therapy

5. Contraindications

   a) Hypersensitivity to amide-type local anesthetics

   b) Second or third degree AV block (unless an artificial pacemaker is present)

6. Patient education

   a) Promptly report unusual bruising or bleeding, signs of infection (fever, chills, sore throat), pulmonary symptoms (cough, exertional dyspnea, wheezing), rash.

   b) May be taken with food/snack to reduce gastrointestinal irritation

   c) Tremor is early sign of toxicity.

h. Flecainide (Tambocor)

1. Inotropic effect

   a) Moderately to markedly negative effect

2. Acute/chronic side effects
Most common side effects are CNS: dizziness, tremor, nervousness, parasthesia, headache, fatigue, visual disturbances
Nausea, abdominal pain, diarrhea, constipation
New first degree AV block in 1/3 of patients, intraventricular conduction disturbances, CHF, dyspnea, chest pain, interference with functioning of artificial cardiac pacing by increasing pacing thresholds
ECG changes include: prolongation of the PR, QRS, and QT intervals, widening of the QT interval (by about 8%) is due to widening of the QRS duration – lengthing of the PR and QRS intervals reflect the pharmacologic effect and do not predict effectiveness or cardiac side effects – caution should be used for PR increases > 30% and QRS > 18%

3. Proarrhythmia
(7%); incidence related to dose and underlying cardiac disease
4. Interactions
   a) Propranolol may be associated with increased plasma levels of both drugs – also found to have additive inotropic effect
   b) Digoxin in combination with flecainide increases digoxin and flecainide plasma levels – prolongation of the PR interval – warrants careful monitoring of digoxin and flecainide levels; may need to decrease digoxin
   c) Phenytoin, phenobarbital, and carbamazepine increase the rate of elimination of flecainide
   d) Digoxin, propranolol, and cimetidine increase flecainide concentration – monitor flecainide plasma levels when digoxin, propranolol, and cimetidine are initiated or discontinued or the flecainide dosage is changed
   e) Verapamil, disopyramide should be avoided due to additive negative inotropic effect
   f) Amiodarone increases plasma flecainide levels significantly – warrants reduction of usual flecainide dosage by 50% and monitoring for signs of toxicity
   g) Pacemakers – flecainide may alter acute and chronic pacing thresholds – best to avoid, or give cautiously in pacemaker-dependent patients
5. Contraindications
   a) Cardiogenic shock
   b) Second or third degree AV block and RBBB associated with a left hemiblock (unless an artificial pacemaker is present)
6. Patient education
   a) Promptly report signs of chest pain or congestive heart failure (shortness of breath, swelling of feet or lower legs), trembling or shaking, yellow eyes or skin; unusual, irregular fast or slow heart beat
   b) Dizziness and blurred vision are the most commonly reported side effects which tend to be mild although may resolve with continued therapy, may require a reduction in the total daily dose
i. Propafanone (Rythmol)
   1. Intropic effects
      a) Moderate negative effects
   2. Acute/chronic side effects:
   Dizziness, blurred vision, tremor, ataxia, parasthesia, slurred speech, headaches, fatigue, alteration of smell Anorexia, nausea, vomiting, abdominal cramps, dry mouth

Angina, exacerbation of CHF, palpitations, first degree heart block, intraventricular conduction disturbances

3. Proarrhythmia
4.7%; the percentage being much higher in patients with a history of CHF

4. Interactions
   a) Digoxin in combination with propafanone increases digoxin levels – does not appear to be the result of renal excretion of digoxin – carefully monitor digoxin plasma levels at the initiation of propafanone and then reduce digoxin if plasma concentrations are relatively high
   b) Warfarin (Coumadin) in combination with propafanone increases propafanone levels and warfarin blood levels – measure prothrombin times frequently when propafanone is begun – appropriately adjust warfarin as indicated
   c) β-blockers and calcium channel blockers potentiate β-blocker effect on heart rate, AV nodal conduction, left ventricular function – increases propranolol levels and elimination half-life of propranolol – propafanone inhibits hydroxyation pathway of propranolol; may warrant a reduction in β-blocker dosage
   d) Quinidine, at small doses, inhibits the metabolism of propafanone – concomitant usage of quinidine is not recommended
   e) Cimetidine in combination with propafanone increases cimetidine and propafanone levels
   f) Local anesthetics in combination with propafanone increase the risk of central nervous system side effects
   g) Pacemakers – propafanone may alter pacing and sensing thresholds of artificial pacemakers – warrants careful monitoring of pacing parameters prior to initiation of propafanone and at regular intervals during therapy

5. Contraindications
   a) Uncontrolled congestive heart failure, cardiogenic shock
   b) Sinoatrial, atrioventricular and intraventricular impulse conduction disorders (sick sinus syndrome, atrioventricular block) in the absence of an artificial pacemaker
   c) Bradycardia
   d) Marked hypotension
   e) Bronchospastic disorders

6. Patient education
   a) Promptly report chest pain or congestive heart failure (shortness of breath, swelling of feet or lower legs), trembling or shaking, fever, chills, unusual, irregular fast or slow heart beat

   b) Side effects are usually mild and often dose related – occur during the first month of therapy in the majority of patients – the most common side effects are cardiovascular, neurologic, and gastrointestinal

4. β-Blockers (Class II)
   a. Propranolol (Inderal)
      1. Intropic effects
         a) moderately to markedly negative effect
      2. Acute/chronic side effects
         Mental depression, hallucinations, emotional lability, clouded sensorium
         Bradycardia, intensification AV block and IVCD, hypotension, development or worsening of CHF
         Nausea, vomiting, diarrhea, hypoglycemia without tachycardia
         Increased airway resistance, pharyngitis
         Agranulocytosis
         Erythematous rash
         Fever
      3. Chronic side effects
         Fatigue, lethary, vivid dreams
         Signs and symptoms of arterial insufficiency and Raynaud's phenomenon
         Alopecia
         Positive ANA
         Lupus-like symptoms with myalgia, arthralgia, and arthritis
      4. Proarrhythmia
         a) low proarrhythmia profile
      5. Interactions
         a) Lidocaine in combination with propranolol decreases lidocaine clearance and increases steady state of lidocaine levels – may require reduction of lidocaine infusion rate – monitor lidocaine levels during concurrent administration with appropriate dosage adjustment
         b) Tubocurarine (Tubarine) in combination with propranolol enhances neuromuscular blockade and hypotension through blocking of the β-adrenergic receptors
         c) Clonidine (Catapres) in combination with propranolol may produce symptoms of sympathetic activity and rapidly elevated blood pressure at the discontinuance of clonidine from comcomitant therapy – may experience rapidly elevated blood pressure with the abrupt discontinuance of beta-blocker therapy – discontinue propranolol well in advance of stopping clonidine therapy – consider substituting cardioselective β-blocker when clonidine will be abruptly discontinued

d) Methyldopa (Aldomet) in combination with IV propranolol can produce severe hypertension – postulated that the β-blockade may allow unopposed α-constrictor response to adrenergic stimulation – methyldopa increases the pressor effects of sympathomimetic amines

e) Prazosin (Minipress) when added to a β-blocking agent can cause acute hypotension and impaired venous return with the first dose – no unusual hypotensive response when the first dose of β-blocker is given to a patient on long term prazosin

f) Cimetidine decreases the hepatic metabolism of propranolol – delays elimination of propranolol – increases propranolol blood levels – monitor patients for signs of enhanced β-blocking activity that may require reduction in propranolol or cimetidine dose – consider ranitidine (Zantac) or famotidine (Pepcid) alternatives to cimetidine or another β-blocking agent

g) Insulin – propranolol blunts the rebound of blood sugar following insulin induced hypoglycemia and blocks clinical signs of hypoglycemia such as sweating and tachycardia – cardioselective agents do not have this reaction

h) Alcohol increases absorption of propranolol – patients should exercise prudence

i) MAOI antidepressants may precipitate severe hypertensive crisis because of unopposed α-adrenergic activity

j) thyroxine causes increased plasma T_4 due to decrease in the conversion of T_4 to T_3

k) Antithyroid drugs or radioiodine increase plasma steady state concentration of propranolol

l) Digitalis glycosides may induce digitalis bradycardia (due to propranolol's membrane stabilizing action)
n.b.: useful combination in controlling arrhythmias not controlled by digitalis alone; propranolol is also useful in controlling arrhythmias due to digitalis toxicity

m) Smoking has a direct adverse effect on the heart which may negate the beneficial effects of propranolol requiring increased propranolol dosages – patients who stop smoking during propranolol treatment may have increased propranolol levels – atenolol or another agent not dependent on liver metabolism may be alternative for patients who smoke

n) Hydralazine in combination with propranolol enhances antihypertensive activity of hydralazine which may cause bradycardia, bronchospasm

o) Epinephrine in combination with propranolol causes an increase in systolic and diastolic blood pressure, and decrease in heart rate – cautious usage of propranolol with sympathomimetic drugs with α-agonist activity which leave vaso-constrictor effects unopposed – a cardioselective β-blocker may be used in place of propranolol, initiated a few days prior to the sympathomimetic drug

p) Ephedrine, isoproterenol, and other β-adrenergic broncho-dilators in combination with propranolol decrease bron-chodilation

q) Theophylline in combination with propranolol increases theophylline levels – patient clinical status as well as the-ophylline levels should be monitored
n.b.: propranolol increases bronchial resistance

r) Aluminum hydroxide decreases bioavailability of proprano-lol by around 60% – separate dosing of aluminum hydroxide product and propranolol as much as possible

s) Chlorpramazine (Chlor-Promanyl) significantly increases the bioavailability of propranolol, increases chlorpromazine levels – monitor both chlorpromazine and propranolol levels

t) Indomethacin (Indocin) may decrease hypotensive effects of propranolol – carefully monitor patient blood pressure – propranolol may need to be increased or indomethacin dis-continued

u) Cholestyramine (Questran) decreases propranolol plasma concentration; may be the result of nonabsorbable complex by both propranolol and cholestyramine – patients on long term propranolol therapy who have cholestyramine added or withdrawn may require adjustment of propranolol

v) Furosemide (Lasix) increases blood levels of propranolol which can be accompanied by an increase in β-blockade – closely monitor patients receiving concomitant therapy and make appropriate dose adjustments

6. Contraindications

a) Bronchospastic diseases

b) Sinus bradycardia, second or third degree heart block, sino-atrial disease

c) Cardiogenic shock

d) Congestive heart failure unless resulting from tachyarrhyth-mia treatable with a β-blocker

e) Severe left ventricular dysfunction

f) Severe peripheral arterial insufficiency

g) Right ventricular failure secondary to pulmonary hyper-tension

h) Concomitant usage of other drugs that may potentiate ad-verse effects of β-blockers (e.g., anesthetics that produce myocardial depression; *before any surgical procedure notify the anesthesiologist that the patient is receiving propranolol*)

7. Patient education
   a) Do not abruptly discontinue
   b) Common signs of hypoglycemia are masked
   c) Take consistently with meals; food increases the absorption of propranolol
   d) Increased sensitivity to the cold is not uncommon — dress warmly during cold weather – avoid prolonged exposure to the cold
   e) Common side effects may occur that usually do not require medical attention and may go away as the body adjusts to the medication – fatigue, lightheadedness, trouble sleeping, drowsiness, decreased sexual ability – report side effects that continue to be bothersome
   f) Promptly report signs of difficulty breathing, coughing or wheezing, irregular, or unusual fast or slow heart beat, chest pain, confusion, or mental depression

5. Drugs that prolong repolarization (class III)
   a. Bretylium
      1. Intropic effect
         a) positive effect
      2. Acute side effects
         Transient sympathomimetic effects (initial release of norepinephrine) soon after onset of administration include: transitory hypertension, aggrevation of the ventricular arrhythmia or may provoke new arrhythmia, tachycardia, flushing, angina
         Other side effects: hypotension, postural hypotension (due to lack of sympathetic influence secondary to sudden drop in peripheral vascular resistance), bradycardia, nausea, vomiting, diarrhea, abdominal pain, hiccoughs, vertigo, dizziness, lightheadedness, syncope, hyperthermia, confusion, paranoid psychosis, emotional lability, lethargy, anxiety, renal dysfunction, erythematous macular rash, diaphoresis, generalized tenderness, shortness of breath, conjunctivitis
      3. Chronic side effects:
         Parotid gland pain and swelling, headache, nasal congestion
      4. Proarrhythmia
         Transient early catacholamine release known to provoke the existing ventricular arrhythmia as well as new arrhythmia; otherwise low proarrhythmia profile – not known to induce torsades de pointes, however, not useful in its treatment
      5. Interactions
         a) Catacholamines (ex. dopamine, norepinephrine) have increased vasopressor effects – dilute solutions should be used – monitor blood pressure closely

      b) Digitalis – digitalis induced arrhythmias may be aggravated by the initial release of norepinephrine by bretylium

      c) Procainamide, quinidine potentiate hypotension

      d) Alcohol increases hypotensive effects

   6. Contraindications

      a) Treatment of digitalis induced arrhythmias unless other antiarrhythmics are ineffective (digitalis toxicity is aggravated by the initial release of norepinephrine by bretylium)

   7. Patient education

      a) Instruct patient to remain in supine position until tolerance to hypotension develops

      b) Instruct patient to report any chest pain, nausea, dizziness, lightheadedness, faintness

b. Amiodarone (Cordarone)

   1. Intropic effects

      a) None to mildly negative effect

   2. Acute side effects

      a) Because of delayed onset of action there are few acute side effects other than cardiovascular – during acute IV administration: bradycardia, hypotension, conduction abnormalities, heart block, QT prolongation, nausea, flushing

   3. Chronic side effects

      a) Deposition of metabolites in fat stores responsible for renowned side effects

         1) Corneal deposits (accumulation of metabolites in the corneal tissue of the eye is inevitable) – 1–2% of patients develop blurred vision when striated pattern falls across the line of direct vision – colored halos around lighted objects in a rainbow of orange, brown, blue – regression of deposits after discontinuation of amiodarone (may take up to 7 months

         2) Sun sensitivity – blue-grey discoloration of the skin (may return to normal pigmentation > 6 months of discontinuation of amiodarone depending upon the length of therapy) – darkened purple patches in more exposed areas such as the hands

      b) The chemical structure of amiodarone, being closely related to thyroxine (T_4, inactive thyroid), interfers with the conversion of T_4 to T_3 (active thyroid) causing borderline hypo/hyperthyroidism – 5–10% of patients require referral to endocrinologist for thyroid correction

      c) 2–7% incidence of pulmonary fibrosis – incidence increases with length of treatment – more prevalent in patients taking > 600 mg/day – symptoms: nonproductive cough, anorexia, weakness, fatigue, dyspnea on exertion, low grade fever, pleural rub and rales, diffuse interstitial infiltrates, and fibrosis on chest x-ray

d) Other side effects

altered liver enzymes, hepatic dysfunction, muscle weakness, peripheral neuropathy, dry eyes, rash, parasthesia, headache, ataxia, nausea, constipation, bradycardia, hypotension, QT prolongation, development of a "U" wave and changes in T wave contour, CHF

4. Proarrhythmia

Low proarrhythmia profile; may induce torsades de pointes

5. Interactions

Because of its extended half-life, the potential for interactions must be considered even after its discontinuance, depending upon the length of amiodarone therapy

a) Warfarin (Coumadin) causes increased prothrombin time – closely monitor prothrombin times especially during initial amiodarone loading

b) Digoxin in combination with amiodarone causes increased digoxin elimination and increased serum digoxin levels – review the need for digitalis at the onset of amiodarone therapy and consider reduction of dosage – warrants careful monitoring of digoxin levels – observe for clinical evidence of toxicity – observe for ECG manifestations such as sinoatrial or atrioventricular depression

c) Quinidine or procainamide in combination with amiodarone may increase plasma levels of quinidine or procainamide – increased side effects – increased potential for proarrhythmia (torsades de pointes) – monitor for QT prolongation

d) Propafanone (Rhythmol) potentiates hypotension and bradycardia – if concomitant propafanone therapy is necessary, initiate at a lower dose

e) Flecainide and encainide potentiate proarrhythmia, bradycardia, and atrioventricular block – increased side effects – if concomitant flecainide or encainide therapy is necessary, initiate at a lower dose

f) β-blockers in combination with amiodarone have an additive negative inotropic and chronotropic response – sinus arrest, sinus bradycardia, heart failure (may have to consider a pacemaker)

g) Calcium channel blockers – sinus arrest, atrioventricular nodal depression (may have to consider a pacemaker)

h) Phenytoin (Dilantin) in combination with amiodarone increases phenytoin serum levels – increases central nervous system side effects

6. Contraindication
   a) Pre-existing bradycardia or sinus node disease, conduction disturbances, second or third degree AV block (unless an artificial pacemaker is present
7. Patient education
   a) Incidence of side effects usually related to dose and duration of therapy – generally reversible when therapy is stopped
   b) Deposits of metabolites of the drug into the fatty tissue of the body account for many of its unusual side effects – side effects may not appear for several days, weeks, or even longer, and usually persist for some time after discontinuing treatment
   c) Corneal deposits are almost inevitable; detectable only by an opthamologist on slit-lamp examination – onset 1–4 months after beginning treatment – rarely interfere with vision
   d) Increased sensitivity of the skin to sunlight – cautious sun exposure; wear sunscreen containing zinc or titanium oxide, and sunglasses – cover skin and wear a wide brimmed hat if you go out into the sun – sensitivity may continue for several months after discontinuing treatment – a burn can occur through a glass window or thin cotton clothing
   e) A blue-gray skin color may develop in exposed areas such as face, hands, and arms following extended treatment – usually fades after discontinuing treatment
   f) Promptly report symptoms of low grade fever, cough, painful breathing, shortness of breath, signs of congestive heart failure, unusual, irregular fast or slow heart beat, difficulty walking, weakness in arms or legs, tremor, dizziness, numbness of fingers or toes, rash
      Chronic side effects: sensitivity to heat, unusual sweating, unusual tiredness, dry eyes, difficulty sleeping, unusual tiredness, blurred vision, blue-green halos around lighted objects, unusual sensitivity to the light, headache, constipation, nausea

c. Sotalol
   1. Intropic effects
      a) Mildly negative effect
   2. Acute/chronic side effects
      a) Shares side effects of other β-adrenergic blocking agents but has less myocardial depressant effects – fatigue, depression, bronchospasm, lipid abnormalities, impotence, cold extremities, chest discomfort, dizziness/lightheadedness, exertional dyspnea, peripheral vascular disorders, insomnia, emotional lability, clouded sensorium, memory loss, hypoglycemia without premonitory symptoms such as tachycardia

      b) Cardiac side effects: marked bradycardia especially in patients with sick sinus syndrome, exacerbation of CHF, QT prolongation

      c) Other side effects: retroperitoneal fibrosis, alopecia, dry mouth, nausea, epigastric distress, diarrhea, constipation, lupus like reactions, psoriasisform rashes, erythematous rash, fever, chills, muscle pain

3. Proarrhythmia
Low proarrhythmia profile; may induce torsades de pointes

4. Interactions
Sotalol information is limited other than the usual interactions of β-blocking drugs) in combination with:

      a) Antihypertensive drugs may augment the action of the antihypertensive drug

      b) Bronchodilators are expected to have reduced bronchodilator action

      c) Antiarrhythmics known to cause QT prolongation would be expected to have an additive effect and therefore increased risk of proarrhythmia

5. Contraindications

      a) Pre-existing bradycardia, second or third degree AV block, sinoatrial disease

      b) Cardiogenic shock

      c) Bronchospastic diseases

      d) Concomitant usage of other drugs that may potentiate the adverse effects of β-blockers (e.g., anesthetics that produce myocardial depression; *before any surgical procedure notify the anesthesiologist that the patient is receiving β-blocker therapy*)

      e) Severe left ventricular dysfunction

6. Patient education

      a) Shares common side effects of β-blocking agents (see propranolol)

6. Calcium channel blockers (class IV)

  a. Verapamil (Calan)

    1. Intropic effects

      a) Decreased inotropic effect – dose related – countered by the reduction of afterload – cardiac index usually not reduced

    2. Acute side effects
CHF, pulmonary edema, bradycardia, first, second, and third degree heart block, worsening of heart block and sick sinus syndrome, tachycardia, hypotension, dyspnea, urinary retention, nausea, flushing, dizziness

    3. Chronic side effects
ankle edema, constipation, elevation of liver enzymes, headache, fatigue

4. Proarrhythmia
No proarrhythmia profile; used in the treatment of supraventricular arrhythmias

5. Interactions
verapamil (Isoptin, Calan) in combination with:

a) Verapamil will increase the digoxin level if the patient is on concomitant digoxin therapy – closely monitor digoxin levels during combined therapy with calcium channel blockers

b) β-blockers cause additive antianginal, antihypertensive effect – increased risk of negative inotropic, chromotropic, dromotropic effects – cautious usage in patients with depressed ventricular function – closely monitor blood pressure, heart rate, clinical status especially at the onset of concomitant therapy

c) Digoxin can cause increased digoxin plasma levels (especially in patients with hepatic cirrosis) – increased risk of digoxin toxicity – frequent digoxin levels and reassessment of daily digoxin dose especially on the discontinuation of verapamil – digitalization dosages should be reduced

d) Antihypertensive agents (vasodilators, angiotensin converting enzyme inhibitors, diuretics, β-blockers) will have an additive effect on lowering blood pressure – closely monitor blood pressure, heart rate, clinical status

e) Prazosin (Minipress) and similar agents that attenuate α-adrenergic function may cause excessive hypotension – increase in peak prazosin levels – monitor for rapid decrease in blood pressure – prazosin dosage may have to be reduced

f) Nitrates have shown beneficial additive antianginal effect

g) Cimetidine may reduce verapamil clearance

h) Lithium in combination with verapamil may decrease lithium levels; may increase sensitivity to the effects of lithium – monitor lithium levels and patients for signs of lithium neurotoxicity if verapamil is added or withdrawn from therapy

i) Carbamazepine causes increased levels of carbamazepine leading to increased side effects such as diplopia, headaches, ataxia, or dizziness

j) Rifampin may markedly reduce bioavailability of verapamil

k) Phenobarbital may increase verapamil clearance

l) Inhalation anesthetics depress cardiovascular activity – titrate the dose of each carefully

m) Curare-like and depolarizing neuromuscular blocking agents prolong neuromuscular blockade – may need to decrease dosage of one or both agents

n) Cyclosporin increases cyclosporin levels

    o) Calcium gluconate causes increased serum calcium levels nullifying the action of verapamil – monitor patients being treated with verapamil when calcium is added or withdrawn for a change in response to verapamil

    p) Theophylline has caused a marked increase in theophylline levels and signs of theophylline toxicity — monitor theophylline levels – may need to decrease theophylline dose

    q) Quinidine has caused significant hypotension in patients with hypertropic cardiomyopathy and should be avoided in these patients – verapamil inhibits the metabolism of quinidine resulting in increased quinidine levels – counteracts the effects of quinidine on AV conduction

    r) Flecainide may have additive effects on myocardial contractility, AV conduction and repolarization

    s) Disopyramide increases the risk of decreased myocardial contraction – disopyramide should not be given 48 hours before or within 24 hours after the administration of verapamil

6. Contraindications
Intravenous and oral

    a) Severe hypotension or cardiogenic shock

    b) Second or third degree AV block, sick sinus syndrome (unless an artificial pacemaker is present)

    c) Severe congestive heart failure (unless secondary to a supraventricular tachycardia treatable with verapamil)

    d) Severe myocardial depression

    e) Recent (within a few hours) intravenous administration of a β-blocker intravenous formulation

    f) Atrial flutter or atrial fibrillation with an accessory bypass tract (Wolff-Parkinson-White, Lown-Ganong-Levine syndromes) may develop ventricular tachycardia/fibrillation

    g) Ventricular tachycardia, wide complex tachycardia (can lead to marked hemodynamic deterioration and ventricular fibrillation)

7. Patient education

    a) It is helpful for patients to learn to take their pulse regularly. If it is much slower than their usual rate they should notify their doctor

    b) Promptly report difficulty breathing, swelling of hands and feet, chest pain, unusual, irregular fast or slow heart beat.

    c) Constipation is a common side effect.

7. General patient drug information

    a. Patients can be of great help in their own care by keeping the physician informed.

1. Allergies to any medications
2. Past medications
   a) Reason they were discontinued if known
3. All current medications including tranquilizers, antacids, diabetic medication, as well as nonprescription drugs
   a) Because some drugs interact, drugs other than those prescribed should not be taken without checking with the doctor
   b) Many cold medications contain sympathomimetics which may aggravate heart irregularities
4. If more than one doctor is treating the patient, it is necessary that each one knows any changes made in drugs and dosages.
5. Other medical problems such as liver or kidney problems, diabetes, glaucoma, prostate problems, bronchitis, emphysema, peripheral vascular disease
6. All unusual side effects
   a) Some may go away during treatment as the body adjusts to the medication, or the doctor may need to adjust the medication dosage
7. Promptly report the development of unusual bruising or bleeding, or signs of an infection such as fever, chills, sore throat; nausea vomiting, diarrhea; pulmonary symptoms such as dyspnea, cough, wheezing; visual disturbances, or unusual, irregular fast or slow heart beat.
8. Tell the doctor or dentist what medications they are on before any kind of surgery, including dental surgery.

b. Patients need to understand what their medications do, and how they should be taken.
   1. Take the medication exactly as prescribed.
      a) Can the medication be taken during waking hours only, or should it be taken at evenly spaced intervals during day and night (e.g., 3 times a day verses every 8 hours)? Taking medication at the same time each day will increase compliance
      b) If they miss a dose to take it as soon as possible. If it is almost time for the next dose, to skip the missed dose and go back to their regular dosing schedule.
      c) Never double their dose
      d) Do not stop taking medication without notifying their physician even if they feel better.
   2. When a new antiarrhythmic is prescribed to replace a current antiarrhythmic, ask how long after the last dose of their current antiarrhythmic they should wait before starting the new drug.

389

Notify their physician promptly of side effects after beginning a new medication

3. If they are a social drinker, how much can they drink?

    a) Alcohol may not directly interact with the medication they are taking but the combined depressant effect on the heart may be dangerous.

4. Know what each medication is for.

    a) The drugs described in this text belong to a group of medicines known as antiarrhythmics. They help stabilize irregular heart beats and maintain normal heart rhythm.

    b) Antiarrhythmics do not cure. It is likely that this type of medication may have to be taken for the rest of their life. There may be alternative therapy available, or that may need to be considered at some later time. They may wish to discuss alternatives with their doctor.

5. Medication to be stored in a tightly closed container and in a dry place.

    a) Medication should not be stored in the bathroom or refrigerator

    b) Store away from heat and direct light

References

Anderson JL. Clinical implications of new studies in treatment of benign, potentially malignant and malignant ventricular arrhythmias. Am J Cardiol. 65:36B–41B. 1990.

Chung EK. Principles of Cardiac Arrhythmias. 4th edition. Baltimore: Williams and Wilkins. 704–738. 1989.

Contemporary Antiarrhythmic Therapy. Conventional vs. Newer Pharmacologic Approaches. Health Scan Inc. 8. 1989.

The Cardiologist's Compendum of Drug Therapy. Core Publishing Division Excerpta Medica, Inc. Cardiovascular: Antiarrhythmics. Chapter 16. 1990–1991.

Grayboys TB. Treating dysrrhythmias: lessons from the CAST. Choices Cardiol. 4:1:4–6. 1990.

Kerin NZ. Crime, misdemeanor, and arrhythmia: decoding CAST. Clin Pharmacol.

Morganroth J. When and how to treat ventricular arrhythmias in light of CAST results. J Myocard Ischemia. 3:5:63. 1991.

Physicians' Desk Reference. Barnhart, Edward R. 45th Ed. 1991.

Podrid PJ. New and investigational antiarrhythmic drugs. Prim Cardiol. 139–151. 1985

Podrid PJ, Beau SL. Antiarrhythmic drug therapy for congestive heart failure with focus on moricizine. Am J Cardiol. 20:56D–64D. 1990.

Podrid PJ, Blatt CM, Amann FW. Investigational antiarrhythmic drugs. Cardiol Pract. 223–234. 1984

Pratt CM. Introduction: the aftermath of the CAST–a reconsideration of traditional concepts. Am J Cardiol. 1–2B. 1990.

Pratt CM, Moye LA. The cardiac arrhythmia suppression trial: backround, interim results and implications. Am J Cardiol. 65:20B–29B. 1990.

Rinkenberger RL, Naccarelli GV, Dougherty AH. New antiarrhythmic agents: part X–safety and efficacy of encainide in the treatment of ventricular arrhythmias. Pract Cardiol. 13:3:1–12. 1987.

Salerno DM. Antiarrhythmic drugs: 1987. Part I: Cardiac electrophysiology, drug classification, methodology, and approaches to management of ventricular arrhythmia. J Electrophysiol. 1:3:217–228. 1987.

Siddoway LA, Schwartz SL, Barbey JT. Clinical pharmacokinetics of moricizine. Am J Cardiol. 20:21D–25D. 1990.

Shinn AF. Evaluations of Drug Interactions. New York: Macmillan Publishing. 1988/89.

U.S. Pharmacopedial Convention, Inc. USP DI 1992. 12th edition. 1992.

Velebit V, Podrid P, Lown B, Cohen BH, Grayboys TB. Aggravation and provocation of ventricular arrhythmias by antiarrhythmic drugs. Circulation. 65:5:889–892. 1982.

CHAPTER 28.B.1

Therapeutic Modalities: Device Therapy
Antitachycardia Pacing

Rosemary S. Bubien

The addition of antitachycardia pacing capabilities to third generation defibrillators has significantly increased the use of and interest in antitachycardia pacing treatment of slower ventricular tachycardias. Conversely, antitachycardia pacing for supraventricular arrhythmias, including that of AV nodal reentrant tachycardia, atrioventricular reentrant tachycardia, and atrial flutter is now less frequently used since radiofrequency ablation is recognized as a primary therapeutic modality. Because atrial reentrant tachycardias in children after operative interventions for congenital heart disease are not generally responsive to ablation therapy and because these arrhythmias are also often refractory to pharmacologic treatment, antitachycardia pacing therapy remains a frequently used modality in this instance. Thus, the principles of antitachycardia pacing and programming options will be discussed in this section. The theoretical basis for arrhythmia termination by antitachycardia pacing applies to all patients, old or young, and to both supraventricular and ventricular tachycardias.

Antitachycardia pacing may also be done to prevent tachycardias when the tachycardia is pause dependent (i.e., torsades de pointes), due to repolarization arrhythmias (i.e., long QT syndrome), or bradycardia dependent (occasionally i.e., atrial fibrillation with sick sinus syndrome [SSS]).

From: Schurig L. *Educational Guidelines: Pacing and Electrophysiology.* Armonk, NY: Futura Publishing Co, Inc, © 1994.

Objectives

1. State indications for antitachycardia pacing therapy.
2. Explain what is meant by the term "peeling back refractoriness."
3. Explain the significance of an excitable gap.
4. Describe common tachycardia detection algorithms.
5. Discuss the operation of scanning, decremental, adaptive, and autodecremental pacing techniques.
6. Identify outcome criteria that you would include in formulating patient education guidelines.

Glossary and Abbreviations

Adaptive pacing: Tachycardia termination algorithm in which the initial pacing cycle length and the coupling interval of the paced beats within the burst are a percentage of the cycle length of the tachycardia.

Autodecremental: Each interval after the first interval in a burst is decremented by a programmed intra-burst step size (from one beat to the next within a burst) which may be either fixed or adaptive.

Automatic gain control: A mechanism that compensates for variations in the amplitude of the cardiac electrogram to maintain an appropriate sensing margin.

Burst pacing: Tachycardia termination algorithm in which multiple extrastimuli are delivered at a rate faster than the rate of a reentrant tachycardia. The length of the cycle burst may be fixed or adaptive to the tachycardia rate.

Cycle length: The interval in milliseconds between cardiac electrical signals or pacing stimuli. This can be calculated by 60,000 divided by the heart rate in beats per minute.

Delta: change

Decremental: When applied to antitachycardia pacing, the term indicates a decrease in either or both the initial coupling interval of the pacing stimulus to the tachycardia or to a decrease in the paced cycle length within or between bursts.

Entrainment: Term established by Waldo to describe the capability of pacing stimuli during rapid pacing to enter the tachycardia circuit and reset the tachycardia in the presence of fusion. Demonstration of the entrainment phenomena includes the fusion of the paced beats and the tachycardia beats during pacing with progressive fusion at faster pacing rates and resumption of the tachycardia with the original morphology and at the rate of the original tachycardia when pacing is terminated.

Excitable gap: A period of time during reentry in which the myocardium is excitable and a pacing wavefront can enter the circuit and depolarize part or all of the circuit earlier than expected.

Extended high rate: When used in tachycardia detection, it functions as an enhancement feature which requires that the heart rate/cycle length designated as being indicative of a tachycardia persists for a specified number of intervals. May also be referred to as a sustained high rate.

Extended high rate/high rate timer: When used as a programmable therapy parameter for certain defibrillators, it causes the device to default to high-energy therapy if a tachycardia is not terminated by less aggressive treatments specified.

Incremental: When applied to antitachycardia pacing, the term indicates an increase in either or both the initial coupling interval of the pacing stimulus to the tachycardia or to an increase in the paced cycle length or between bursts.

Incremental burst pacing: The cycle length of a pacing burst is decreased by a selected size in a step wise manner.

Intraburst step: Used in tachycardia termination algorithms, it refers to the amount that each pacing interval will be decreased or increased within a given burst.

Non-invasive programmed stimulation (NIPS): Programmed electrical stimulation is performed by an implanted device.

Overdrive pacing: Tachycardia termination algorithm in which the heart is paced at a rate 20–30% faster than the rate of the tachycardia.

Peeling back refractoriness: Mechanism of tachycardia termination in which multiple stimuli enter the refractory zone. This shortening of the refractory period allows excitability to occur at narrower coupling intervals, culminating in block of the tachycardia circuit.

Programmed extrastimuli: early paced beat.

Ramp pacing: Pacing technique in which the paced rate is progressively increased within a burst.

Rate detection: The heart rate chosen to define the presence of an abnormal heart rhythm.

Rate stability: A tachycardia detection enhancement feature that requires a specified minimum deviation in consecutive sensed electrogram intervals before a tachycardia is recognized. The smaller the change or the greater the number of intervals the harder the criterion is to be satisfied. This algorithm may be beneficial in patients with atrial fibrillation.

Scanning: A tachycardia termination algorithm which incorporates burst pacing. The term is used to describe an automatic change in cycle length of the extrastimulus (i) with successive attempts to terminate a tachycardia. Options available include decreasing or increasing the cycle length of a burst while maintaining a constant cycle length within a burst, varying the cycle length within a burst, and varying the initial coupling interval.

Sudden onset: Tachycardia detection criterion. There must be a sudden change (δ) in heart rate by a programmable amount. The programmable amount is the minimal difference that must exist between the first two consecutive high-rate intervals and the preceding intervals. This is used to differentiate sinus tachycardia from a pathological tachycardia. The greater the delta the less likely that a tachycardia will be detected.

Sustained high rate: Tachycardia detection criterion. The high rate must be sustained for a programmed duration or number of intervals. See extended high rate.

Trains: Single burst of paced stimuli.

Underdrive pacing: Asynchronously delivered paced beats at a rate slower than the tachycardia. It may be effective in slow (less than 150 bpm) hemodynamically well-tolerated tachycardias. It can also be done with certain pacemaker pulse generators that revert to the asynchronous pacing mode with magnet application.

Education Content

A. Device Therapy

  1. Antitachycardia pacing

    a. Indications

      1. Treatment of reentrant tachycardias, i.e., ventricular tachycardia, type I atrial flutter, atrioventricular reentrant tachycardia, and AV nodal reentrant tachycardia

      2. Hemodynamically stable tachycardia

      3. Clinical tachycardia is inducible

      4. Tachycardia can be reliably terminated by pacing

      5. Lack of efficacy and/or intolerance of antiarrhythmic agents

  2. Contraindications

    a. Acceleration of the tachycardia with pacing, i.e., acceleration to ventricular fibrillation or atrial fibrillation

    b. Hemodynamically unstable tachycardia

    c. Incessant tachycardia

    d. Severely symptomatic tachycardia

    e. Non-inducible tachycardia

    f. Tachycardia termination is not reproducible

    g. Wolff-Parkinson-White syndrome with rapid antegrade conduction over an accessory pathway, i.e., rapid pacing or acceleration could produce ventricular fibrillation

    h. Rapid pacing rates necessary to interrupt the tachycardia are poorly tolerated

  3. Complications

    a. All complications that may occur with an implanted lead system – refer to Part Two, Chapter 18, i.e., lead fracture, insulation failure, dislodgement

    b. All complications that may occur with an implanted pulse generator system – refer to Part Two, Chapter 18 and Part Three, Chapter 28.B.2.

    c. Device – device interactions – refer to Part One, Chapter 8.

  4. Principles of antitachycardia pacing

    a. Tachycardia mechanism is reentry (with an excitable gap) that exhibits

      1. Reproducible initiation and termination of the tachycardia

      2. Resetting of the tachycardia cycle length (extrastimuli alter the cycle length without tachycardia termination.)

      3. Entrainment – 4 criteria

    b. Factors that affect termination

1. Intrinsic factors
    a) Duration of the tachycardia's refractory period within the circuit
    b) Length of the tachycardia circuit
    c) Conduction velocity of the circulating impulse
    d) The tachycardia cycle length or rate
2. Extrinsic factors
    a) Strength of the pacing impulse
    b) Proximity of the pacing stimulus to the region of slow conduction in the excitable gap
    c) Conduction velocity and refractoriness of the tissue between the reentrant circuit and the pacing stimulus
c. Conditions required for termination
    1. Pacing wavefront must conduct to the reentrant circuit
    2. "Peeling back refractoriness"
        a) Each paced beat advances the pacing wavefront
        b) Depolarization or greater activation of the atrium or ventricle with each beat
        c) Multiple paced beats usually more effective than single beats
        d) Refractory zone is penetrated
    3. Excitable gap
        a) Properties
            1) Window of excitable myocardium within the circuit by which a pacing wavefront can enter the circuit and activate a portion of the circuit earlier than expected
            2) Zone of slow conduction
        b) Duration of the gap
            1) Typically varies with the tachycardia cycle length, generally slow tachycardia – wide gap fast tachycardia – narrow gap
            2) May affect the ease of termination, generally wide gap – easier to terminate– narrow gap – more difficult to terminate
    4. Mechanism of termination
        a) Pacing wavefront encounters the refractory period
        b) Failure to propagate through the reentrant circuit
        c) Unidirectional block occurs in both limbs of the reentrant circuit
5. Device operation
    a. Tachycardia recognition – is based upon predefined criteria or algorithms to differentiate whether or not a tachycardia is pathological
        1. Rate

    2. Sudden onset

    3. Rate stability

    4. Extended high rate

    5. Combinations of 1–4 (trade off between sensitivity and specificity – the greater the specificity the greater the risk of failure to detect)

  b. Tachycardia termination – antitachycardia pacing relies on predefined algorithms for

    1. Timed single extrastimulus

    2. Timed multiple extrastimuli

    3. Underdrive pacing

    4. Burst or overdrive pacing

      a) Fixed cycle lengths

      b) Scanning burst

      c) Decremental burst

      d) Decremental/incremental combination

      e) Autodecremental pacing (variable cycle lengths within a burst)

      f) Adaptive (percentage of the tachycardia cycle length and coupling interval)

      g) Ramp pacing

  c. Technical considerations – implantable pulse generators

    1. Auto adjustment rather than fixed gain sensitivity electrogram amplitude changes between sinus rhythm and tachyarrhythmias

    2. Tachycardias shift the strength duration curve to the right

      a) Greater voltage required

      b) Longer pulse width may be required

    3. Microprocessor based memory systems

      a) Stored electrograms

      b) Number of tachycardias detected

      c) Number of antitachycardia pacing attempts

      d) Whether the primary or secondary modality was successful

6. Patient management

  a. Approach

    1. Requires electrophysiologic testing

    2. Determine arrhythmia mechanism

    3. Assess tachycardia response to pacing

    4. Assess risk of tachycardia acceleration

    5. Determine most reliable antitachycardia pacing algorithm

    6. Determine most reliable detection criteria

  b. Factors affecting modality selection

1. Same or variable rate of clinical tachycardia (Patients may demonstrate a wider range of tachycardia rates during their usual daily activities.)
2. Adaptive pacing mode may be preferable with a variable tachycardia rate
3. The nature of a reentrant tachycardia may change over time
4. Drugs alter the rate of the tachycardia and affect the response to pacing, necessitating additional testing
5. Underlying structural cardiac condition may change
6. The termination algorithm may become ineffective or dangerous
7. Out-patient adjustment may be done with NIPS (non-invasive programmed electrical stimulation)
8. Tachycardia acceleration may occur, particularly with more aggressive therapies

References

Brugada P, Wellens HJ. Entrainment as an electrophysiologic phenomenon. J Am Coll Cardiol. 3:451–454. 1984.

Camm AJ, Davies DW, Ward DE. Tachycardia recognition by implantable electronic devices. PACE. 10:1175–1190. 1987.

Gillette PC, Garson A. Pediatric Arrhythmias: Electrophysiology and Pacing. Philadelphia: WB Saunders Co. 1990.

Gillette PC, Zeigler VL, Case CL, Buckles DS. Atrial antitachycardia pacing in children and young adults. Am Heart J. 122:844–849. 1991.

Guarnieri T, Ellenbogen KA. Antitachycardia pacing and the implantable cardioverter defibrillator. In Ellenbogen, KA (Ed.) Cardiac Pacing. Boston: Blackwell Scientific Publications. 1992.

Henthorn RW, Okumura K, Olshansky B, et al. A fourth criterion for transient entrainment: the electrogram equivalent of progressive fusion. Circulation. 77:1003–1012. 1988.

Josephson ME. Evaluation of electrical therapy for arrhythmias. In Clinical Cardiac Electrophysiology. 2nd ed. Philadelphia: Lea & Fabiger. 683–725. 1993.

Kay GN, Bubien RS. Clinical management of cardiac arrhythmias. Gaithersburg: Aspen Publishers. 1992.

Kay GN, Mulholland DH, Epstein AE, Plumb VJ. The effect of pacing rate on the human atrial strength-duration curve. J Am Coll Cardiol. 15: 1618–1623. 1990.

Rosenthal ME, Josephson ME. Current status of antitachycardia devices Circulation. 82:1889–1899. 1990.

Saksena S, Goldschlager N. Electrical Therapy for Cardiac Arrhythmias Pacing, Antitachycardia Devices, Catheter Ablation. Philadelphia: WB Saunders Co. 1990.

Waldo AL, Mac Lean WAH, Kouchoukos NT. et al. Entrainment and interruption of atrial flutter with atrial pacing. Circulation. 56:737–745. 1977.

CHAPTER 28.B.2

Therapeutic Modalities: Device Therapy

Implantable Cardioverter Defibrillator

Lois Schurig

Historically, the use of electrical current as a treatment for tachyarrhythmias began in 1899 by Prevost and Bittelli. In 1947, Beck defibrillated a patient with the open chest technique. Nine years later, Zoll published the first report of successful closed chest defibrillation in man. The method became acceptable for the treatment of hemodynamically unstable tachyarrhythmias.

Mirowski, in 1967, proposed the idea of implanting such a device in man for arrhythmia management. The idea was not well received. It was inconceivable to implant this large, powerful device in humans. Mirowski was not discouraged by the negative response and continued his work on the automatic implantable defibrillator.

Device therapy for the management of cardiac arrhythmias now includes the implantable cardioverter defibrillator (ICD). The ICD monitors cardiac rhythm for rate and rate/morphology. When the device recognition criteria have been met to diagnose ventricular tachycardia (VT) or ventricular fibrillation (VF), the generator charges to a preset energy level and discharges to convert the arrhythmia. It will recycle four or five times to deliver additional shocks if the arrhythmia is not converted. The ability of an implanted device to shock abnormal rhythms has also been incorporated in devices capable of tiered therapies (bradycardia pacing, antitachycardia pacing, cardioversion, and then defibrillation). Algorithms are programmed in the device giving it recognition criteria and options in a sequence to chose for treatment. Still the device does not prevent the arrhythmia. Tiered therapy devices have gained

From: Schurig L. *Educational Guidelines: Pacing and Electrophysiology.* Armonk, NY: Futura Publishing Co, Inc, © 1994.

credibility as a method of treatment and are currently undergoing several studies which will facilitate definition of their role in arrhythmia management.

Objectives

1. Identify indications for device therapy.
2. Assess patient/device interaction post implantation.
3. Application of scientific knowledge to implementation of device therapy in clinical practice.
4. Define standards of care.
5. Plan for management of the patient receiving device therapy.
6. Recognize complications with device therapy.
7. Select safety precautions for the patient receiving device therapy.
8. Identify the long-term needs of the ICD patient population.

Glossary and Abbreviations

Active mode: The device will be able to detect (sense) a life-threatening arrhythmia, charge to a preset energy level and terminate the arrhythmia.

Capacitor: A device for storing an electrical charge.

Charge time: The time required to charge the ICDs capacitors to a level sufficient to deliver a therapeutic shock.

Defibrillation threshold (DFT): The minimal amount of electrical energy required to successfully convert an arrhythmia.

Double counting: Abnormal response of the ICD to pacemaker artifacts. The ICD counts the pacing artifact and the intrinsic rate for recognition criteria. (The device may also triple count with dual chamber pacemakers.)

External cardioverter/defibrillator (ECD): The device used during implant to check defibrillation thresholds and mimic the device to be implanted.

EMI: Electromagnetic interference.

EP mode: The mode during which the device is active but unable to sense an arrhythmia. This mode is used to test the device post-implant.

ERI: Elective replacement indicator

ERT: Elective replacement time

Implantable cardioverter defibrillator (ICD): An implanted device designed to recognize life-threatening arrhythmias, charge and deliver a sequence of shocks. Some devices incorporate antitachycardia pacing.

Inactive mode: The device is turned off.

Joule: A unit of electrical current delivered by a defibrillator, sometimes stated as watts/second.

Magnet: A device used to temporarily inactivate a device implanted for defibrillation. (The same device is used with pacemakers to temporarily convert them to asynchronous pacing.)

Misdirect: The charge from the device during testing is directed to the patient, not to the device.

Patch: The term used to describe the defibrillator electrode. It is the same concept as defibrillator paddles. Delivers electrical current from one point to another through the heart.

Probability density function (PDF or morphology detection): One of the criteria the ICD uses to detect arrhythmias. The device monitors the QRS morphology, calculates the amount of time the complex spends on or near the baseline (isoelectric segments), and decides if the rhythm is a shockable rhythm with its analysis. The PDF is satisfied more quickly by rhythms with a sinusoidal configuration.

Programmer: An external device used to communicate with the ICD. It interrogates the unit for information stored in its memory regarding arrhythmia recognition and treatment sequences and based on review of the data operational settings of the device are non-invasively changed.

Pulses: Term used to describe the shocks delivered to the patient by the defibrillator.

Rate cut-off (rate criterion): The rate limit set in the device to determine delivery of shocks.

Recycling: The ICD is programmed to deliver up to four or five shocks in a sequence. When the initial shock fails to terminate the arrhythmia, the device will automatically recharge to deliver the additional shocks.

Redirect: Application of the magnet over the device for a few seconds causes the charge to be dumped internally.

Rescue shock: Shocks given to the patient by an external defibrillator.

Spurious shock: Inappropriate shocks delivered to the patient.

Tiered therapy: The ability of a device to deliver multiple arrhythmia treatments determined by preset algorithms, combinations of pacing and defibrillation.

Sudden cardiac death (SCD): An unwitnessed death, or a death within 1 hour from onset of symptoms, either of natural causes or from cardiac origin.

Education Content

A. Indications
1. Sudden cardiac death from VT, VT/VF or VF
2. Drug refractory sustained VT or VF
3. Resuscitated out of hospital cardiac arrest
4. Long QT syndrome resuscitated from SCD
5. Also being evaluated for patients with NS (non-sustained) VT, low ejection fraction (EF) and patients at high risk for SCD (cardiomyopathy, etc.)

B. Considerations for Implantation of an ICD
1. Event not associated with myocardial infarction (MI)
2. Response to antiarrhythmic therapy
3. Failures with serial electrophysiology testing
4. Long-term prognosis
5. Frequency of arrhythmia
6. Occurrence of non-sustained VT (NSVT)
7. Patient compliance with treatment
8. Uncontrolled congestive heart failure (CHF)
9. Patient acceptance of the device (psychological instability)

C. Diagnostic Evaluation
1. Electrophysiologic study
   a. Inducible VT
   b. Rate of VT
   c. Morphology of VT
   d. Effect of antiarrhythmic agents
   e. Site(s) of origin of VT
   f. Same review for SVT
2. Intraoperative mapping (during surgery)
3. Cardiac catheterization (potential to evaluate presence of coronary artery disease (CAD) and LV function)
4. Holter monitoring
5. Stress testing for maximum sinus heart rate, other arrhythmias triggered by the exercise or presence of myocardial ischemia.
6. Signal averaged ECG (SAECG)
7. Echocardiography

D. Life-Threatening Arrhythmias (review from other text)
1. Premature ventricular contractions (relationship to VT)

   2. Ventricular tachycardia
      a. Sustained
         1. Monomorphic
         2. Polymorphic
      b. Non-sustained
   3. Ventricular fibrillation
   4. VT/VF combination

E. ICD Candidate Demographics
   1. Usually male
   2. 55 years of age
   3. Ejection fraction < 35%
   4. Failed trials of 3–5 antiarrhythmic drugs
   5. 1–3 episodes of SCD
   6. Primary cardiac diagnosis
      a. Coronary artery disease
      b. Cardiomyopathy
      c. Prolonged QT syndrome
   7. New York Heart Association class III or IV
   8. Approximately 18% of patients have had previous cardiac surgery

F. Admission Evaluation and Patient Preparation
   1. Laboratory exams
      a. CBC and differential
      b. Electrolytes
      c. Antiarrhythmic drug levels
      d. Type/cross-match blood
      e. Coagulation studies and platelet count
      f. Arterial blood gasses
      g. Magnesium level
      h. BUN and creatinine
   2. Chest x-ray – rule out CHF (treat any CHF)
   3. Pulmonary function evaluation – rule out Amiodarone toxicity
   4. Informed consent
   5. Anesthesia evaluation
   6. 12 lead ECG
   7. SAECG (if not done)
   8. Off anticoagulants for 1 week
   9. Discontinue antiplatelet agents
   10. Antimicrobial washes daily

11. Avoid causing anterior skin lesions with cardiac monitoring electrodes
12. Examine potential pocket location
    a. Skin lesions or rashes
    b. Anatomy
    c. Consider special conditions such as the patient's occupation or paraplegia
13. Evaluate pacemaker implants – must be a bipolar device
14. Financial review
15. Anesthesia evaluation
16. Preparation for additional operative procedures
    a. Resection of arrhythmogenic substrate
    b. Coronary bypass
    c. Valve repair/replacement
    d. Aneurysmectomy
    e. Other

G. ICD Technology
   1. Lead system
      a. Superior vena cava spring defibrillation lead
      b. Bipolar right ventricle sensing lead
      c. Myocardial sensing leads
      d. Epicardial defibrillation patch combinations
      e. Subcutaneous or submuscular defibrillation patches
      f. Transvenous lead
   2. Generators
      a. CPI
         1. Ventak 1500-1510-1520
         2. Ventak 1550
         3. Ventak – P 1600
         4. PRX – 1700
         5. PRX II
      b. Teletronics
         1. Guardian 4202/4203
         2. Guardian 4210
      c. Medtronic
         1. PCD 7216A
         2. PCD 7217, 7217B
         3. Jewel PCD 7219D, 7219C
      d. Intermedics – Res Q

     e. Ventritex – Cadence

     f. Siemens-Pacesetter – Siecure

3. Device Programmability (varies with device)

     a. Mode active/inactive

     b. Rate criteria

     c. PDF on/off

     d. Shock delay

     e. Shock energy

     f. Number of shocks in a series

     g. Tiered therapy criteria

     h. VVI pacing parameters

     i. Device test sequences

          1. Defibrillation test

          2. Manual shock (emergency shock)

          3. Pacer cell impedance

          4. Lead impedance

          5. Lead threshold test

     j. Telemetry

          1. Arrhythmia conversion history

          2. Charge times

          3. Test data

          4. Diagnostic data

          5. Device settings

          6. Intercardiac electrograms

          7. Event markers

4. Cycle of operation – varies with device implanted

     a. Recognition

     b. Delay (confirmation)

     c. Charge

     d. Discharge

     e. Recycle

     f. Delivery of complete shock sequence if needed

     g. Utilizations of tiered therapy

5. Magnet operation – varies with device implanted

     a. Activate/deactivate

     b. EP mode

     c. Redirect

     d. Verification of sensing

     e. Disable tachyarrhythmia functions

          1. Pacing

     2. Shock therapy

     3. Antitachycardia pacing

H. ICD Complications

  1. Operative death

  2. Lead migration

  3. Lead fracture

  4. Spurious shocks

  5. Infections

  6. Pacemaker interactions

     a. Detection inhibition

     b. Multiple counting

     c. Sensing errors

  7. EMI

  8. Component failure

  9. Radiation effects

  10. Bleeding

  11. SVC thrombosis

  12. Pneumothorax

  13. Cerebrovascular accident

  14. Erosion of a coronary artery by the patch

  15. Pocket erosion

  16. Psychosocial effects

  17. Acceleration of VT

  18. Skin potentials

  19. Device interactions

  20. Malsensing

  21. Arrhythmias

  22. Loose connections

  23. Threshold alterations

  24. Cardiac perforation

  25. Phrenic nerve damage with extrapericardial patch

I. Troubleshooting an ICD

  1. Inadequate DFT (defibrillation thresholds)

     a. Air between patch and heart

     b. Remove chest retractor

     c. Insulated side of patch sewn against heart

     d. Reposition defibrillation patches

     e. Try new lead configuration

      f.   Reverse polarity with patch-patch configuration
      g. Change patch size
      h. Evaluate drug levels
      i.   Evaluate anesthetic agent

2.   Non-detection
      a. Is ICD activated?
      b. Detection criterion for arrhythmia – rate or rate/morphology
      c. Is heart rate > rate criterion of device
      d. EMI
      e. PDF off, is the R wave > 5 mV and QRS duration < 100 msec
      f.   Evaluate pacemaker interaction
      g. Confirm battery status

3.   ICD non-conversion (pocket open)
      a. Place generator in pocket
      b. Does DFT exceed setting of the device?
      c. Reconfirm lead integrity and interface with ICD
      d. Isolate ICD and leads from monitoring system
      e. Is device active?

4.   ICD non-conversion (pocket closed)
      a. Pericardial effusion
      b. Lead fracture
      c. Are connector pins visible in connector jacks?
      d. Migration of spring lead
      e. Evaluate drug treatment
      f.   Is device active?
      g. Evaluate recovery time from EP mode
      h. Evaluate potential for threshold variations
      i.   What is joule setting of the device?

5.   Spurious (inappropriate) shocks
      a. Is there 30 second ECG recording before a shock? Evaluate for bursts of non-sustained VT.
      b. Did the heart rate exceed the rate criterion?
      c. Are the beeping tones indicating ICD sensing R-wave synchronous?
      d. Are the beeping tones R-wave synchronous during movement?
      e. Asynchronous beeps may be due to lead fracture.
      f.   Is the ICD double or triple counting?
           1. Sensing pacemaker spikes
           2. T wave sensing
           3. EMI

6. Programming problems
    a. Programmer malfunction
    b. Accessory connection
    c. Check software module
    d. EMI
    e. Incorrect use of the programmer (read instructions)
    f. Use of a magnet for deactivation during a programming session
    g. Using EP test mode
    h. Low battery
    i. Position of programming wand
    j. Settings requested not in device's range
    k. Pacemaker interaction with the ICD
    l. Depth of the implanted device

J. Interactions
    1. Pharmacological
        a. Alteration in DFT
        b. Alteration in VT cycle length
        c. Alteration in frequency of events
        d. Alteration in morphology
        e. Control of atrial arrhythmias
        f. Decrease or eliminate non-sustained VT events
        g. Cause conduction disturbances
        h. Proarrhythmia
    2. Physiological and psychological
        a. Skin potentials
        b. Alteration of body image
        c. Erosions
            1. Skin
            2. Myocardium under patches
            3. Coronary vessels
        d. Suicide potential
        e. Inability to adapt to lifestyle changes
        f. Fear of defibrillation or failure of device
        g. Infections
        h. Physical symptoms related to procedures performed
        i. Imagined shocks
        j. Dependency
    3. Devices
        a. Pacemakers

411

      1. Single chamber
      2. Dual chamber
      3. Rate modulated
  b. External defibrillators
  c. Electrocautery
  d. Diathermy
  e. Lithotripsy
  f. Magnetic residence imaging
  g. Ionizing (therapeutic) radiation
  h. RF transmitters
  i. Arc welding equipment
  j. Running motors
  k. Transformers
  l. Monitoring equipment – interfere with normal pulse operation
  m. Any devices with magnets or that generates a magnetic field during operation

K. Patient Education (Review Part One, Chapter 7, Patient Education)
  1. Patient assessment
    a. Attitude
    b. Current status – knowledge base for events in progress
    c. Ability to learn
    d. Motivation
    e. Impediments to learning
    f. Concept of quality of life
    g. Support system
  2. Education – phase I – pre-implantation
    a. Cardiac anatomy and conduction system
    b. Cardiac arrhythmias
    c. Drug management, conventional and investigational
    d. Electrophysiology
      1. Electrophysiology study procedure
      2. Post-care
      3. Emergency procedures
      4. Study results
      5. Treatment options
    e. Cough version
    f. Cardioversion
    g. External defibrillation
    h. CPR

    i. Preoperative instructions for ICD
        1. Review of previous material
        2. Benefits of the ICD
        3. Realistic expectations of the ICD
        4. Operation of the ICD
        5. Video – "A Gift of Time" or internally generated video
        6. Patient manual
        7. Patient interview for lifestyle
        8. Operative procedure
        9. Prevention of respiratory complications
        10. Initiate instruction on early ambulation
        11. Complications associated with ICD

3. Education – phase II – post-implantation
    a. Review of preoperative instructions
        1. Prevention of respiratory complications
        2. Early ambulation
    b. Wound care
    c. Medications
        1. Antiarrhythmics
        2. Antibiotics
        3. Cardioactive drugs
        4. K^+ (potassium) supplements
    d. Patient monitoring
    e. Postoperative course
    f. Activation of the device
    g. Follow-up EPS to evaluate the ICD
    h. Discharge planning (continuing care)

4. Education – phase III – long term or discharge planning
    a. Self care instructions
    b. Activity instructions
    c. Function of the ICD – treatment not prevention
    d. Therapy diary (events surrounding a treatment episode – acitivity, surroundings, etc.)
    e. Actions for return of symptoms
    f. Home emergency plan
    g. Wound care for healing and prevention of infection
    h. Diet and medications
    i. Do not omit K^+ supplements
    j. Avoid magnets
    k. Equipment to avoid

      l. Driving
      m. Travel
      n. Return to work
      o. Weights (lifting)
      p. Monitor heart rate and physical status
      q. Identification card
      r. Medic alert ID
      s. Instruction letter to health care personnel
      t. Warranty
      u. Cardiac rehabilitation
      v. Transtelephonic monitoring
      w. ICD replacement
      x. Clinic visits
      y. Required ICD follow up
      z. Local support groups

5. Resources for patient education
      a. The education team members
      b. ICD video
      c. Photo tour of the procedure
      d. ICD models
      e. Written instruction material
      f. Warranty
      g. ID card
      h. Medic alert order form
      i. Therapy diary
      j. Emergency letter

L. Operative Management – Implantation of an ICD
  1. Implant approach
      a. Transvenous leads via jugular, cephalic or subclavian
      b. Left lateral thoracotomy
      c. Median sternotomy
      d. Subxiphoid
      e. Subcostal
      f. Other
  2. EP preparation
      a. Monitoring system – minimum 4 channels
         1. Rate sensing lead electrogram
         2. Morphology-sensing/defibrillating lead electrograms

        3. EP test event markers

        4. Surface ECG

   b. External cardioverter defibrillator (ECD) or other testing device (Some units act as their own test device)

        1. Test ECD prior to use

        2. Hook up of ECD

        3. Operation of ECD

        4. Arrhythmia analysis with ECD

        5. Equipment

            a) Recording cables

            b) ECD test lead

            c) ECD user manual

            d) Spring clips – 2

   c. Threshold evaluations

        1. Defibrillation threshold

            a) VT

            b) VF

        2. Rate sensing

            a) Amplitude

            b) Duration

            c) Placement

        3. Morphology

        4. Standard pacing thresholds

        5. Pacemaker interactions if the patient also has a pacemaker (Evaluate longevity of the device and utilization of the ICD pacing functions)

3. Operating room

   a. Operating room supplies

        1. ICD system – consider having spare generator and leads on hand

        2. Appropriate company equipment to check device and record thresholds

        3. Example equipment list, have one available for each type of device implanted in the facility – *sterile*

            a) Bipolar cable to ECD

            b) Adapter pins – 2

            c) High-voltage cable to ECD

            d) Monitoring leads with 0 rings (1 red, 1 black, 2 silver)

            e) Magnets

            f) Model 6577 programming wand (6575 cannot be sterilized)

            g) Accessory kit

      h) Rings

      i) Cap driver

      j) Hex wrench

   4. ICD programmer

      a) Programming module for device to be implanted

      b) External wand

      c) EGM cable

   5. Sterile internal and external defibrillator paddles

   6. Equipment from surgeons' preference lists for the case

b. Case preparation

   1. Interrogate device prior to implant

   2. Be sure device is inactive until ready to test it

   3. Be sure ECD or other testing devices are fully charged

   4. Test this equipment before the case

   5. Check programmer prior to case

   6. Sterilize all equipment needed to be placed in the operative field

   7. Review inventory prior to case for availability of accessories or frequently needed replacement items

   8. Complete an electrical safety check of the area prior to implantation

   9. Emergency equipment on stand-by

   10. Bypass pump on stand-by

   11. Perfusionist on stand-by

c. Patient material

   1. ID card enclosed with the ICD

   2. Patient education book enclosed with ICD

   3. Warranty

d. Case documentation

   1. Thresholds

   2. Device tests (ICD, ECD, programmer)

   3. Conversion tests

   4. Generator/lead data (registration form)

   5. Medications

   6. Standard procedure documentation

   7. Final device settings

M. Patient Management

   1. Patient education – section k.

   2. Standards of care

a. The facility will design and implement the policies, procedures, and protocols necessary to define care of the patient with an ICD.

b. Monitor/assess the following parameters with the ICD patient. The frequency will be determined by the patient's condition and guidelines in their facility

   1. Arterial blood pressure – invasive or non-invasive

   2. Venous monitoring – Swan Ganz system

   3. ECG

   a) Rate

   b) Rhythm

   c) Morphology

   d) Ectopy

   e) Ischemia

   4. Temperature

   5. Urine output

   6. Chest tube drainage

   a) Color

   b) Amount

   c) Type of drainage

   d) System patency

   7. Respiratory status

   a) Rate

   b) Rhythm

   c) Depth

   d) Lung sounds

   e) Ventilator settings until patients are on their own

   8. Heart sounds

   a) Present

   b) Audible

   c) Abnormal sounds (rubs, etc.)

   d) Rate/rhythm/frequency/pitch

   9. Neurological

   a) Level of consciousness

   b) Orientation

   c) Awareness of environment

   d) Pupillary reaction

   10. Perfusion – capillary refill test

   11. Dressings

   12. Device

   a) Active/inactive

      b) Rate cutoff

      c) Treatment cycles

      d) PDF on/off

  13. Back-up temporary pacing (transvenous or transcutaneous in addition to the ICD)

      a) Ventricular

      b) AV sequential

      c) DDD

  14. Pain interventions

c. Assess the patient's condition/environment for events which could precipitate arrhythmias.

  1. Identify events

      a) Decreased circulating volume

      b) Pain

      c) Anxiety

      d) Hypoxemia

      e) Decreased cardiac output

      f) Sepsis

      g) Drugs

      h) Ischemia

      i) Atelectasis

      j) Metabolic imbalances

      k) Electrolyte imbalances – potassium, magnesium

  2. Anticipate treatment

      a) Lidocaine as first drug of choice

      b) Other antiarrhythmics

      c) Permit ICD to act if active

      d) CPR

      e) Treatment of other causes

      f) Bradycardia pacing

d. Monitor/assess the patient for postoperative complications in addition to those related to the ICD. Monitor for the following

  1. Pneumothorax

  2. Tamponade

  3. Hypovolemia

  4. Altered ventricular compliance

  5. Coronary artery spasm

  6. Pulmonary edema

  7. Drug reactions

  8. Bleeding

e. Incorporate into the plan of care the following considerations
  1. Status of the device
  2. Safety precautions
  3. Minimize the number and duration of invasive lines
  4. Record any/all shock events with interventions
    a) ICD
    b) Rescue shocks
    c) Drug therapy
    d) Patient symptoms
f. Initiate appropriate interventions for actual or potential problems determined from the assessment.
g. Design a plan of care to identify and manage actual or potential problems for the patient with an ICD. Appropriate nursing diagnoses are:
  1. Activity intolerance
  2. Anxiety
  3. Alterations in cardiac output – decreased
  4. Ineffective individual coping
  5. Ineffective family coping
  6. Alterations in health maintenance
  7. Knowledge deficit
  8. Non-compliance
  9. Disturbance in self concept
  10. Impairment of skin integrity
h. Design and implement a plan of care for the patient with an ICD to result in positive patient outcomes and safe discharge.
i. Evaluate the plan of care for the ICD patient on a regular basis.
j. Complete documentation during the length of stay for the ICD patient
  1. Patient monitoring
  2. Patient assessment
  3. Plan of care
  4. Interventions
  5. Outcomes
  6. Evaluations
  7. Discharge planning
  8. Recommendations
  9. Follow-up care
3. Long-term patient follow-up
  a. Schedule
  b. Procedure considerations

    c. Protocol
    d. Programming
    e. ERI/replacement determination
  4. Safety program
    a. Physical environment
    b. Electrical safety
    c. Hospital environment
    d. Emergency planning
  5. Discharge
    a. Prescriptions
    b. Clinic appointments
    c. Diet
    d. Activity
    e. Referrals
       1. Home care
       2. Rehabilitation
       3. Social services
       4. Psychiatric
       5. Support groups
       6. Other

N. Documentation
  1. Patient care policies, procedures or protocols
  2. Standards of care
  3. Patient management
  4. Patient education
  5. Implantation and operative management
  6. Anesthesia evaluation
  7. Implant and device tracking
  8. Equipment inventory
  9. Follow-up
  10. Arrhythmia evaluation for implantation

O. Emergency Actions with an ICD
  1. CPR
  2. Treatment of arrhythmias
  3. Activation and deactivation of device
  4. Magnet maneuvers with an ICD
  5. Management of pacemaker interactions
  6. Transport of an ICD patient

References

Belder MS, Camm AJ. Implantable cardioverter-defibrillators (ICDs) 1989: how close are we to the ideal device? Clin Cardiol. 12:339–345. 1989.

Bigger JT. Future studies with the implantable cardioverter defibrillator. PACE. 14:883–889. 1991.

Brodsky AM, Miller MH, Cannom D, Ilvento JP, Mirable G, Carillo R. Survey highlights psychosocial adaptation to the AICD: AICD Advances, third quarter:4–5. 1988.

Cannom DS. Support group benefits patients, spouses, physicians and nurses. AICD Advances, third quarter:2–4. 1988.

Cannom DS, Winkle RA. Implantation of the automatic implantable cardioverter/defibrillator. In Tilkian AG, Daily EK, (Eds.) Cardiovascular Procedures, Diagnostic Techniques and Therapeutic Procedures. St. Louis: Mosby, 314–326. 1986.

Cooper DK, Luceri RM, Thurer RJ, Myerburg RJ. The impact of the automatic implantable cardioverter defibrillator on quality of life. Clin Prog Electrophysiol Pacing. 4:4:306–309. 1986.

Debasio N, Rodenhausen N. The group experience: meeting the psychological needs of patients with ventricular tachycardia. Heart Lung. 13:6:597–601. 1984.

Gottlieb CD, Horowitz LN. Potential interactions between antiarrhythmic medication and the automatic implantable cardioverter defibrillator. PACE. 14:898–904. 1991.

Higgins CA. The AICD: a teaching plan for patients and family. Crit Care Nurse. 10:6:69–74. 1990.

Lehmann MH, Steinman RT, Schuger CD, Jackson K. The automatic implantable defibrillator as antiarrhythmic treatment modality of choice for survivors of cardiac arrest unrelated to acute myocardial infarction. Am J Cardiol. 62:803–805. 1988.

Manolis AS, Rastegar H, Estes M. Automatic implantable cardioverter defibrillator – current status. JAMA. 262:10:1362–1368. 1989.

McCrum AE, Tyndall A. Nursing care for patients with implantable defibrillators. Crit Care Nurse. 9:9:48–65. 1989.

Menard-Rothe K, Callahan CM. Cardiac rehabilitation and the automatic implantable defibrillator patient: is it appropriate? J Cardiopulmon Rehab. 6:400–408. 1986.

Moser SA, Crawford D, Thomas A. Caring for patients with implantable cardioverter defibrillators. Crit Care Nurse. 8:2:52–64. 1988.

Myerburg RJ, Kessler KM, Castellanos A. Pathophysiology of sudden cardiac death. PACE. 14:935–943. 1991.

Panidis IP, Morganroth J. Sudden death in hospitalized patients. Prim Cardiol. 11:6:55–71. 1985.

Reid PR, Griffith L, Mower MM, et al. Implantable cardioverter-defibrillator: patient selection and implantation protocol. PACE. 7:1338–1343. 1984.

Saksena S, Lindsay BD, Parsonnet V. Developments for future implantable cardioverters and defibrillators. PACE. 10:1342–1358. 1987.

Tomaselli G, Guarnieri T. The technique of automatic implantable cardioversion/defibrillation. J Crit Ill. 3:3:87–95. 1988.

Winkle RA. State of the art of the AICD. PACE. 961–966. 1991.

CHAPTER 28.C

Therapeutic Modalities:
Endocardial Catheter Ablation

Karen Belco

Ablation is a technique, which interrupts or modifies tachyarrhythmia foci or pathways by delivering energy to a localized area of cardiac tissue. The first intentional catheter ablation, to create complete AV block, was in 1982, following an unintentional ablation with accidental D/C cardioversion shock delivered through an electrode catheter in 1979. The role of catheter ablation in the treatment of tachyarrhythmias has grown rapidly and has been proven wise and effective in certain applications, especially with the advent of radiofrequency techniques. This has saved many patients from open chest surgical procedures.

Objectives

1. Identify the indications for endocardial catheter ablation.
2. Understand methods of catheter ablation.
3. Recognize complications associated with catheter ablation.
4. Define standards of care for patients undergoing catheter ablation.
5. Identify safety precautions for the patient undergoing catheter ablation.
6. Set up electrophysiology lab with appropriate equipment for catheter ablation.

From: Schurig L. *Educational Guidelines: Pacing and Electrophysiology*. Armonk, NY: Futura Publishing Co, Inc, © 1994.

Glossary and Abbreviations

Accessory pathway: Myocardial fibers connecting the atrium and ventricle apart from the normal conduction system.

Antidromic reciprocating tachycardia: Anterograde conduction to the ventricle via the accessory pathway, and retrograde conduction through either the normal conducting system or another accessory pathway.

Concealed bypass tract: An accessory pathway that conducts from the ventricle to the atrium only and, therefore, is not seen on 12 lead ECG recording, because the ventricle is not pre-excited.

Delta wave: "Slurring" of the QRS on 12 lead ECG representing pre-excitation of the ventricle.

Direct current: High-energy counter shock with sinusoidal pulse waveform delivered from a standard external defibrillator.

Dual AV nodal pathways: An extra conduction pathway located within or near the AV node. In most patients, anterograde conduction travels via the slow pathway and retrograde conduction goes over the fast pathway (substrate for AV nodal reentry tachycardia).

High-energy D/C shocks: Electrical catheter ablation by flow of a defibrillator impulse between electrodes or electrode and surface patch.

Kent potential: Impulse representing an accessory pathway during electrophysiologic recording.

Orthodromic AV reciprocating tachycardia: Anterograde conduction over the AV node – His axis with retrograde conduction over the accessory pathway.

Orthodromic reciprocating tachycardia: Reentry circuit tachycardia involving anterograde conduction through the AV node to the ventricle, and retrograde conduction through the accessory pathway causing the atria to contract after the ventricles.

Pace mapping: Catheter manipulation with ventricular pacing to assist in the localization of arrhythmogenic focus. Pacing near this focus will produce a similar QRS morphology to that of the ventricular tachycardia.

Radiofrequency: Alternating current with a frequency of 100–500 kHz. Tissue damage is caused by thermal injury.

Transcoronary chemical ablation: Introduction of chemicals (i.e., ethanol or phenol) by selective catheterization of a small coronary artery, supplying blood to an arrhythmogenic area, or tachycardia pathway for tissue destruction. Also this method is not used clinically at this time.

Education Content

A. Methods (Energy Sources)
1. High-energy D/C shocks (very seldom used)
   a. Flow of current across the myocardium between electrodes.
   b. Lesion formed from disruption of myocardial membrane by intense electrical field.
2. Radiofrequency waves
   a. Generator of heat at electrode-tissue interface

B. Anatomical Locations for Catheter Ablation
1. AV junctional ablation
   a. Indications
      1. Patients with atrial arrhythmias that use the AV node as an obligatory common pathway.
      2. Patients with atrial arrhythmias who are refractory to or intolerant of drug therapy and refractory to ablation specific to the arrhythmia.
         a) Atrial fibrillation/flutter
         b) Ectopic atrial tachycardia
   b. Technique – destruction
      1. Catheter placed against the RV apex for ventricular pacing
         a) Ablating catheter is inserted and positioned to record the largest His and atrial electrogram
         b) Catheters visualized by fluoroscopy
         c) Energy delivered via His catheter
         d) In some 5–10% of patients, the His bundle is ablated using a left heart (retrograde aortic) approach
         e) Accelerated junctional rhythm at onset of energy application is an indicator of successful ablation resulting in AV block
   c. Goals
      1. Complete AV block requiring permanent pacing
   d. Complications
      1. Ventricular arrhythmias (early and late), including sudden cardiac death
      2. Myocardial perforation resulting in cardiac tamponade (not with radiofrequency)
      3. Refer to Part Three, Chapter 24 for complications of routine EPS
      4. Pacemaker complication in those with previously implanted pacemakers
         1) Pacemaker malfunction

   2) Venous complications

   3) Pulmonary emboli

   4) Refer to complications in Part Two, Chapter 18

2. AV junction modification

 a. Indications

  1. AV nodal reentry tachycardia

 b. Techniques

  1. Catheter placement

   a) Right ventricle

   b) Coronary sinus for reference

   c) HIS bundle

   d) Ablation (mapping) catheter

  2. Energy delivered via large tipped ablation catheter

  3. Programmed stimulation performed to determine efficacy of ablative procedure

 c. Goals

  1. Eliminate conduction in one limb of the AV node, usually the slow pathway

  2. Eliminate the fast pathway which is manifest by elimination in alteration of retrograde conduction and prolongation of the AH by 250%.

  3. Non-inducibility of AV nodal reentry tachycardia

 d. Complications

  1. Complete heart block requiring permanent pacing

  2. See complications of routine Part Three, Chapter 24

3. Accessory pathway

 a. Indications

  1. Symptomatic reentrant tachycardia

  2. Potential for life-threatening episodes of atrial fibrillation

 b. Technique

  1. Catheter placement:

   a) Coronary sinus

   b) Right atrium

   c) Right ventricle

   d) His

   e) Mapping catheter

  2. Accessory pathway is typically located along the mitral or tricuspid annulus.

  3. Patient with a δ wave can be mapped during sinus rhythm using accessory pathway potential recordings on the shortest AV interval

4. Mapping retrograde activation during orthodromic tachycardia or ventricular pacing is helpful, especially for patients with concealed WPW

5. Success is usually achieved at the site of earliest retrograde atrial activity

6. Recording a retrograde accessory pathway potential is helpful, but not always possible

7. Characteristics of successful ablation sites
    a) AP potential recorded
    b) Local AV interval less than 70 msec in most patients with δ wave present
    c) Local VA less than 90 msec in most patients
    d) Successful accessory pathway ablation can be achieved at sites of early atrial or ventricular activation where no accessory pathway potential is seen in some patients
        1) Stability of atrial/ventricular electrogram
        2) Closest AV interval

8. Programmed stimulation performed to determine efficacy of ablative procedure.

c. Goals
    1. Disappearance of δ wave
    2. Inability to induce reentry tachycardia

d. Complications
    1. Coronary sinus or other perforation
    2. Coronary artery spasm
    3. Complete AV block
    4. Pericardial tamponade
    5. Ventricular arrhythmias
    6. Refer to complications of routine EPS in Part Three, Chapter 24

e. Advantages of catheter ablation for SVT
    1. Effective
    2. Low morbidity
    3. Low mortality
    4. Cost-effective

4. Ventricular
   a. Indications
      1. Recurrent symptomatic VT, which is drug refractory, not amenable to defibrillator or surgical therapy
      2. Ventricular tachycardia is inducible by programmed stimulation and is tolerated hemodynamically so that the ventricle can be mapped
      3. Bundle branch reentrant VT

b. Contraindications
   1. Hemodynamically unstable VT
   2. Multiple morphologies of VT
   3. Presence of LV thrombus
c. Technique
   1. VT foci is identified via mapping techniques
   2. Arterial access may be required if origin of VT is in the left ventricle
   3. Localization of the earliest site of activation (before the QRS complex on surface ECG), by manipulating the catheter during ventricular pacing (pace mapping)
   4. Energy delivered to endocardium via catheter
   5. Programmed stimulation performed to determine efficacy of ablative procedure
d. Goals
   1. Non-inducible VT
   2. Decreased episodes of spontaneous VT
   3. Drug controllable VT
   4. VT may be inducible immediately post-ablation, but non-inducible several days later (late success)
   5. Non-clinical VT induced post-ablation does not predict long-term outcome
e. Complications
   1. Myocardial perforation
   2. Tamponade
   3. Worsening of ventricular arrhythmias
   4. Refer to complications of routine EPS in Part Three, Chapter 24

C. Special Equipment
   1. Radiofrequency generator
   2. Patient grounding pad
   3. Large tipped steerable catheters
   4. Arterial pressure monitoring
   5. 12 Lead ECG capability
   6. Anesthesia equipment (optional)

References

Braunwald E. Heart Disease: A Textbook of Cardiovascular Medicine. Philadelphia: WB Saunders Co, 1988.

Cain M, Luke R, Lindsay B. Diagnosis and localization of accessory pathways. PACE. 15:801–824. 1992.

Calkins H, Sousa J, El-Atassi R, Rosenheck S, et al. Diagnosis and cure of the Wolff-Parkinson-White syndrome or paroxysmal supraventricular tachycardias during a single electrophysiologic test. N Engl J Med. 324: 1612–1618. 1991.

Chen SA, Tsang WP, Hsia CP. Catheter ablation of free wall accessory atrioventricular pathways in 89 patients with Wolff-Parkinson-White syndrome – comparison of direct current and radiofrequency ablation. Eur Soc Cardiol. 13:1329–1338. 1992.

Chen SA, Tsang WP, Wang DC, et al. Safety and efficacy of a modified catheter-mediated ablation of accessory pathways. Jpn Heart J. 13:303–326. 1992.

Chen XU, Borggrefe M, Shenasa M, Haverkamp W. Characteristics of local electrogram predicting successful transcatheter radiofrequency ablation of left-sided accessory pathways. J Am Coll Cardiol. 20:656–665. 1992.

Epstein LM, Scheiman MM. Modification of the atrioventricular node: a new approach to the treatment of supraventricular tachycardias. Cardiol Clin. 8:567–574. 1990.

Fontaine G, Scheinman M. Ablation in cardiac arrhythmias. Mt Kisco, New York: Futura Publishing Co, Inc., 1987.

Goy JJ, Fromer M, Schlaepfer J, Kappenberger L. Clinical efficacy of radiofrequency current in the treatment of patients with atrioventricular node reentrant tachycardia. J Am Coll Cardiol. 16:418–423. 1990.

Haissaguerre M, Gaita F, Fischer B, et al. Elimination of atrioventricular nodal reentrant tachycardia using discrete slow potentials to guide application of radiofrequency energy. Circulation. 85:2162–2175. 1992.

Haissaguerre M, Montserrat P, Warin JF, et al. Catheter ablation of left posteroseptal accessory pathways and of long RP tachycardias with a right endocardial approach. Eur Soc Cardiol. 845–859. 1991.

Jackman W, Wang X, Friday K, et al. Catheter ablation of accessory atrioventricular pathways (Wolff-Parkinson-White syndrome) by radiofrequency current. N Engl J Med. 324:1605–1611. 1991.

Josephson ME. Clinical Cardiac Electrophysiology Techniques and Interpretations. 2nd Edition. Philadelphia: Lea and Febiger. 1993.

Langberg J, Calkins H, Kim Y. et al. Recurrence of conduction in accessory atrioventricular connections after initially successfully radiofrequency catheter ablation. J Am Coll Cardiol. 19:1588–1592. 1992.

Langberg J, Chin M, Rosenqvist M, et al. Catheter ablation of the atrioventricular junction with radiofrequency. Circulation. 80:1527–1535. 1989.

Langberg J, Kim YN, Goyal R, et al. Conversion of typical to "atypical" atrioventricular nodal reentrant tachycardia after radiofrequency catheter modification of the atrioventricular junction. J Am Coll Cardiol. 69: 503–508. 1992.

Lee M, Morady F, Kadish A, et al. Catheter modification of the atrioventricular junction with radiofrequency energy for control of atrioventricular nodal reentry tachycardia. Circulation. 83:827–835. 1991.

Lesh M, Van Hare G, Schamp D, et al. Curative percutaneous catheter ablation using radiofrequency energy for accessory pathways in all locations: results in 100 consecutive patients. J Am Coll Cardiol. 1303–1309. 1992.

Levy S, Scheiman MM. Cardiac arrhythmias from diagnosis to therapy. Mt Kisco: Futura Publishing Co, Inc., 1984.

Luderitz B, Saksena S. Interventional electrophysiology. Mt Kisco: Futura Publishing Co, Inc., 1991.

Milstein S, Sharma A, Guiraudon G. An algorithm for the electrocardiographic localization of accessory pathways in the Wolff-Parkinson-White syndrome. PACE. 15:801–823. 1992.

Natale A, Wathen M, Yee R, et al. Atrial and ventricular approaches for radiofrequency catheter ablation of left-sided accessory pathways. J Am Coll Cardiol. 70:114–116. 1992.

Platia EV. Management of Cardiac Arrhythmias. The Nonpharmacologic Approach. Philadelphia: JB Lippenncott, 1987.

Saul J, Hulse J, De W, et al. Catheter ablation of accessory atrioventricular pathways in young patients: use of long vascular sheaths, the transseptal approach and a retrograde left posterior parallel approach. J Am Coll Cardiol. 21:571–583. 1993.

Scheinman M, Wang YS, Van Hare G, et al. Electrocardiographic and electrophysiologic characteristics of anterior, midseptal and right anterior free wall accessory pathways. J Am Coll Cardiol. 20:1220–1229. 1992.

Schluter M, Kuck KH. Catheter ablation from right atrium of anteroseptal accessory pathways using radiofrequency current. J Am Coll Cardiol. 19: 663–670. 1992.

Sousa J, El-Atassi R, Rosenheck S, et al. Radiofrequency catheter ablation of the atrioventricular junction from the left ventricle. Circulation. 84: 567–571. 1991.

Szabo T, Klein G, Guiraudon G. Localization of accessory pathways in the Wolff-Parkinson-White syndrome. PACE. 12:1691–1705. 1989.

Wathen M, Natale A, Wolfe K, et al. An anatomically guided approach to atrioventricular node slow pathway ablation. Am J Cardiol. 70:886–889. 1992.

Wu D, Yeh SJ, Wang CC, et al. Nature of dual atrioventricular node pathways and the tachycardia circuit as defined by radiofrequency ablation technique. J Am Coll Cardiol. 20:884–895. 1992.

Zardini M, Leitch J, Guiraudon G, Klein G, et al. Atrioventricular nodal reentry and dual atrioventricular node physiology in patients undergoing accessory pathway ablation. Am J Cardiol. 66:1388–1389. 1990.

Zipes D, Jalife J. Cardiac electrophysiology from cell to bedside. Philadelphia: WB Saunders Co, Inc., 1990.

CHAPTER 28.D

Therapeutic Modalities:
Surgical Therapy

Michelle G. Tobin

Subsection:
1. Methods
2. Anatomical Locations
3. Special Equipment
4. Complications
5. Patient Education

Surgical intervention has been a standard therapy for patients with ectopic atrial tachycardia, Wolff-Parkinson-White syndrome, and ventricular tachycardia. Some of these procedures can be done without the use of cardiopulmonary bypass and cardioplegia, which has the following advantages: 1) continuous monitoring of cardiac electrical activity, 2) immediate assessment of ablation results, 3) diminished trauma and morbidity. Cardiopulmonary bypass is used when the patient becomes hemodynamically unstable, seen more often in intraoperative ventricular tachycardia mapping and resections. The role of surgery has diminished with the emergence of radiofrequency ablation, but will continue to be the therapy of choice for those patients requiring concomitant surgery such as valvular replacement and/or repair, and coronary bypass grafting.

The associated professional's role may include patient education pre- as well as postoperatively, securing specialized equipment necessary for the procedure, assuring safety, assist and/or operate equipment during the procedure, and other duties per hospital policy.

From: Schurig L. *Educational Guidelines: Pacing and Electrophysiology.* Armonk, NY: Futura Publishing Co, Inc, © 1994.

Objectives

1. List four accessory pathways of Wolff-Parkinson-White syndrome.
2. Describe the surgery used to treat AV nodal reentrant tachycardia.
3. List three disadvantages regarding safety and effectiveness of laser ablation.
4. Assemble the proper equipment for an intraoperative ventricular tachycardia mapping.

Glossary and Abbreviations

Ablation: Eradication. Removal of a part by cutting, freezing or heat.

Atrial fibrillation: Atrial arrhythmia characterized by rapid randomized contractions of the atrial myocardium, causing a totally irregular, often rapid ventricular rate.

Atrial flutter: A condition of cardiac arrhythmia in which the atrial contraction are rapid, but regular. In many instances a circus pathway is present. The ventricles are unable to respond to each atrial impulse, so that a partial block usually is present.

AV groove: Atrioventricular linear depression. Coronarius cordis.

AV nodal reentrant tachycardia: Based on reentrant mechanism within the atrioventricular node.

Cardiopulmonary bypass: Diversion of the flow of blood from the entrance of the right atrium directly to the aorta, usually via pump oxygenator, avoiding both the heart and the lungs.

Ectopic atrial tachycardia: Arises anywhere in the atrial myocardium. A distinguishing features on an electrocardiogram is an abnormal P-wave morphology.

VT: Abbreviation for ventricular tachycardia.

WPW: Abbreviation for Wolff-Parkinson-White syndrome, defined as a congenital heart disease resulting from an accessory atrioventricular connection, generally located in the atrioventricular sulcus and consisting of normal working myocardium.

Education Content

A. Methods

1. Resection – removing tissue in this case, that is the origin of the arrhythmia

2. Cryotherapy – destroying tissue by the use of extreme cold. Source is nitrous oxide to -60 to $-70°C$

3. Incision – cutting tissue to destroy arrhythmogenic foci

4. Laser – destroying tissue by the use of immense heat and power at close range. Source is argon using wavelengths of 1064 nM and a power of 20–25 W

5. Ancillary surgical procedures – procedures that accompany surgical ablations such as coronary bypass grafting, valvular replacement/repair, aneurysmectomy

B. Anatomical Locations/Indications

1. Atria

   a. Ectopic atrial tachycardia

      1. Preoperative mapping in the electrophysiology lab to localize the ectopic foci

      2. Intraoperative mapping is often difficult because of the inability to induce the tachycardia following general anesthesia

      3. Surgical treatment is done by either: incising the focus area and then applying cryotherapy or excising the abnormal focus and placing cryolesions around the edges of the dissection

   b. Paroxysmal atrial flutter/fibrillation

      1. Preoperative EPS

      2. Intraoperative mapping to identify the slow conduction area and fragmented potentials

      3. Surgical treatment – Maze procedure using cryotherapy in combination with numerous incisions to ablate abnormal pathways

2. AV node

   a. AV nodal reentry tachycardia

      1. Preoperative EPS to assess ventricular/atrial conduction. Intervals less than 70 msec can be seen

      2. Intraoperative mapping

      3. Surgical treatment by: cryolesions applied around the AV node from the right atrial surface in the triangle of Koch, or by dissection at the area where the earliest retrograde atrial activation was identified during tachycardia

      4. Results may produce complete heart block and require temporary

433

pacing assistance for a short time, but patient should be prepared for the possibility of permanent pacing

3. Accessory pathways

  a. Pre-operative EPS to determine WPW diagnosis

  b. Intraoperative mapping along AV groove to determine earliest activation. This is accomplished by using a roving probe or by using a computerized mapping system. Multiple pathways may be identified

  c. Surgical treatment can be done by two approaches

    1. Endocardial technique for left or right free wall pathways involves opening the appropriate atrium, incising above the affected valve and then dissecting the AV groove. Cardioplegia is required.

    2. Epicardial approach involves incising and dissecting the AV groove from the epicardial surface. Following dissection, cryotherapy is performed at the junction of the atria and ventricular myocardium to the valve.

4. Ventricles

  a. Ventricular tachycardia and subendocardial resections

    1. Pre-operative mapping – VT is usually easier to induce in the EPS lab and if stable is vital for surgical resection.

    2. Intraoperative mapping is done to localize the site of VT origin. This is achieved by using a roving probe or by a computerized mapping system. Mapping is done in sinus rhythm and during programmed ventricular stimulation.

    3. Surgical treatment is to resect the mapped area seen as a fibrous scar 3–5 cm in diameter. If no scar seen at the site of the origin of arrhythmia, cryotherapy or laser therapy is used

  b. Ischemic ventricular tachycardia

    1. Pre-operative mapping

    2. Intraoperative mapping (as above)

    3. Surgical treatment is a partial encircling endocardial myotomy, which encompasses the internal left ventricle circumference partially, mostly at the septum, but encircles the arrhythmogenic tissues completely

    4. In areas unfit for incision or resection, ablation is done using cryodestruction or laser therapy.

    5. Coronary bypass grafting accompanies this procedure

C. Special Equipment

  1. Cryomachine

  2. Cryoprobes – numerous sizes 3–10 mm and a diamond tip

  3. Laser – i.e., ND-Yag laser

4. Pacing electrodes
5. Recording monitor – capable of recording surface as well multiple intracardiac electrograms
6. Programmable stimulator – able to deliver sensed and paced extrastimuli
7. Lead switch box or junction box
8. Computerized mapping system–that has the ability to record multiple sites simultaneously; therefore, observing earliest ectopic activations quicker
9. Compatible mesh electrodes and latex balloons for computerized mapping system – comes in various sizes and shapes depending on the areas to map

D. Complications
1. Complete heart block
2. Infection
3. Risks given with any cardiac surgical procedure/or anesthetic risk
4. Death

E. Patient Education
1. Pre-operatively the risks of surgery are discussed with the patient and family with the surgical team
2. Intraoperatively the cardiology and surgical team work together to locate the area of origin of the tachycardia
3. An ablating technique is then performed at the discretion of the team and may include: incising, resecting, cryodestruction or laser therapy
4. Postoperative stay is usually 5–7 days
5. At discharge, patients are reminded of the possibility of reoccurrence, and encouraged to call their cardiologist if symptoms should arise
6. Patients return for postoperative EPS evaluation in approximately 6 weeks. If the study proves negative, resumption of all activity is encouraged.

References

Cox J. Surgical management of cardiac arrhythmias. In El-Sherif T, Samet P. (Eds.) Cardiac Pacing & Electrophysiology. Philadelphia: WB Saunders Co, 436. 1991.

Kay GN, Bubien RS. Clinical Management of Cardiac Arrhythmias. Gaithersburg: Aspen, 99, 123, 189. 1992.

Kaushik RR. Risk factors in antiarrhythmic surgery. In Luderitz B, Saksena S. (Eds.) Interventional Electrophysiology. Mt Kisco: Futura Publishing Co, Inc., 489. 1991.

Bredikis JJ, Benetis R, Bredikis AJ, et al. Closed heart antiarrhythmic surgery in supraventricular tachycardia (except surgery on conduction pathways). In Luderitz B, Saksena S. (Eds.) Interventional Electrophysiology. Mt Kisco: Futura Publishing Co, Inc., 495. 1991.

Guiraudon GM, Klein GJ, Yee R. Surgical ablation of supraventricular arrhythmias in Wolff-Parkinson-White syndrome. In Luderitz B, Saksena S. (Eds.) Interventional Electrophysiology. Mt Kisco: Futura Publishing Co, Inc., 507. 1991.

Breithardt G, Borggrefe M, Hief C, et al. Indications for nonpharmacological therapy in patients with sustained ventricular tachycardia or fibrillation. In Luderitz B, Saksena S. (Eds.) Interventional Electrophysiology. Mt Kisco: Futura Publishing Co, Inc., 517. 1991.

Gielchinsky I. Endocardial resection for ventricular tachycardia and its limitations. In Luderitz B, Saksena S. (Eds.) Interventional Electrophysiology. Mt Kisco: Futura Publishing Co, Inc., 529. 1991.

Ostermeyer J, Borggrefe M, Breithardt G, et al. Circumcisional techniques for ablation of arrhythmogenic tissues underlying malignant ischemic ventricular tachycardia. In Luderitz B, Saksena S. (Eds.) Interventional Electrophysiology. Mt Kisco: Futura Publishing Co, Inc., 539. 1991.

Saksena, S. Intraoperative laser ablation in malignant ventricular tachycardia. In Luderitz B, Saksena S. (Eds.) Interventional Electrophysiology. Mt Kisco: Futura Publishing Co, Inc., 545. 1991.

Marchlinski FE, Josephson ME. Appropriate diagnostic studies for arrhythmia surgery. PACE. 902–916. 1984.

Svenson RH, Selle JG, Gallagher JJ, et al. Neodymium: YAG laser photocoagulation: a potentially useful method for intraoperative ablation of arrhythmogenic foci. In Fontaine G, Scheinman MM. (Eds.) Ablation in Cardiac Arrhythmias. Mt Kisco: Futura Publishing Co, Inc., 379. 1987.

Narula OS. Laser catheter technique for induction of AV nodal delays: possible applications for management of supraventricular tachyarrhythmias. In Fontaine G, Scheinman MM. (Eds.) Ablation in Cardiac Arrhythmias. Mt Kisco: Futura Publishing Co, Inc., 405. 1987.

Mesnildrey P, Laborde F, Bruneval P, et al. Therapeutic and prophylactic surgical treatment of ventricular tachycardia by Nd-YAG laser irradiation. In Fontaine G, Scheinman MM. (Eds.) Ablation in Cardiac Arrhythmias. Mt Kisco: Futura Publishing Co, Inc., 429. 1987.

CHAPTER 29

Research Guidelines

Margaret Millis Faust

Subsection:
A. Study Design
B. Regulatory Process
C. Financial Considerations
D. Documentation
E. Patient Concerns and Outcomes
F. Role of the Non-Physician Health Provider

As the field of clinical research changes to meet the demands of biotechnologic advancement and socioeconomic change, the role of non-physician health providers in research is expanding. Frequently the non-physician health provider is involved in many facets of clinical research. Duties and responsibilities may include but are not limited to: study design and development; budget development; patient recruitment; data collection and interpretation; patient, family and staff education; and performing life science procedures related to research protocols. The non-physician health provider who has experience in clinical research will become involved in originating new research and research funding.

The field of modern clinical research is vastly different from medical experimentation in the past. Few medical advances occurred from the age of Hippocrates to the end of the eighteenth century. During the eighteenth century there are isolated reports of human experimentation using prisoners and children. The nineteenth century was an era of "auto-experimentation;" experiments were performed by physicians upon themselves or families. This auto-experimentation continued to be practiced well into the twentieth century. Indeed, right heart catheterization was performed as an auto-experiment in 1929 by Werner Forssmann. Dr. Forssmann received the Nobel Prize in 1956 for demonstrating that right heart catheterization could be performed safely. The twentieth century has witnessed the most rapid growth in clinical

From: Schurig L. *Educational Guidelines: Pacing and Electrophysiology.* Armonk, NY: Futura Publishing Co, Inc, © 1994.

research; this is largely due to advances in the pharmaceutical industry. Synthetic pharmaceuticals have been available only during the last two decades of the twentieth century; prior to the appearance of synthetic pharmaceuticals, drug therapy connoted quackery.

The advent of modern drug therapy stimulated the modern era of human experimentation. The magnitude of human experimentation caused a great deal of public concern and around 1931, steps were implemented to institute guidelines for human experimentation. These guidelines are very similar to the code of conduct used today; informed consent and prior animal testing were major principles of the guidelines. At the same time, Nazi medical experiments were being conducted on prisoners in concentration camps during World War I. The Nurenberg Code resulted from the prosecution of those involved in the Nazi experiments. According to Norman Howard-Jones, the Nurenberg code is very similar to the guidelines set forth by the Germans in 1931. The Nurenberg trials forced the world's medical community to examine ethical values in human experimentation; the World Health Organization's "Declaration of Helsinki" in 1964 (revised in 1975) addressed concerns regarding medical experimentation on human subjects.

Blatant examples of unethical experimentation are known to have occurred in the United States as late as 1972. The most well-known example of unethical experimentation is the "Tuskegee Syphilis Study" (1932–1972). The National Commission for the Protection of Human Subjects of Biomedical and Behavioral Research was formed in 1974 to address ethical principles and develop guidelines for biomedical research involving human subjects. The regulations set forth in 1974 were revised in 1981 and continue to be examined by various branches of the United States government. The regulations are designed to protect human rights and assure institutional review of research by a committee of peers. The non-physician health providers will be affected by these regulations in every aspect of their practice.

Objectives

1. Identify study designs commonly utilized.
2. Identify study phases of pharmacologic research.
3. Recognize study phases for device research.
4. Organize components that should be included in a study budget.
5. Recognize patient concerns for financial responsibility in research endeavors.
6. Recognize current difficulty with third party payment for research-related reimbursement.
7. Name the documents required while conducting clinical research.
8. List the components of informed consent.

9. Review the historical perspectives involved in current protection of human rights.
10. Plan for patient and family education regarding research protocol and human rights.
11. Recognize role of AP in educating medical and ancillary staff about research protocol and patient recruitment.
12. Plan for patient right of confidentiality in research.
13. Plan for emotional support of patient and family participating in research.
14. Recognize need of patient and family to be informed of outcomes of study.

Education Content

A. Study Design

    1. Time dimensional designs

        a. Prospective

        b. Retrospective

    2. Experimental study design

        a. Randomized clinical trials

            1. Researcher blinded to group receiving treatment

            2. Control groups used to compare results

            3. Placebo can be used to "blind" patient and investigator

            4. Trial can be investigator blind, double blind (both patient and investigator) or non-blind

        b. Surveys

            1. Used to collect data

            2. No independent variable utilized

            3. Example: pacemaker registry, Catheter ablation registry

        c. Descriptive design

            1. No manipulation of variables

            2. Investigator bias is a problem

        d. Correlational design

            1. Relationship between variables within an identified situation

            2. Variance is controlled

            3. Correlation does not establish cause

B. Overview of the Regulatory Process

    1. Research study phases – drugs

        a. Phase I – new drug to man, usually healthy volunteers

        b. Phase II – trials on limited number of subjects for disease control or prophylaxis

        c. Phase III – safety and efficacy in a specific population, long-term effects

        d. Phase IV – marketed product studies

    2. Research study phases – devices

        a. Devices subject to general controls applicable to all devices, Ex: standard manufacturing practices, labeling, safety, etc.

        b. Devices with previously established performance standards, devices are more complicated and can involve a higher degree of risk associated with use.

        c. Devices which pose the greatest potential hazard to the user and require pre-market approval and must undergo scientific evaluation prior to general use.

C. Financial Considerations
  1. Designing study budget
     a. Personnel costs
        1. Principal investigator
        2. Co-investigator
        3. Study coordinator
        4. Study personnel
        5. Consultants
           a) Includes consultants for data analysis
           b) Specialists needed for study
     b. Procedures costs
     c. Laboratory costs
     d. Equipment (that which needs to be purchased for study)
     e. Supplies
     f. Travel
        1. Patient
        2. To meetings if multicenter study
        3. Patient care cost
           a) Co-payments of deductibles if third party payment is option
           b) Cost for procedures, hospitalization, instrumentation if no insurance coverage expected.
  2. Patient concerns
     a. Personal expenditure
        1. Examples
           a) Unreimbursed travel
           b) Portion of bill not covered by insurance
           c) Uninsured individuals
     b. Insurance coverage is usually limited for research devices and procedures
     c. Uninsured individuals
  3. Funding sources
     a. Grants
     b. Contracts
     c. Fellowships
     d. Foundations/guilds
     e. Cooperative agreements

D. Documentation
  1. Documents required to be on file
     a. Study protocol
     b. Informed consent form
     c. Form FD-1572 to sponsor of study (reflects adherence to federal code of regulation, Title 21, Part 56). The purpose of this regulation is to ensure that an IRB is responsible for initial and annual review approval of the study.
     d. Curriculum vitae
        1. Principal investigators
        2. Co-investigators
     e. Study budget
     f. Laboratory normal ranges for tests performed as part of the protocol
        1. Laboratory license and certification
     g. Radiotherapy dosages (if applicable)
     h. Institutional review board correspondence
        1. Copy of approved protocol, approved consent form
        2. Copy of approved amendments
        3. Copy of adverse experiences
        4. Copy of any advertisements, brochures or literature for the study
        5. Annual review of protocol
     i. Sample case report forms
     j. Enrollment log
     k. Drug packing slips
     l. Drug inventory list
     m. Study supplies invoices
     n. Study monitor visit log
     o. All correspondence regarding study
        1. Sponsor generated
        2. Investigator generated
        3. Contributing pharmaceutical and device companies
  2. Informed consent-required components
     a. Basic elements
        1. Purpose of the study
        2. Number of subjects involved in study
        3. Procedures to be followed
        4. Clear statement identifying which parts of the study are experimental
        5. Approximate duration of the study

6. Risks or discomforts that can be reasonably expected
7. Possible benefits to the patient
8. Statement regarding confidentiality of records and data
9. Statement that participation is voluntary and that refusal to participate will involve no loss of benefit or penalty to subject. Statement must also include subject's right to withdraw from study without prejudice.
10. Statement addressing compensation or if medical treatments are available if injury occurs as a result of research involving more than minimal risk.
11. Explanation of who to contact with questions relating to the research or patient rights or research related injury.

   b. Additional elements (optional or included only if applicable)

1. Any circumstances which might cause the investigator to discontinue patient's participation without consent (termination criteria).
2. Additional costs which may be incurred related to participation in the research.
3. Statement that findings from research will be provided to the patient.
4. Consequences to patient for withdrawal from study.
5. Statement relating to effects of research on embryo or fetus if subject may become pregnant (if applicable).

3. Reporting requirements
   a. Institutional review board
      1. Composition
         a) Multidisciplinary
            1) Includes "non-scientific" members (lawyers, clergy, etc.)
         b) Duties
            1) Perform initial review of proposed research
            2) Review research in an ongoing fashion with review of protocol amendments, periodic review
            3) Prompt review of unanticipated problems or adverse effects related to research.
            4) Report and respond to Food and Drug Administration

   b. Sponsor
      1. Timely completion of all study data forms
      2. Prompt notification of unanticipated problems related to research
      3. All correspondence should be in files
   c. Food and Drug Administration (United States)

    1. FDA may audit investigator records at any time during the study.

    2. Documents needed for FDA audit
      a) IRB correspondence
      b) All study data forms
      c) Medical records of study patients and enrollment log
      d) Drug inventory records
      e) All correspondence to and from sponsor
      f) Other documents as requested by FDA inspector

4. Results of study
   a. Case report forms (CRFs)
     1. Use black ball point pen
     2. Draw a line through error and initial the correction
     3. Fill in *all* spaces; leave no missing data
     4. CRFs must remain on file for 2 years
     5. Check data for validity, congruency
   b. Types of data forms commonly requested
     1. Enrollment
     2. Clinical history and physical
     3. Clinical test results
     4. Efficacy report
     5. Adverse effects reports
     6. Event forms
     7. Follow-up
   c. Establish a publication policy prior to completion of study design.
     1. Discuss primary, secondary and last author listing on publications

E. Patient Concerns
   1. Education
     a. Assist with ensuring patient understanding of informed consent
     b. Assist with ensuring patient and family understanding of disease and treatment process.
     c. Development of patient literature can be helpful
   2. Confidentiality
     a. All patient data used in publication of results will be referred to by patient number only
     b. All study data will be confidential
       1. FDA is the only exception to this rule; they may examine all CRF's
   3. Follow-up

    a. Stress importance of keeping scheduled visits
    b. Stress importance of compliance
    c. Inform patient on mechanism of scheduling interim visits
  4. Emotional support
    a. Reassure patient and family that the research is legitimate and carefully monitored
    b. Act as a liaison between patient, patient's family and the health care team
    c. Educate the patient and/or patient's family as the study outcome is learned

F. Role of the Non-Physician Health Provider
  1. Patient recruitment
    a. Perform screening of patient populations for potential participants in clinical trials
    b. Dispel fears regarding participation in clinical trials
  2. Collaboration with physician for maximal data collection
    a. Frequent patient contact
  3. Study implementation
    a. "Hands-on" participation
  4. Patient concerns
    a. Education
    b. Assist with ensuring patient understanding of informed consent
    c. Assist with ensuring patient and family understanding of disease and treatment process.
    d. Development of patient literature can be helpful
  5. Organization of the project
    a. Scheduling
      1. Admissions
      2. Tests
      3. Follow-up
    b. Monitoring and documenting adherence to schedule
      1. Scheduled visits
      2. Missed tests/visits
      3. Protocol deviations
    c. Establish communication system
      1. Multidisciplinary approach
    d. Data management
      1. Organize data collected by patient
      2. Protocol and update notebook
        a) IRB approval

        b) Annual review
        c) Correspondence from and to sponsor
   3. Pharmaceutical research
        a) Pill counts
        b) Save shipping labels
6. Educating public
   a. Regarding importance and benefits of clinical trials
   b. Patient and family education about specific protocols
7. Publications
   a. Data analysis
   b. Manuscript preparation
   c. Abstract/poster presentations

References

Howard-Jones N. Human experimentation in historical and ethical perspective. Soc Sci Med. 16:1429–1448. 1982.

Thomas SB, Quinn SC, Public Health Then and Now. Am J Pub Health. 81: 1498–1505. 1991.

National Commission for the Protection of Human Subjects of Biomedical and Behavioral Research. The Belmont Report. FR Doc 79–12065. 2–8. Filed 4/7/79.

United States. Code of Federal Regulations. Title 21, Parts 1–99. 217–231. Government Printing Office, Washington, DC. 1989.

United States. Code of Federal Regulation. Title 21. Parts 300–499. 85–91. Government Printing Office, Washington, DC. 1989.

Suggested Reading

Jones J. Bad Blood: The Tuskegee Syphilis Experiment – A Tragedy of Race and Medicine. New York: The Free Press. 1981.

Engel King C. Facilitating Clinical Trials: The Expanding Role of the Nurse. Cancer. 67:1793–1797. 1991.

FDA. Answers to frequently asked questions – IRB. Department of Health and Human Resources. Rockville: April, 1984.

Code of Federal Regulations. Food & Drugs, Book 21, Parts 800 to 1299, Subsection 1000.1, Subchapter J – Radiological Health, Part 1000 General, Subpart C – Radiation Protection Recommendations. 438–445. 1991.

Code of Federal Regulations. Public Welfare, Book 45, Parts 1 to 199, Subsection 36.1, Part 46 – Protection of Human Subjects. 117–136. 1991.

Code of Federal Regulations. Food & Drugs, Book 21, Parts 1 to 99, Subsection 25.50, Part 50 – Protection of Human Subjects. 217–225. 1991.

Code of Federal Regulations. Food & Drugs, Book 21, Parts 1 to 99, Subsection 56.102, Part 56 – Institutional Review Boards. 225–233. 1991.

Code of Federal Regulations. Food & Drugs, Book 21, Parts 300 to 499, Subsection 310.545, Part 312 – Investigational New Drug Application. 61–95. 1991.

Code of Federal Regulations. Food & Drugs, Book 21, Parts 300 to 499, Subsection 312.160, Part 314 – Applications for FDA Approval to Market a New Drug or an Antibiotic Drug. 95–138. 1991.

CHAPTER 30

Electrophysiology: Patient Education

Tomas P. Ozahowski

Once a patient has been admitted for a serious arrhythmia problem, it is important to utilize assessment skills to determine if and how a patient can learn. Inquiring about what has brought the patient into the hospital can help determine his/her capabilities to learn. It is also very important to include spouses and/or significant others in the educational process, if appropriate. Many patients and families do not understand why they have been transferred or their expectations are inaccurate, possibly due to anxiety, fear, or denial. If the patient is unable to comprehend why he/she is in the hospital, all further teaching will be difficult.

Another problem that can arise is seen in the patient who is being treated for more than one problem. For example, a post-infarct patient whose hospitalization has been complicated by unstable angina and complete heart block, has the unfortunate experience of cardiac arrest. This patient will have difficulty determining what has happened and will need capable, clear and simple explanations in order to sort out the differences. The focus should be on what the patient needs to know to progress once discharged.

Patients learn differently because of their past experiences, age, knowledge base, social and demographic situation, intelligence level, problem-solving ability, and motivational factors. We also need to take into consideration the patient's anxiety levels and memory capabilities. Once we have assessed this, we can determine what and how much teaching is appropriate. It is important to note that knowledge of the medical condition does not increase compliance, but knowledge of the regimen does. Therefore, the primary focus on educating the arrhythmia patient should include what is needed to treat and/or control the rhythm problem.

From: Schurig L, et al. *Educational Guidelines: Pacing and Electrophysiology*. Armonk, NY: Futura Publishing Co, Inc, © 1994.

Objectives

1. Describe information that should be included in a patient education program for patients undergoing electrophysiology studies.
2. List additional teaching responsibilities for electrophysiology patients when preparing for discharge.
3. Discuss the role for follow-up patient education post-discharge and the feasibility of an in-hospital self-administration drug program.

Education Content

If patients understand what has happened to them and they are motivated to learn, a description of the following is in order prior to the electrophysiology study.

A. Electrophysiology Content for Patient Education

   1. Simple description of the conduction system of the heart.

   2. State the suspected cause of the arrhythmia problem and where it occurs.

   3. Describe symptoms of recurrence and/or hemodynamic compromise of the arrhythmia and appropriate actions to take.

   4. Have the patient describe how he/she felt during the episode.

   5. Explain the purpose of a routine primary electrophysiology study.

   6. Give a simple explanation of the study. A written booklet, for example such as Dartmouth's Electrophysiology Studies, *What It's All About*, should also be presented so that the patient can review and also share this information with family members. Video tapes are also available and can be useful for patients who cannot read.

   7. Identify major events which will occur in order to prepare for the electrophysiology study.

      a. NPO

      b. Preparation

      c. Sedation

      d. Need to come off current antiarrhythmic medications. This can be scary for some patients.

   8. State potential complications of an electrophysiology study.

      a. Hematoma at catheter site

      b. Infection

      c. Thromboembolus/phlebitis

      d. Pneumothorax (rare)

      e. Perforation of right ventricle – possible cardiac tamponade

      f. Syncope – not really a complication, but needs to be explained to the patient

   9. State the major care events which will occur after the study.

      a. Vital signs

      b. Bedrest/resumption of activity

      c. Resumption of meals

      d. Intravenous status

      e. Effects of sedation (if used)

    f. Positioning

    g. Frequent groin and/or antecubital, I.J. or subclavian checks

10. State time and expected length of electrophysiology study. This is very important for type "A" personalities.

11. Discuss potential need for sleep medications if required.

12. Discuss potential problems during EPS

    a. Back discomfort

    b. Shoulder discomfort

    c. Urinary urgency

13. Discuss need for follow-up studies.

B. Techniques for Enhancing Compliance and Reinforcing Education

    1. In-hospital self-administered drug program

        a. Possible step-by-step approach on a telemetry monitored floor by staff nurses

        b. Descriptions of levels

            1. First level – nursing staff is responsible for medication administration, and function as a resource explaining the drugs and dosage schedule

            2. Second level – the patient is responsible for the timing of the medication. Nursing staff administers drugs

            3. Third level – the patient is responsible for both the timing and the proper administration. End of day pill counts are done by the nursing staff

        c. Advantages

            1. Patients are less dependent, more trustful, and have greater autonomy

            2. Less disruption in the patient's pattern or daily activities

            3. Provides the patient with positive feedback

            4. Nurses will be better able to assess compliance

            5. Considered safe: possible mistakes can be made in a safe environment

        d. Disadvantages

            1. Patients may not be ready to deal with taking their medications or are unable to

            2. Spouse involvement may be difficult

            3. Potential cancellation of an EP study due to patient's omittance of a dose

            4. Greater chance of error

    2. Utilization of major manufacturer's excellent teaching tools

        a. Video

 b. Handouts

 c. Models

3. Incorporation of a schedule with follow-up telephone calls included in discharge teaching guidelines

 a. Advantages

 1. Reinforcement and assessment of patient's ability to retain information on the medical, surgical and/or device-related regime

 2. Flexibility in time frame for making calls

 3. Convenience for patients, reduction of anxiety levels, allows verbalization which patient and/or spouse may not be able to discuss in person

 4. Allowance of time to review potential complications of EP study and drug side effects

 5. Probability of no cost to patient

 b. Disadvantages

 1. Inability to perform "hands on" care and visualization

 2. Elimination of therapeutic touch responses

 3. Hospital financial concerns; patients probably won't be billed for phone calls

4. Miscellaneous educational components for EP patients

 a. One person CPR teaching for spouse and/or significant others

 b. Local EMS should be notified

 1. External cardioverter/defibrillator should be available

 c. Pulse taking should be taught

 d. Discuss potential problems when switching from brand name to generic antiarrhythmic medications

 1. Patient should know state law regulations regarding the dispensing of either of these drugs

References

Grubb BP. Recurrence of ventricular tachycardia following conversion from proprietary to generic procainamide. Am J Cardiol. 63:1532–1533. 1989.

Nolan PE. Generic substitution of antiarrhythmic drugs. Am J Cardiol. 64: 1371–1377. 1989.

CHAPTER 31

Surface ECG

Rosemary Fabiszewski-Volosin

Subsection:
A. Signal Averaged Electrocardiogram

Research is being done to develop and assess new techniques for identifying patients at increased risk for sustained ventricular tachycardia. Non-invasive identification of these patients would facilitate patient management. The signal averaged ECG is a sensitive non-invasive method for risk stratification of patients recovering from myocardial infarction.

Clinical studies using mapping techniques during sinus rhythm have shown that patients with prior MI who develop sustained VT have a greater number of ventricular sites demonstrating abnormal and fragmented electrograms than patients with prior MI without sustained VT. The term *late potential* has been applied to these delays in conduction. A late potential is thought to originate from areas of delayed ventricular depolarization. These late potentials represent derangement of ventricular conduction and thus an electrophysiologic substrate conducive to the development of ventricular arrhythmias. Late potentials are microvolt level, high-frequency waveforms that are continuous with the QRS complex and persist for tens of milliseconds into the ST segment.

Most patients who have sustained ventricular tachycardia have coronary artery disease and/or depressed left ventricular function. Many have PVCs or ventricular tachycardia post-myocardial infarction.

In patients with ventricular tachycardia, the initial portion of the filtered QRS of the SAECG is similar to normals, but there is a *tail* of low amplitude signal that is not present in patients without ventricular tachycardia (VT).

Results of published studies show that 14–29% of patients recovering from myocardial infarction (MI) who have abnormal SAECGs will have sus-

From: Schurig L. *Educational Guidelines: Pacing and Electrophysiology.* Armonk, NY: Futura Publishing Co, Inc, © 1994.

tained ventricular tachycardia within the first year.[1] The predictive accuracy of the SAECG is increased when results are combined with measures of left ventricular function. However, it has not been determined how long after MI the SAECGs should be obtained during the second week after MI for predictive accuracy for arrhythmic episodes.

The surface ECG represents the summation of the heart's total electrical activity. Because the amplitude of late potentials is typically under 1 mV when measured directly, conventional surface ECGs cannot detect these signals reliably because they are masked by noise.

Consequently, late potentials may be present but are buried within the ECG signal. Surface signal averaging has been developed as a technique for extracting this concealed, but clinically important information. Signal averaging is a computer based technique used to reduce random noise in the ECG and to enhance the detection of low-amplitude signals, thereby allowing the detection of late potentials. The process averages together multiple samples of a repetitive waveform, then high-pass filters them to reduce or cancel random noise. With averaging of successive cycles, random electrical events (such as respiration and environmental activity) will be diminished and the desired signal will accumulate.

Objectives

1. Define ventricular late potential and recognize significance of its presence in a post-MI patient.
2. Recognize value of signal averaging as a tool for identifying high-risk patients in this population (post-MI patients).
3. Recognize indications for signal averaging.
4. Identify and differentiate types of noise which may interfere with data acquisition and know ways to eliminate random noise.
5. Understand criteria used for determining presence of a ventricular late potential (VLP).

Glossary and Abbreviations

D-40: A measurement of time that the QRS complex remains below 40 microvolts.

High-frequency QRS duration (HFQD): Represents the high-frequency QRS duration, or the duration of the QRS after it has been filtered.

Noise reduction: Noise can be physiologic or electronic, and must be reduced as much as possible while acquiring the SAECG. Noise reduction can be facilitated by the type of filters in the SAECG machine by acquiring an adequate number of beats for averaging and by controlling the environmental noise before data acquisition. The patient's skin should be prepared with alcohol to decrease impedance. Any noise in the room should be eliminated or kept at a minimum.

QRS duration (QRSD): Represents the total duration of the QRS complex.

RMSA: The root mean square voltage of the terminal 40 msec of the filtered QRS.

Ventricular late potential (VLP): Abnormal late potential arising from areas of slow conducting myocardium. They are the result of delayed and fractionate electric wavefronts through the myocardium. They reflect depolarization activity (non-repolarization) and are more reflective of endocardial activity than epicardial activity. The purpose for using VLPs is to develop a non-invasive marker which may function as a screening test for EPS testing and may detect patients at high risk of sudden death or recurrent VT.

Education Content

A. Indications for use of SAECG in Patients

    1. Sustained ventricular tachycardia – There are both retrospective and prospective studies that conform the increased risk of sustained ventricular tachycardia or sudden death in post-MI patients who have an abnormal SAECG. For risk stratification in these patients, the SAECG is independent from left ventricular function or the presence of complex ectopy.[1]

    2. Non-sustained ventricular tachycardia – Studies have shown that patients with old MI, non-sustained VT and abnormal SAECG are more prone to inducible sustained VT. The SAECG may be useful for risk stratification and management of these patients.

    3. Syncope – Clinical use of the SAECG in this group of patients has not been determined. Some studies have shown that patients with syncope and an abnormal SAECG are more prone to inducible sustained VT during programmed stimulation.

B. Data Analysis

    1. Criteria for determining late potential using time-domain analysis – The definition of a late potential and the determination of an SAECG as normal or abnormal has not yet been standardized at this time.

        a. Criteria which may be considered standard are

            1. The use of a high-pass corner filter frequency of 25 Hz or 40 Hz; and

            2. Using a Butterworth filter, a noise cutoff of 1 microvolt using 25 Hz or .7 microvolts at 40 Hz.

        b. Criteria for a positive late potential which may be used are

            1. A filtered QRS (HFQD) greater than 114 msec.

            2. A D-40 greater than 38 msec.

            3. A root mean square amplitude (rmsa) less than 20 microvolts.

        c. Individual laboratories should determine their own normal values for a late potential.

    2. Factors which will affect the quality of the SEACG tracing

        a. Environmental noise (i.e., other equipment in room, monitors, vibration of bed or floor.

        b. Lead placement and skin contact – leads should be placed in same spot for serial acquisitions and good electrode skin contact maintained.

C. Domains for Obtaining SAECG

    1. Time domain – Analysis of a vector magnitude of the filtered QRS complex. Standards for time domain analysis are listed in section B of this chapter.

2. Frequency domain – Using the fast fourier transform, the ECG can be represented in the frequency domain. The fourier transform is a complete description of the ECG and contains information that may not be seen in the output of a particular fixed-band filter.

References

Breithardt G, et.al. Standards for analysis of ventricular late potentials using high-resolution or signal-averaged electrocardiography. J Am Coll Cardiol. 17:5:999–1006. 1991.

Vatterot JP, Hammill SC, Bailey KR, Berbari EJ, Matheson SJ. Signal-averaged electrocardiography: a new noninvasive test to identify patients at risk for ventricular arrhythmias. Mayo Clin Proc. 63:931–942. 1988.

Engel TR. High-frequency electrocardiography: diagnosis of arrhythmia risk. Prog Cardiol. 18:1302–1316. 1989.

Flowers NC. Signal averaging as an adjunct in detection of arrhythmias. Circulation. 75(suppl.111): 78:1985.

Simson MB. Signal averaging. Circulation. 75(suppl.111):111:69–73. 1985.

Breithardt G, Borggrefe M. Recent advances in the identification of patients at risk of ventricular tachyarrhythmias: role of ventricular late potentials. Circulation. 75:6:1091–1096. 1987.

El-Sherif N, Gomes JAC, Restivo M, Mehra R. Late potentials and arrhythmogenesis. PACE. 8(Part 1):1091–1096. 1985.

CHAPTER 32.A

Other Diagnostic Modalities
Tilt Table Testing

Kathleen Ruggiero

Head up tilt table testing is currently one of many diagnostic procedures used in determining etiology of syncopal attacks. Specifically, tilt table testing identifies syncopal episodes that occur as a result of neurally mediated hypotension and/or bradycardia. This phenomenon is also sometimes called malignant vasodepressor/vasovagal syndrome.

Not all patients would be considered appropriate candidates for tilt table testing. Contraindicated patients would include those with recent myocardial infarctions, unstable angina, congestive heart failure, and hemodynamic instability. Precautions in performing the test would have to be applied in elderly patients and those with known coronary artery disease.

The tilt table test procedure takes approximately 60 to 80 minutes. It is performed after patients are free of vasodilator medications for at least 5 half-lives and are in a fasting state. A consent should be obtained prior to testing once the procedure has been thoroughly explained. Equipment required includes the tilt table itself, draw sheets or Velcro straps to safely secure the patient on the table, intravenous equipment including a pump for medication administration, blood pressure monitoring equipment and a cardiac monitor. A crash cart should also be on hand and stocked with emergency medications and equipment. Atropine, in particular, should be readily accessible.

Once the consent has been signed and the equipment has been gathered, the test begins. With the patient securely on the tilt table and connected to cardiac and blood pressure monitoring equipment, he/she is maintained in the supine position for approximately 15 minutes. Vital signs should be documented throughout the entire procedure. The patient is then tilted upright at approximately 70° for 30 to 45 minutes. A positive response includes presyncope (warmth, lightheadedness, nausea) or syncope in conjunction with

From: Schurig L. *Educational Guidelines: Pacing and Electrophysiology*. Armonk, NY: Futura Publishing Co, Inc, © 1994.

significant hypotension and/or bradycardia. If the test is negative, the patient is returned to the supine position and, unless contraindicated, the same procedure may be repeated while isoproteronol infuses at titrated rates. The isoproteronol infusion is started at 1 μg/minute and is continued at that rate for approximately 5 minutes while the patient remains supine. The patient is then tilted upright at 70° for 5 to 10 minutes while the Isuprel infuses. If the results remain negative, the process is repeated as the Isuprel is increased by 1 μg/minute at a time. The patient should be placed supine at each titration and then re-tilted. If the patient has been tilted for approximately 10 minutes with the Isuprel infusion at 5 μg/minute without significant hypotension/bradycardia, this is considered a negative test. It should be noted that the use of isoproteronol provocation in tilt table testing is controversial in that it is felt by some to elicit false-positive results.

Endpoints of tilt table testing besides a positive response or a negative result at peak Isuprel infusion (5 μg/minute) include severe headache, nausea, chest pain, ST depression, and heart rate > 150 beats per minute. In patients who are elderly or who have known coronary artery disease, the endpoints should be altered in that the maximum dosage of Isuprel may be 2 to 3 μg/minute rather than 5 μg/min and the maximum desired heart rate may be 120–130 rather than 150. If a positive response is elicited at any time, the patient must be immediately returned to the supine position and if isoproteronol is infusing, it should be immediately discontinued and the line flushed with normal saline. With these measures, the patient should quickly regain consciousness and have symptoms subside. Additionally, blood pressure will quickly normalize once the patient is supine and bradydysrhythmias/asystolic episodes should dissipate. If asystole or significant symptomatic bradycardias persist, atropine should be quickly administered.

The tilt table test can also be done with the addition of esmolol (an intravenous β-blocker). The purpose of this approach would be to test the efficacy of a β-blocker as the treatment of choice for the patient. A patient who has a positive tilt table test with or without isoproteronol can have the test repeated with esmolol infusing. If the results are negative with the addition of esmolol, the treatment of choice for the patient would be oral β-blockers to prevent further vasodepressor episodes. If the test is still positive with esmolol infusing, chances are good that the patient would not respond to oral β-blockers and another treatment plan would be chosen for the patient.

Various other treatment protocols for patients who demonstrate a positive response to tilt table testing include flourinef, elastic stockings, disopyramide, theophylline and vagolytic agents such as transdermal scopolamine. Re-testing can be performed with these individual pharmacologic agents in use to determine efficacy of treatment. In isolated cases where a positive tilt table response is associated with significant ventricular asystole, a dual chamber pacemaker may be necessary. In cases such as these, the DDI mode with hysteresis is indicated. It should be noted, however, that the use of dual chamber pacing for the prevention of neurocardiogenic syncope is controversial in that the hypotensive response in these patients almost always precedes the bradydysrhythmia. The pacemaker does not prevent the hypotension and may, therefore, not prevent future syncopal episodes.

Educational points for patients undergoing tilt table testing include explanation of the procedure and risks involved prior to testing. If a patient is found to have a malignant vasodepressor syndrome, they should be instructed in the use and importance of elastic stockings. They should also be instructed to avoid standing for long periods of time and to quickly sit or recline should prodromal symptoms occur. Newly prescribed medications, including their actions and possible side effects, should be reviewed with these patients. Additionally, patients who require implantation of a permanent pacemaking device as a course of treatment will require further instructions specific to these devices.

Objectives

1. Identify indications for tilt table testing.
2. Identify contraindications to tilt table testing.
3. Recognize basic pathophysiology involving neurocardiogenic syncope.
4. Demonstrate proper equipment set up and performance of tilt table test.
5. Recognize endpoints for termination of tilt table testing.
6. Describe the pharmacologic effects of isoproterenol and esmolol and their use in tilt table testing.
7. Explain various pharmacologic treatment protocols including mechanisms of action.
8. Evaluate treatment plan for each individual patient.
9. Identify when a pacemaker is indicated as choice of treatment.
10. Identify educational points for the tilt table/neurocardiogenic syncope patient.

Glossary and Abbreviations

Asystole: Cardiac standstill or arrest – absence of heart beat.

Catecholamine: One of a group of similar compounds having a sympathomimetic action.

Hysteresis: Escape interval is significantly longer than automatic interval.

Mechanoreceptor: A receptor that is excited by mechanical pressures or distortions as those responding to sound, touch, and muscular contraction.

Neurally mediated: Originating from the nervous system

Prodrome: A premonitory symptom or precursor

Syncope: Temporary suspension of consciousness due to generalized cerebral ischemia.

Vagolytic: Having an effect resembling that produced by interruption of impulses transmitted by the vagus nerve.

Vasodilator: An agent that causes dilation of blood vessels.

Education Content

A. Indications for Tilt Table Testing

    1. Syncope of undetermined etiology

    2. Pre-syncope of undetermined etiology

    3. Patients with prodrome prior to syncope

B. Contraindications to Tilt Table Testing

    1. Recent myocardial infarction

    2. Unstable angina

    3. Congestive heart failure

    4. Hemodynamic instability

C. Pathophysiology of Neurally Mediated Bradycardia/Hypotension

    1. Activation of myocardial mechanoreceptors (C fibers) due to increased myocardial contractility may override normal baroreceptor reflex in standing patients.

    2. Sympathetic tone is inhibited by activation of these mechanoreceptors

    3. Parasympathetic tone is increased due to activation of these mechanoreceptors

    4. Peripheral vasodilation, hypotension, and bradycardia result from this decrease in sympathetic tone and increase in parasympathetic tone resulting in syncope

    5. This response is abnormal as compared to the average person whose arterial pressure is normally maintained when standing due to a baroreceptor-reflex mediated increase in sympathetic tone which causes enhanced cardiac contractility, increased heart rate and peripheral vasoconstruction

D. Tilt Table Procedure

    1. Obtain informed consent

    2. Equipment necessary

        a. Tilt table with safety straps

        b. Intravenous equipment, including medication pump

        c. Blood pressure equipment

        d. Cardiac monitor

        e. Emergency cart and medications

    3. General procedure protocol

    4. Isoproteronol protocol

    5. Esmolol protocol

    6. Termination endpoints

    a. Positive response

    b. Chest pain

    c. Severe headache

    d. Nausea

    e. ST depression

    f. Heart rate > 150 beats/min

    g. Reaching peak Isuprel rate of 5 μg/min without eliciting positive response

7. Alterations in tilt table procedure

    a. Caution to be used with elderly patients

    b. Caution to be used in patients with known coronary artery disease

8. Intervention for positive response

    a. Return patient immediately to supine position

    b. Discontinue Isuprel infusion if infusing

    c. Administer atropine for persistent symptomatic bradydysrhythmias only

E. Treatment Plan

  1. β-blocker therapy; may lower discharge frequency of mechanoreceptors and also leaves α-receptors unopposed, causing peripheral vasoconstriction

  2. Disopyramide – has peripheral vasoconstrictor effects, anticholinergic effects and negative inotropic effects

  3. Transdermal scopolamine – vagolytic action

  4. Theophylline – acts by blocking the uptake of endogenous adenosine

  5. Flourinef – sodium supplement

  6. Elastic stockings

  7. Dual chamber pacemaker

F. Evaluation of Treatment Plan

  1. Repeat testing with pharmacologic agent instituted

  2. Negative test on pharmacotherapy indicates appropriate intervention for this patient.

  3. Positive test on pharmacotherapy indicates inappropriate intervention and an alternate pharmacologic agent or intervention must be chosen and tested.

G. Educational Guidelines

  1. Explain tilt table testing to patient.

  2. If patient response is positive for malignant vasodepressor syndrome

    a. Basic pathophysiology should be explained to patient

b. Patient should be discouraged from standing for long periods

c. Patient should be encouraged to lie or sit at first signs of symptoms

d. Elastic stockings and their purpose should be encouraged

e. Review medications including dosage, frequency and side effects to patient

f. Pacemaker teaching for those patients who require insertion of dual chamber pacemaker for therapeutic intervention.

References

Almquist A, Goldenberg IF, Milstein S, et al. Provocation of bradycardia and hypotension by isoproterenol and upright posture in patients with unexplained syncope. N Engl J Med. 320:6:346–351. 1989.

Chang-Sing P, Peter T. Syncope: evaluation and management. Cardiology Clinics. Acute Cardiac Care. 645–647. 1991.

Grubb B, Temesy-Armos P, Hahn H, Elliott L. Utility of upright tilt table testing in the evaluation and management of syncope of unknown origin. The Am J Med. 90:6–10. 1991.

Grubb B, Temesy-Armos P, Moore J, Wolfe D, Hahn H, Elliott L. Head-upright tilt-table testing in evaluation and management of the malignant vasovagal syndrome. Am J Cardiol. 69:904–908. 1992.

Fitzpatrick A, Theodorakis G, Ahmed R, Williams T, Sutton R. Dual chamber pacing aborts vasovagal syncope induced by head-up 60° tilt. PACE. 14:13–19. 1991.

Hammill S, Holmes D, Wood D, et al. Electrophysiologic Testing in the upright position: improved evaluation of patients with rhythm disturbances using a tilt table. J Am Coll Cardiol. 4:1:65–71. 1984.

Kligfield P. Tilt table for the investigation of syncope: there is nothing simple about fainting. J Am Coll Cardiol. 17:1:131–132. 1991.

Pavlovic S, Kacovic D, Djordjevic M, et al. The etiology of syncope in pacemaker patients. PACE. 14:2086–2091. 1991.

Schaal S, Nelson S, Boudoulas H, Lewis R. Current Problems in Cardiology: Syncope. XVII:4:245–249. 1992.

Sheldon R, Killam S. Methodology of isoproterenol–tilt-table testing in patients with syncope. J Am Coll Cardiol. 19:4:773–779. 1992.

Sra J, Murthy V, Jazayeri M, et al. Use of intravenous esmolol to predict efficacy of oral β-adrenergic blocker therapy in patients with neurocardiogenic syncope. J Am Coll Cardiol. 19:2:402–408. 1992.

Sra J, Jazayeri M, Avitall B, et al. Comparison of cardiac pacing with drug therapy in the treatment of neurocardiogenic (vasovagal) syncope with bradycardia or asystole. N Engl J Med. 328:115:1085–1090. 1993.

CHAPTER 32.BCD

Other Diagnostic Modalities
Holter Recording, Stress Testing, Echocardiography

Beverly Taibi

Ambulatory electrocardiographic monitoring is an essential tool in the diagnostic evaluation of patients with bradyarrhythmias and supraventricular and ventricular tachyarrhythmias. It is helpful in assessing the patient's symptoms, especially if there are complaints of dizziness, palpitations, pre syncope, or syncope. If the episodes are frequent in nature, the Holter monitor will provide information as to the type of arrhythmia, the mechanism of onset, the duration and the termination of the arrhythmia. Holter recordings are usually obtained over a 24-hour period. However, when symptoms do not occur on a daily basis, recordings over a 48-hours period may be obtained.

Many physicians obtain a Holter recording within the first week or two after implantation of a pacemaker since this is the most likely time for lead dislodgement. Holter monitoring is also valuable in assessing the patient for pacemaker syndrome, device malfunction, evaluating patient-device interaction, and assessing the efficacy of antiarrhythmic drug and device therapy.

If patient symptoms are transient and occur on a less frequent basis, an endless-loop event recorder would be an effective diagnostic tool. The event recorder is usually issued on a 30-day basis and the heart rhythm is continually *dumped* until the patient has symptoms and presses the record button. The heart rhythm is then saved and transmitted for interpretation.

Exercise tolerance testing is widely used in the detection of ischemic heart disease, sinus node response to exercise, effect of exercise on pre-existing

From: Schurig L, et al. *Educational Guidelines: Pacing and Electrophysiology*. Armonk, NY: Futura Publishing Co, Inc, © 1994.

arrhythmias, and for evaluation of exercise-induced arrhythmias. It is also very useful in evaluating a patient's exercise capacity.

Stress testing prior to pacemaker implantation will guide the physician in appropriate device selection and determination of the optimal upper rate limit for programming. Patients receiving antitachycardia devices and implantable cardioverter defibrillators should have exercise tolerance tests performed to assess the maximum sinus rate achieved during exercise, or the maximum ventricular response with underlying atrial fibrillation. The device should then be programmed to avoid shocks and antitachycardia pacing during sinus tachycardia and atrial fribrillation with rapid AV conduction.

Recent advances in the field of cardiac nuclear medicine has enabled the physician to perform more sensitive non-invasive screening for ischemic heart disease than is possible with treadmill testing alone. The recent FDA approval of intravenous dipyridamole permits application of nuclear sensitivity in a much broader patient population, specifically to those patients unable to perform maximal treadmill exercise due to physical disabilities, pulmonary disease, peripheral vascular disease, chronotropic incompetence, or rate suppression due to therapy with β-blockers. These patients are prime candidates for either dipyridamole thallium imaging or atrial paced thallium imaging. Patients with false positive treadmill tests can be identified with exercise radionuclide imaging, reducing the need for unnecessary coronary angiography. The addition of radionuclide imaging also adds important prognostic information in coronary heart disease patients and those with left or right ventricular failure. Through radionuclide angiography, the physician is able to identify high-risk patients by measuring left and right ventricular ejection fractions, as well as diastolic performance, at rest and with exercise.

Although this chapter does not cover the subject of positron emission tomography (PET) scanning, it should be noted here that through PET with metabolic (i.e., fluorodeoxyglucose) imaging, patients who would benefit from coronary artery bypass grafting or percutaneous transluminal coronary angioplasty can be identified and unnecessary procedures can be avoided in patients with no viable tissue. Positron emission tomography scanning can provide metabolic information which may be helpful to differentiate stunned, hibernating and ischemic from irreversibly damaged, necrotic myocardium.

Echocardiography has many clinical applications in pacing and electrophysiology. Cardiac anatomy and physiology can be defined through use of M-mode and two-dimensional echocardiography, whereas cardiac blood flow is assessed by means of Doppler echocardiography. Color flow mapping occurs when pulsed Doppler and two-dimensional data are superimposed.

It is important to evaluate left ventricular function in patients with ventricular arrhythmias. A patient is at a much greater risk of sudden death when ventricular tachycardia is combined with poor left ventricular function. Ejection fractions and wall motion abnormalities can be readily determined by means of echocardiography.

Data obtained through echocardiography is used to diagnose and manage patients with cardiac structural anomalies, valvular heart disease, systolic and diastolic dysfunction, cardiomyopathies, endocarditis, intracardiac masses, and pericardial disease. It has been also proven to be very helpful in aiding the physician's evaluation of patients pre- and post-pacemaker implantation.

Objectives

1. Identify indications for use of Holter monitoring versus the use of an endless-loop event recorder.
2. Identify pseudomalfunction associated with Holter monitor recording.
3. Identify indications for treadmill exercise testing.
4. Recognize when radionuclide exercise testing would be a more appropriate diagnostic tool.
5. Be aware of the non-invasive methods available for use in the evaluation of ischemic heart disease and the functional capacity of the heart.
6. Understand the common endpoints for termination of exercise testing.
7. Understand the proper procedure used in preparing the patient for exercise tolerance testing.
8. Be aware of the diagnostic value of two-dimensional echocardiography with color flow mapping.
9. Be able to determine when echocardiography may be used in the management of patients with arrhythmias and in patients receiving permanent pacemakers.
10. Recognize the complications of pacing which can be detected by echocardiography.
11. Understand the application of stress echocardiography through rapid atrial pacing in the diagnosis of corornary artery disease.

Glossary and Abbreviations

Akinetic: Absence of movement.

Dyskinetic: Fragmentary or incomplete movement.

Ejection fraction: The relation of left ventricular stroke volume to end diastolilc volume. Normal 60–70%

Hemopericardium: An effusion of blood within the pericardium.

Hibernating myocardium: Mechanical complication of an ischemic process which is not transient, but chronic in nature.

Hyperkinetic: Abnormally increased activity.

Hypokinetic: Abnormallly decreased activity.

Myocardial ischemia: Deficiency of blood supply to the heart muscle due to constriction or obstruction of the coronary arteries.

Maximal treadmill exercise: The ability to exercise until the age predicted maximum heart rate is attained.

Pacemaker syndrome: A syndrome which may occur during cardiac pacing when loss of AV synchrony is present. The patient may or may not exhibit retrograde activation of the atrium. Symptoms include pounding in the neck and chest, cannon A waves, shortness of breath, fatigue, dizziness, and a drop in blood pressure during cardiac pacing. Other causes include fixed rate pacing resulting in a restricted cardiac output during exercise.

Pseudomalfunction: Having the appearance of malfunction when in fact, normal pacemaker operation is maintained.

Radionuclide: A radioactive nuclide, capable of existing for a measurable lifetime (generally greater than 10 to the -10 seconds).

Stunned myocardium: Dysfunctional myocardium which has contractile abnormalities with systolic bulging and wall thinning. Ischemic myocardial dysfunction without necrosis.

Education Content

A. Holter Monitoring

    1. Indications

        a. To assess the frequency and nature of arrhythmias

            1. Symptoms suggestive of possible arrhythmia

            2. To assess efficacy of antiarrhythmic drug and device therapy

            3. Post-MI patients with documented PVCs

            4. Assess frequency and nature of suspected or known arrhythmias

        b. Assessment of pacemaker function

            1. Post-implant

            2. Suspected device malfunction

                a) Suspect lead

                b) Abnormally high- or low-lead impedance

                c) Post-MI

                d) Post-open heart surgery

                e) Patient symptoms

                f) Syncope of unknown etiology

                g) High-capture threshold

                h) Poor sensing

            3. Effect of antiarrhythmic drugs on pacing system

            4. Patient-device interactions

                a) Determine normal operation

                b) Frequency and nature of arrhythmia

                c) Environmental effects on device

        c. Assessment of pacemaker dependency – frequency of pacing

            1. Evaluation of pacemaker syndrome

        d. Monitoring of rate adaptation during activities of daily living

            1. Chronotropic incompetence

            2. Programmed pacing parameters

        e. Monitoring for EMI during specific patient activity

            1. Work environment

            2. Hobbies

        f. Assessment of heart rhythm to verify frequent PVCs or upper rate limit behavior as indicated by pacemaker telemetry and/or event record.

    2. Patient instruction

        a. Importance of accurate diary

        b. Ensuring electrodes, cable remain intact

        c. Importance of performing usual activities of daily life, being active

    d. Performance of specific activities usually associated with symptoms

    e. Depressing event marker when symptoms occur and noting symptoms in diary

    f. Do not shower or take a tub bath with Holter on

3. Considerations for easier interpretation of Holter monitor recordings

    a. Proper skin preparation

        1. Cleanse with alcohol, shave area and gently scrape with sandpaper prior to placing electrodes

        2. Ensure firm contact of skin and electrode

        3. Obtain a sample rhythm strip in several leads after electrodes are in place

        4. Check recordings for presence of artifacts with patient activity

        5. Follow manufacturer's guidelines in placement of electrodes

    b. Obtain baseline 12 lead ECG and submit to physician with Holter report.

    c. Document list of patient medications.

    d. Document patient diagnosis and reason for Holter.

    e. Submit patient diary with Holter report.

    f. If the patient has a pacemaker

        1. Program to unipolar pacing configuration when possible and if appropriate during Holter recording (do not program unipolar with an ICD)

        2. Submit pacemaker programmed parameters at the time of the Holter with the report.

        3. Indicate manufacturer and model of pacemaker implanted as well as the mode of operation

            a) A-A versus V-V based timing cycle

            b) Specific device behavior and idiosyncracies

4. Follow-up of Holter monitor report

    a. Medical interventions

        1. Antiarrhythmic therapy

        2. Medication changes

        3. Further clinical evaluation

        4. Further diagnostic studies when indicated

            a) Electrophysiology study

            b) Signal averaged ECG

            c) Echocardiography

            d) Exercise tolerance testing

    b. Reprogramming of device as needed

        1. Pacemaker

      2. Defibrillator

      3. Tiered therapy device

   c. Restriction of specific patient activity

   d. Documented device malfunction

      1. Surgical intervention

         a) Lead replacement

         b) Generator replacement

         c) Upgrade of device

      2. Avoidance of specific sources of EMI

      3. Device reprogramming

 5. Identification of pseudomalfunction associated with Holter monitor recording

   a. Artifact

      1. Minimize with good skin prepping and electrode placement

   b. Inappropriate timing of Holter recording due to slowing or stop and go malfunction of recording device

      1. Reel to reel

      2. Cassette

      3. Battery malfunction

      4. Proper maintenance of equipment

   c. Holter with separate channel for detection of pacemaker output pulses

      1. Inappropriate identification of pacemaker stimuli

         a) Multiple stimuli indicated

         b) Inappropriate timing of stimuli

B. Stress Testing

 1. Indications

   a. Exercise ECG stress test

      1. Asymptomatic patient with multiple risk factors

      2. Evaluation of exercise capacity

      3. Assessment of sinus node response to exercise

      4. Determination of maximum heart rate attained with exercise

         a) Defibrillator patients

         b) Patients with antitachycardia devices

         c) Determination of upper rate limit for pacemaker programming

         d) Maximum rate of AV conduction with underlying atrial fibrillation

      5. Effect of exercise on pre-existing arrhythmias

      6. Evaluation of exercise-induced arrhythmias

    7. Device selection pre-pacemaker implantation
       a) Chronotropic response
       b) Evaluation of AV conduction defects with increases in the sinus rate
    8. Post-MI patients
    9. Patients experiencing near sudden death
b. Exercise radionuclide imaging
    1. Patients with positive exercise ECG stress tests
    2. Pre- and post-coronary artery bypass grafting
    3. Pre- and post-percutaneous transluminal coronary angioplasty
    4. Patients with resting ECG abnormalities
       a) Digitalis effect
       b) Bundle branch blocks
       c) Dependent pacemaker rhythms
       d) ST segment abnormalities
       e) Mitral valve prolapse
    5. Evaluation of extent of known CAD
       a) Stable angina
       b) Unstable angina
       c) Post-MI
    6. Pre- and post-thrombolytic therapy
c. Dipridamole radionuclide imaging
    1. Patients unable to perform maximal treadmill exercise
       a) Peripheral vascular disease
       b) Pulmonary disease
       c) Physical disabilities
       d) Recent stroke
       e) Chronotropic incompetence
       f) Rate suppression due to therapy with β-blockers
    2. Avoidance of rapid heart rate associated with exercise in high-risk patients
       a) Post-MI
       b) Recent cardiac surgery
       c) Significant aortic stenosis
d. Atrial paced radionuclide imaging
    1. Patients unable to perform maximal treadmill exercise
       a) Same as dipridamole radionuclide imaging
    2. Patients who are dependent on their implanted pacemaker
       a) Gradually increase the pacemaker rate through programming until the target heart rate is attained

        1) Monitor blood pressure at each stage during the test

        2) Monitor patient for ECG changes

        3) Inject with radionuclide when target heart rate is achieved

        4) Frequently ask the patient if any symptoms are present

        5) Proceed with routine imaging

2. Patient preparation

    a. Baseline 12 lead ECG

    b. Current history and physical

    c. Evaluation of patient symptoms

    d. List of current medications

        1. Test to be performed on or off medications per physician discretion

    e. Explain procedure to patient and ensure understanding.

    f. Obtain written consent.

    g. Prepare skin and perform proper electrode placement.

    h. Inspect equipment for faulty cables/leads.

    i. Check to see if recording is free of artifacts.

    j. Start IV when appropriate.

    k. Ensure patient is wearing comfortable shoes and clothing.

3. Endpoints for termination of exercise stress testing

    a. Atainment of at least 85% of age-predicted maximum heart rate

    b. Inability of the patient to continue with exercise

    c. Significant ventricular ectopy or ventricular tachycardia

    d. Greater than 3 mm of ST segment depression or elevation with or without symptoms

    e. A systolic blood pressure drop of greater than 20 mm Hg

4. Follow-up of stress test results

    a. Medical treatment

    b. Coronary angiography

        1. PTCA when indicated

        2. CABG when indicated

    c. Reduction in risk factors

    d. Cardiac rehabilitation program to increase exercise capacity

    e. No restrictions with absence of CAD

    f. Pacemaker device selection

    g. Reprogramming of antitachycardia and defibrillator devices as indicated

    h. Reprogramming of optimal upper rate limit in dual chamber pacemakers and maximum sensor rate in rate adaptive devices

C. Echocardiography (ECHO)
  1. Use of echocardiography as a diagnostic tool
   a. Assessment of valvular heart disease
    1. Use of two-dimensional ECHO to assess structural valvular abnormalities
      a) Aortic stenosis
        1) Valvular aortic stenosis
        2) Subvalvular aortic stenosis
        3) Supravalvular aortic stenosis
      b) Mitral stenosis
      c) Tricuspid stenosis
      d) Pulmonary stenosis
      e) Identification of presence of prosthetic valves
    2. Doppler studies for diagnosing valvular insufficiency
      a) Aortic regurgitation
      b) Mitral regurgitation
      c) Tricuspid regurgitation
      d) Pulmonary regurgitation
      e) Prosthetic valve regurgitation
   b. Endocarditis
    1. Detection of vegetation
    2. Evidence of perivalvular infection
    3. Doppler methods to assess the hemodynamic effects of the infective process
   c. Assessment of the left ventricle
    1. Evaluation of left ventricular size
      a) Detection of left ventricular hypertrophy
    2. Determination of global left ventricular systolic function
      a) Calculation of ejection fraction (EF)
    3. Evaluation of left ventricular wall motion
      a) Detection of regional wall motion abnormalities
        1) Normal function
        2) Hyperkinetic
        3) Hypokinetic
        4) Akinetic
        5) Dyskinetic
      b) Detection of myocardial wall thinning
   d. Detecting cardiomyopathies
    1. Hypertrophic cardiomyopathy

   a) Inappropriate thickening of the myocardium
   b) Normal or enhanced systolic function
   2. Congestive cardiomyopathy
      a) Ventricular dilitation
      b) Systolic dysfunction
      c) Right ventricular involvement
   3. Restrictive cardiomyopathy
      a) Impaired diastolic ventricular filling
         1) Idiopathic restrictive
         2) Endomyocardial fibrosis
 e. Intracardiac masses
   1. Thrombi
   2. Cardiac tumors
 f. Evaluation of the pericardium
   1. Pericardial effusion
   2. Cardiac tamponade – presence of pericardial fluid
   3. Pericardial cyst
   4. Congenital absence of the pericardium
 g. Congential heart disease
   1. Evaluation for systemic venous abnormality prior to electrophysiology study
2. Echocardiographic evaluation of pacemakers. (Adapted from Barold SS. *Modern Cardiac Pacing*. 1985:920. With permission of Futura Publishing Co, Inc., and Donald F. Switzer, MD.)
 a. Definition of anatomy prior to pacemaker implantation
   1. Venous anomalies
   2. Diagnosis of atrial septal defect, ventricular septal defect, tricuspid stenosis
   3. Quantification of right ventricular enlargement
   4. Localization of the subclavian vein
 b. Location of leads
   1. Intracardiac position of catheter tip
   2. Guidance for lead manipulation and positioning
 c. Diagnosis of lead complications
   1. Perforation of right ventricular free wall or septum
   2. Hemopericardium
   3. Lead displacement
   4. Thrombosis
   5. Vegetation on lead or tricuspid valve
 d. Tricuspid trauma

1. Flail or torn tricuspid valve
2. Evaluation of tricuspid insufficiency by Doppler
   e. Hemodynamics in dual chamber pacing
      1. Left atrial contraction and quantification of flow with atrial systole
      2. Relative stroke volume and cardiac output in VVI versus DVI pacing, DDD or rate adaptive pacing
      3. Altered hemodynamics in "pacemaker syndrome"
   f. Atrial pacing in the diagnosis of coronary artery disease
   g. Other potential applications
      1. Lead fracture
      2. Identification of fluid or pus at the generator site
3. Stress echocardiography in the diagnosis of coronary artery disease
   a. Detection of wall motion abnormalities which are secondary to coronary artery disease
      1. Limitations of exercise two-dimensional ECHO:
         a) Requires skilled ECHO technician
         b) Motion artifact secondary to hyperventilation or chest wall motion
         c) Exercise-induced wall motion abnormalities resolve quickly with cessation of exercise
      2. Use of atrial-paced transesophageal ECHO (TEE) in the diagnosis of coronary artery disease
         a) Able to obtain target heart rate without associated motion artifacts caused by hyperventilation and chest wall motion seen with exercise
         b) Reliable alternative for patients unable to perform maximal exercise, or patients with bundle branch block
         c) High quality echocardiographic images
         d) Allow for continuous imaging through each stage of exercise
         e) Permits evaluation of wall motion abnormalities during exercise and through the entire recover period
         f) Highly specific and sensitive technique for detection of CAD
         g) Patient discomfort is possible due to echoscope
4. Clincial application of echocardiography
   a. Evaluation of left ventricular function prior to initiation of antiarrhythmic drugs
      1. Negative inotropic drugs can further depress cardiac function and predispose the patient to congestive heart failure.
      2. Proarrhythmia effect is greater in patients with poor ejection fraction.

      3. Tachycardias can be detrimental in patients with poor ejection fractions.

        a) SVT

        b) VT

  b. Evaluation of the left ventricle in patients with congestive heart failure

    1. Assess systolic function

    2. Rule out diastolic dysfunction as cause of failure

  c. Determining patient overall prognosis post-MI

    1. Extent of myocardial damage

    2. Presence of aneurysmal dilatation of the left ventricle

  d. Determine candidacy for revascularizatioon procedures.

    1. Identify high-risk patients

      a) PTCA

      b) CABG

  e. Determine candidacy for cardioversion of atrial fibrillation

    1. Left atrial size

    2. Atrial movement post-cardioversion (silent atrium)

  f. Assessment of atrial rhythm

    1. Presence of atrial capture with atrial paced output

    2. Atrial fibrillation or flutter versus sinus rhythm

    3. Atrial standstill

References

Barold SS. Modern Cardiac Pacing. Mt. Kisco: Futura Publishing Co, Inc., 1985.

Feigenbaum H. Echocardiography. 4th edition. Philadelphia: Lea & Febiger. 1986.

Furman S, Hayes D, Holmes DR. A Practice of Cardiac Pacing. Mt. Kisco: Futura Publishing Co, Inc., 1989.

Gerson MC. Cardiac Nuclear Medicine. 2nd edition. New York: McGraw-Hill. 1991.

Hurst JW, Schlant RC, Rackley CE, et al. The Heart: Vol I and II. New York: McGraw-Hill. 1990.

Janosik R, Buckingham B, Wiens K. Utility of ambulatory electrocardiography in detecting pacemaker dysfunction in the early post-implanatation period. Am J Cardiol. 60:13:1030–1035. 1991.

Lacroix D, Dubuc M, Kus T, et al. Evaluation of arrhythmic causes of syncope: correlation between holter monitoring, electrophysiologic testing, and body surface potential mapping. Am Heart J. 122:5:1346–1354. 1991.

Lambertz H, Kreis A, Trumper HL, et al. Simultaneous transesophageal atrial pacing and transesophageal two-dimensional echocardiography: a method of stress echocardiography. J Am Coll Cardiol. 16:5:1143–1153. 1990.

Leff AR. Cardiopulmonary Exercise Testing. Grune & Stratton. 1986.

Leah MD, Langberg JJ, Griffin JC, et al. Pacemaker generator pseudomalfunction: an artifact of Holter monitoring. PACE. 14:Part 1:854–857. 1991.

Miller DD, Burns RJ, Gill JB, Ruddy D. Clinical Cardiac Imaging. New York: McGrraw-Hill. 1988.

Saksena S, Goldschlager N. Electrical therapy for cardiac arrhythmias: pacing, antitachycardia devices, catheter ablations. Philadelphia: WB Saunders Co. 1990.

Zipes DP, Jalife J. Diagnositic studies: Long-term (Holter) electrocradiogram recordings. In Cardiac Electrophysiology from Cell to Bedside. Zipes DP, Jalife J, (Eds.) Philadelphia: WB Saunders, Co., 791–797. 1991.

Index

NOTES

NOTES

NOTES

NOTES

NOTES